Fauber's
Radiographic
Imaging
and Exposure

Fauber's
Radiographic
Imaging
and Exposure

Terri L. Fauber, EdD, RT(R)(M)

Professor Emeritus of Radiation Sciences
Department of Radiation Sciences
College of Health Professions
Virginia Commonwealth University
Richmond, Virginia

Section Editor

Randy Griswold, MPA, RT(R), FWSRT

Faculty, Northeast Wisconsin Technical College
Program in Biomedical Engineering
Adjunct Faculty, Radiography Program
Fellow Wisconsin Society of Radiologic Technologists
Green Bay, Wisconsin

ELSEVIER

Seventh Edition

Elsevier
3251 Riverport Lane
St. Louis, Missouri 63043

FAUBER'S RADIOGRAPHIC IMAGING AND EXPOSURE, SEVENTH EDITION   ISBN: 978-0-443-11450-2

Previous editions copyrighted 2021, 2017, 2013, 2009, 2004, 2000.

Content Strategist: Meg Benson
Content Development Specialist: Dominque McPherson
Publishing Services Manager: Deepthi Unni
Project Manager: Gayathri S
Design Direction: Amy Buxton

Printed in India

Last digit is the print number: 9   8   7   6   5   4   3   2   1

Working together to grow libraries in developing countries

www.elsevier.com • www.bookaid.org

Chad Dall, DHSc, RT(R), MR
Assistant Professor
Director of Outreach and Engagement
Bellin College
Green Bay, Wisconsin

REVIEWERS

Vesna Balac, EdD, RT(R)(MR)(ARRT)
Assistant Professor, Radiography Program Director,
    and Radiologic Sciences Department Chair
Radiologic Sciences
Indiana University Northwest
Gary, Indiana

Scott Haglund, MA Ed, RTR, ATC
Radiography Program Director
St. Catherine University
St. Paul, Minnesota

Tamara E. Janak, MTD, BSRS, RT(R)(M)(ARRT)
Program Director, Associate Professor
Radiologic Technology Program
College of Southern Idaho
Twin Falls, Indiana

Evan Nielsen, BSc, MRT
Faculty Instructor
British Columbia Institute of Technology
Vancouver, British Columbia, Canada

Richard Sanders, MSRS, RT(R)(CT)
Senior Clinical Education Specialist
Indian Trail, North Carolina

Bethany Stearns, BS, RT(R)(MR)(CT)(ARRT)
Medical Radiography Faculty
ECPI University
Manassas, Virginia

Leslie Townsend Whalley, EMHA, RT(R)(ARRT)
Radiography Instructor and Clinical Coordinator
AdventHealth University
Orlando, Florida

Jamie S. Tucker, RT(R)(CT)(ARRT), EdD
Program Director Radiography
Trinity College of Nursing and Health Science
Rock Island, Illinois

Fauber's Radiographic Imaging and Exposure takes a unique and more effective approach to teaching imaging and exposure by focusing on the practical fundamentals. With a topic such as radiographic imaging, it is impossible to entirely depart from theoretic information, and we do not want to do so. A concerted effort was made to present the most important and relevant information on radiographic imaging and exposure, particularly as it relates to digital imaging technology. This book highlights the practical application of theoretical information to make it more immediately useful to students and practicing radiographers alike. Our ultimate goal is to provide the knowledge to effectively solve problems for consistently producing quality radiographic images in a clinical environment.

WHO WILL BENEFIT FROM THIS BOOK?

Fauber's Radiographic Imaging and Exposure provides a fundamental presentation of topics that are vital for students to master to be competent radiographers. Moreover, radiographers will benefit from the practical approach to the topics of imaging and exposure presented here.

ORGANIZATION

Fauber's Radiographic Imaging and Exposure begins with a description of Wilhelm Conrad Roentgen's discovery of x-rays in 1895 and the excitement it first caused among the members of the 19th-century society, who feared that private anatomy would be exposed for all to see! The introductory chapter moves into the realm of radiologic science with discussions of x-rays as energy, the unique characteristics of x-rays, and the fundamentals of radiation protection. Chapter 2 provides a discussion of the fundamentals of radiation production and the x-ray circuitry of modern x-ray generating systems. Chapter 3 continues the topic of radiation production to focus on the x-ray beam. The subsequent chapters describe image formation and radiographic quality (see Chapter 4); digital image characteristics, receptors, and image acquisition (see Chapter 5); digital image processing, display, and health information management

(see Chapter 6); exposure technique factors (see Chapter 7); and scatter control (see Chapter 8). Chapter 9 focuses on the tools available to assist radiographers in selecting appropriate exposure techniques, such as automatic exposure control devices, anatomically programmed techniques, and exposure technique charts. Chapter 10 discusses the components of fluoroscopic units, fluoroscopic features, and recording and viewing systems, with an expanded discussion on the digital fluoroscopic technology in use today.

Radiation exposure and imaging continues to be a complex subject even in the digital age. This text provides a thorough yet practical level of imaging and exposure to equip radiographers with the knowledge they need to produce high-quality images on the first attempt.

DISTINCTIVE FEATURES

Radiographic imaging and exposure is a complex topic, and a mastery of the fundamentals is necessary to become competent, whether you are a student or a practicing radiographer. Three special features have been integrated within each chapter to facilitate the understanding and retention of the concepts discussed and to underscore their applicability in a clinical setting. In addition, these special features give the practicing radiographer quick visual access to fundamental information that they need every day. Each feature is distinguished by its own icon for easy recognition.

Important Relationships summarize the relationships being discussed in the text, as each one occurs, for immediate summary and review. The topic of radiographic imaging and exposure is replete with fundamental, important relationships, and they are emphasized in short, meaningful ways at every opportunity.

Mathematical Applications demonstrate the importance of mathematical formulas. Radiographic imaging also has a strong quantitative component, and this feature helps accustom readers to the necessity of mastering mathematical formulas. Because the formulas are presented with clinical scenarios, immediate applications and explanations of the formulas are provided.

⚠ **Radiation Protection Alerts** emphasize the imaging and exposure variables that can have an impact on radiation exposure to patients and others. Because computer processing can mask exposure errors, it is even more important for radiographers to comprehend how their exposure technique choices can affect the patient.

NEW TO THIS EDITION

The radiation physics content has been expanded into two chapters to include the fundamentals of the x-ray circuitry to enhance the students understanding of x-ray production. Radiographers will benefit from knowledge about the basics of radiographic image interpretation, and therefore introductory information about the keys to imaging for pathology has been added to Chapters 4 and 7. Chapter 4 relates tissue absorption to visualizing the five anatomic tissue opacities, and Chapter 7 emphasizes the importance of exposure technique selection to improve visualization of soft tissue opacities that may indicate an underlying pathology. In select instances, simple analogies in the form of a *mind image* are used to help in the comprehension of concepts.

An underlying theme throughout this edition is that exposure technique selection still plays an important role in producing quality images regardless of the equipment's automation and computer processing advancements. As in previous editions, emphasis is placed on the responsibilities radiographers have in limiting the radiation exposure to their patients.

The seventh edition of *Fauber's Radiographic Imaging and Exposure* includes the following:

1. Expanded coverage of radiation physics to include the fundamentals of the x-ray circuitry
2. An introduction to imaging for pathology and visualizing the five basic tissue opacities as an interpretive aid.

LEARNING AIDS

One of the primary goals of *Fauber's Radiographic Imaging and Exposure* is to be a practical textbook that prepares student radiographers for the responsibilities of radiographic imaging in a clinical setting. Every effort has been made to make the material easily accessible and understandable, while remaining thorough.

- The writing style is straightforward and concise, and the textbook includes numerous features to aid in the mastery of its content, including *Important Relationships, Mathematical Applications,* and *Radiation Protection Alerts.*
- All the *Important Relationships, Mathematical Applications,* and *Radiation Protection Alerts* are also collected in separate appendices for quick reference and review and are organized by chapter.
- *Fauber's Radiographic Imaging and Exposure* also includes traditional learning aids. Each chapter begins with a list of objectives and key terms and concludes with a set of multiple-choice review questions, which help readers to evaluate whether they have achieved the chapter's objectives. An answer key is provided in the back of the book.

ANCILLARIES FOR INSTRUCTORS

Evolve Resources is an interactive learning environment designed to work in coordination with *Fauber's Radiographic Imaging and Exposure*, 7th edition. It includes laboratory activities, PowerPoint slides, mathematical worksheets, an image collection of approximately 260 images, two practice tests with 60 questions each, and a Test Bank with more than 600 questions.

The ancillary material on Evolve is useful for both practiced and novice educators. The laboratory exercises accommodate different available resources and instructor preferences for varying the recommended laboratory activities. Additional mathematical worksheets are included for educators to provide more practice for students if required.

Instructors may also use Evolve to provide an Internet-based course component that reinforces and expands the concepts presented in class. Evolve may be used to publish the class syllabus, outlines, and lecture notes; set up "virtual office hours" and e-mail communication; share important dates and information through the online class calendar; and encourage student participation through chat rooms and discussion boards. Evolve allows instructors to post examinations and manage their grade books online. For more information, visit http://evolve.elsevier.com/Fauber/radiographic/ or contact an Elsevier sales representative.

ACKNOWLEDGMENTS

I am honored to have my name added to the title of this seventh edition. This journey of creating a thorough but practical textbook on radiographic imaging and exposure has truly been a remarkable experience. A project of this magnitude and scope could not be accomplished without many knowledgeable and dedicated people. New to this edition and one of the most knowledgeable people I know on the topic of radiographic imaging and exposure is Randy Griswold. Randy graciously agreed to collaborate with me on this new edition, and I am forever thankful for his contributions, most notably in adding the x-ray circuitry content and introduction to imaging for pathology. Randy's expertise ranges from biomedical physics to radiographic image interpretation. He has served many roles in our profession from educator to program director, x-ray equipment application specialist to equipment salesperson, and more recently continues to be a highly sought after lecturer on a variety of topics in the radiation sciences. His contribution to this edition is immeasurable and I am truly grateful for his time and effort and dedication to achieving the most current and accurate information on radiographic imaging and exposure.

The publishing team from Elsevier has gone above and beyond for this seventh edition. Meg Benson, Content Strategist-Education, has been a delight to work with. Her enthusiasm and commitment to this edition has made the process seamless. In addition, Dominque McPherson, Content Development Specialist, has guided both Randy and me throughout each stage of revision. Her dedication to ensuring we have all the information and tools we need to streamline our efforts has been phenomenal. I have much gratitude for the Elsevier team and their support and encouragement throughout this seventh edition.

I am also thankful for the reviewers' feedback on this seventh edition. As our technology develops, so do the uncertainties of traditional exposure technique theory. The reviewers inspired us to be innovative in how we present exposure technique selection given the advanced capabilities of digital image processing.

The unique role of radiographers has not changed throughout our history. In addition to quality patient care that all health care professionals provide, we produce quality radiographic images for diagnostic interpretation while optimizing radiation protection. This skill remains unique among all the health care professions.

Terri L. Fauber

CONTENTS

Radiation and Its Discovery

CHAPTER OUTLINE

OBJECTIVES

After completing this chapter, the reader will be able to perform the following:

1. Define all the key terms in this chapter.
2. State all the important relationships in this chapter.
3. Describe the events surrounding the discovery of x-rays.
4. List the properties of x-rays.
5. Describe the dual nature of x-ray energy.
6. State the characteristics of electromagnetic radiation.
7. Differentiate among the units of measurement for ionizing radiation.
8. Recognize the fundamentals of radiation protection.

KEY TERMS

absorbed dose
air kerma
ALARA
equivalent dose
effective dose

electromagnetic radiation
exposure
fluorescence
frequency
photon

quantum
radioactivity
wavelength

X-rays were discovered in Europe in the late 19th century by the German scientist Dr. Wilhelm Conrad Roentgen. Although Roentgen discovered x-rays by accident, he proceeded to study them so thoroughly that within a very short time, he identified all the properties of x-rays that are recognized today. Roentgen was more interested in the characteristics of x-rays as a form of energy than their practical application. X-rays are classified as a specific type of energy termed *electromagnetic radiation (EMR)*, and like all other types of electromagnetic energy, x-rays act like both waves and particles.

DISCOVERY

X-rays were discovered on November 8, 1895, by Dr. Wilhelm Conrad Roentgen (Fig. 1.1), a German physicist and mathematician. Roentgen studied at the Polytechnic Institute in Zurich. He was appointed to the faculty of the University of Würzburg and was the director of the Physics Institute at the time of his discovery. As a teacher and researcher, his academic interest was the conduction of high-voltage electricity through a low-vacuum tube. A low-vacuum tube is simply a glass tube from which a certain amount of air is evacuated.

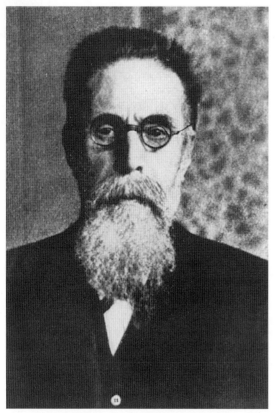

Fig. 1.1 Dr. Wilhelm Conrad Roentgen. (From Glasser O. *Wilhelm Conrad Roentgen and the Early History of the Roentgen Rays.* 1933; Courtesy Charles C. Thomas, Springfield, IL.)

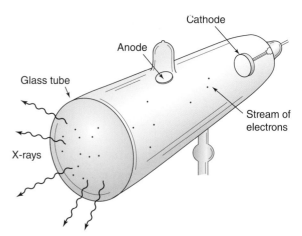

Fig. 1.2 A Crookes tube as used by Roentgen to discover x-rays.

coming from the barium platinocyanide–coated paper. He concluded that the energy emanating from his tube was causing this paper to produce light, or fluoresce. Fluorescence refers to the instantaneous production of light resulting from the interaction of some type of energy (in this case x-rays) and some element or compound (in this case barium platinocyanide).

Roentgen was understandably excited about this apparent discovery; however, at the same time, he was cautious not to make any early assumptions about what he had observed. Before sharing information about his discovery with colleagues, Roentgen spent time meticulously investigating the properties of this new type of energy. Of course, this new type of energy was not new at all; it had always existed and had likely been produced unknowingly by Roentgen and his contemporaries who were also involved in experiments with electricity and low-vacuum tubes. Knowing that others were doing similar research, Roentgen worked in earnest to exactly determine the nature of this energy.

Roentgen spent the next several weeks working feverishly in his laboratory to investigate as many properties of this energy as he could. He noticed that when he placed his hand between his energized tube and the barium platinocyanide–coated paper, he could see the bones of his hand glow on the paper, with this fluoroscopic image moving as he moved his hand. Curious about this, he produced a static (stationary) image of his wife Anna Bertha's hand using a 15-minute exposure. This became the world's first radiograph (Fig. 1.3). Roentgen gathered other materials and interposed them

The specific type of tube that Roentgen was working with was called a *Crookes tube* (Fig. 1.2).

At the end of his workday on November 8, Roentgen prepared his research apparatus for the next experimental session to be conducted when he would return to his workplace. He darkened his laboratory to observe the electrical glow (cathode rays) that occurred when the tube was energized. This glow from the tube would indicate that the tube was receiving electricity and was ready for the next experiment. That day, Roentgen covered his tube with black cardboard and again electrified it. By chance, he noticed a faint glow coming from a certain material located several feet from his electrified tube. The source was a piece of paper coated with barium platinocyanide. Not believing that the cathode rays could reach that far from the tube, Roentgen repeated the experiment. Each time Roentgen energized his tube, he observed this glow

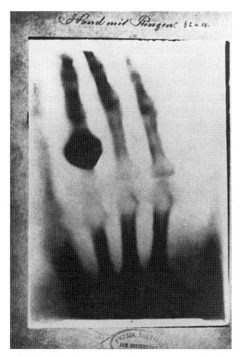

Fig. 1.3 The first radiograph that demonstrates the bones of the hand of Roentgen's wife, Anna Bertha, with a ring on one finger. (From Glasser O. *Wilhelm Conrad Roentgen and the Early History of the Roentgen Rays.* 1933; Courtesy Charles C. Thomas, Springfield, IL.)

between his energized tube and the fluorescent paper. Some materials, such as wood, allowed this energy to pass through and caused the paper to fluoresce, whereas some materials, such as platinum, did not.

In December 1895, Roentgen decided that his investigations of this energy were sufficient to inform his physicist colleagues of what he now believed to be the discovery of a new form of energy. He called this energy *x-rays*, with *x* representing the mathematical symbol for the unknown. On December 28, 1895, Roentgen submitted a scholarly paper on his research activities to his local professional society, the Würzburg Physico-Medical Society. Written in his native language, German, his article was titled "On a New Kind of Rays," and it caused a buzz of excitement in the medical and scientific communities. Within a short time, an English translation of this article appeared in the journal *Nature*, dated January 23, 1896.

Although Roentgen deemed his discovery important, he also considered it to have primarily academic value. His concern was in the x-ray itself as a form of energy and not in its possible practical applications. Others quickly began assembling their own x-ray–producing devices and exposed inanimate objects as well as tissue, both animal and human and both living and dead, to determine the range of use of these x-rays. Their efforts were driven largely by skepticism rather than belief that x-rays could do what had been claimed. Skepticism eventually gave way to productive curiosity as investigations concentrated on ways of imaging living human bodies for medical benefits.

As investigations into legitimate medical applications of the use of x-rays continued, the nonmedical and nonscientific communities began taking a different view of Roentgen's discovery. An x-ray-proof underwear was offered as protection from these rays, which were known to penetrate solid materials, and a New Jersey legislator attempted to enact legislation that would ban the use of x-ray–producing devices in opera glasses. Both these efforts were presumably aimed at protecting an individual's private anatomy from unscrupulous users of x-rays. The public furor reached such a height that a London newspaper, the *Pall Mall Gazette*, offered the following editorial in 1896: "We are sick of Roentgen rays. Perhaps the best thing would be for all civilized nations to combine to burn all the Roentgen rays, to execute all the discoverers, and to corner all the equipment in the world and to whelm it in the middle of the ocean. Let the fish contemplate each other's bones if they like, but not us."

In a similar vein but in a more creative fashion, another London periodical, *Photography*, in 1896 offered the following:

Roentgen Rays, Roentgen Rays?
What is this craze?
The town's ablaze
With this new phase
Of x-ray ways.
I'm full of daze, shock and amaze,
For nowadays
I hear they'll gaze
Through cloak and gown and even stays!
The naughty, naughty Roentgen rays!

Fortunately, despite these public distractions, the scientific applications of x-rays continued to be investigated for the benefit of society. Roentgen's discovery was lauded as one of great significance to science and medicine, and Roentgen received the first Nobel Prize presented for physics in 1901. The branch of medicine that was concerned with the use of x-rays was called *roentgenology*. A unit of radiation exposure was called the *roentgen*. X-rays were, at one time at least, called *roentgen rays*.

Excitement over this previously undiscovered type of energy was tempered by the realization in 1898 that x-rays could cause biological damage. This damage was first noticed as a reddening and burning of the skin (called *erythema*) of individuals who were exposed to large doses of x-rays required at that time. More serious effects, such as the growth of malignant tumors and chromosomal changes, were attributed in later decades to x-ray exposure. However, despite these disturbing findings, it was realized that x-rays could be used safely. When radiation protection procedures to safeguard both the radiographer and the patient are followed, x-rays can assist medical diagnosis by imaging virtually every part of the human body.

PROPERTIES OF X-RAYS

X-rays are known to have several characteristics or properties. These characteristics are briefly explained here and presented in Box 1.1.

- *X-rays are invisible.* In addition to being unable to see x-rays, one cannot feel, smell, or hear them.
- *X-rays are electrically neutral.* X-rays have neither a positive nor a negative charge; they cannot be accelerated or made to change direction by a magnet or electrical field.
- *X-rays have no mass.* X-rays create no resistance to being put into motion and cannot produce force.

BOX 1.1   Characteristics of X-rays

- Are invisible
- Are electrically neutral
- Have no mass
- Travel at the speed of light in a vacuum
- Cannot be optically focused
- Form a polyenergetic (heterogeneous) beam
- Can be produced in a range of energies
- Travel in straight lines
- Can cause some substances to fluoresce
- Can penetrate the human body
- Can be absorbed or scattered in the human body
- Can produce secondary radiation
- Can cause damage to living tissue

- *X-rays travel at the speed of light in a vacuum.* X-rays move at a constant velocity of 3×10^8 m/s or 186,000 miles/s in a vacuum.
- *X-rays cannot be optically focused.* Optical lenses have no ability to focus or refract x-ray photons.
- *X-rays form polyenergetic (heterogeneous) beams.* The x-ray beam that is used in diagnostic radiography is composed of photons that have many different energies. The maximum energy that a photon in any beam may have is expressed by the kilovoltage peak (kVp), which is set on the control panel of the radiographic unit by the radiographer.
- *X-rays can be produced in a range of energies.* These are useful for different purposes in diagnostic routine radiography. The medically useful diagnostic range of x-ray energies is 30 to 150 kVp.
- *X-rays travel in straight lines.* X-rays used in diagnostic radiography form a divergent beam in which each individual photon travels in a straight line.
- *X-rays can cause certain substances to fluoresce.* When x-rays strike certain substances, the substances produce light. These substances are used in some types of image receptors.
- *X-rays can penetrate the human body.* X-rays have the ability to pass through the body based on the energy of the x-rays and on the compositions and thicknesses of the tissues being exposed.
- *X-rays can be absorbed or scattered by tissues in the human body.* Depending on the energy of an individual x-ray photon, that photon may be absorbed in the body or made to scatter, moving in another direction.
- *X-rays can produce secondary radiation.* When x-rays are absorbed as a result of a specific type of interaction with matter (photoelectric effect), a secondary or characteristic photon is produced.
- *X-rays can cause chemical and biologic damage to living tissue.* Through excitation and ionization (removal of electrons) of atoms comprising cells, damage to the cells (mainly through ionization of water in the body) can occur.

X-RAYS AS ENERGY

Energy is the ability to do work, and it can exist in different forms, such as electrical energy, kinetic energy, thermal energy, and electromagnetic energy. Energy can also be transformed from one form to another, for instance, the electrical energy applied to a stove is changed into heat (thermal energy). Similarly, the electrical energy applied to an x-ray tube is transformed into heat and x-rays.

X-radiations, or x-rays, are a type of electromagnetic radiation (EMR). Electromagnetic radiation refers to radiation that has both electrical and magnetic properties. All radiations that are electromagnetic make up a spectrum (Fig. 1.4).

In the academic discipline of physics, energy can generally be described as behaving according to the wave or the particle concept of physics. X-rays have a dual nature: they behave like both waves and particles. Higher-energy electromagnetic radiation, such as x-rays, tends to exhibit more particle-like characteristics, and lower-energy electromagnetic radiation, such as radiowaves, tend to exhibit more wave-like characteristics.

 IMPORTANT RELATIONSHIP

The Dual Nature of X-ray Energy

X-rays act like both waves and particles.

X-rays can be described as waves because they move in waves that have wavelength and frequency. Looking at a sine wave (Fig. 1.5), one can see that the wavelength represents the distance between two successive crests or troughs. Wavelength is represented by the Greek letter lambda (λ), and its values are given in units of angstroms (Å). An angstrom is a metric unit of length equal to one ten-billionth of a meter, or 10^{-10} m. X-rays used in radiography range in wavelength from approximately 0.1 to 1.0 Å. Another unit of measurement for wavelength is nanometer (nm); 1 Å equals 0.1 nm, which equals 10^{-9} m.

The sine wave (Fig. 1.5) also demonstrates that frequency represents the number of waves (cycles) passing a given point per given unit of time (second). Frequency is represented by a lowercase f or by the Greek letter nu (ν), and its values are given in units of Hertz (Hz). One Hertz is equal to one cycle per second. X-rays used in radiography range in frequency from approximately 3×10^{19} to 3×10^{18} Hz. Wavelength

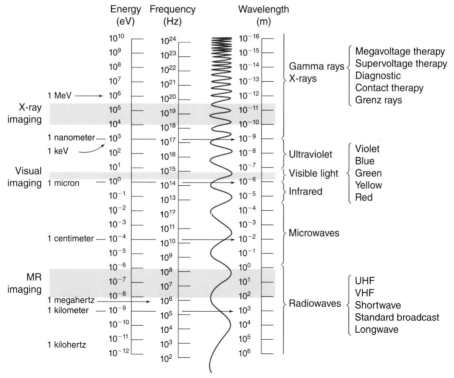

THE ELECTROMAGNETIC SPECTRUM

Fig. 1.4 Electromagnetic spectrum. Radiowaves are the least energetic on the spectrum, and gamma rays are the most energetic. *MR,* Magnetic resonance; *UHF,* ultra high frequency; *VHF,* very high frequency.

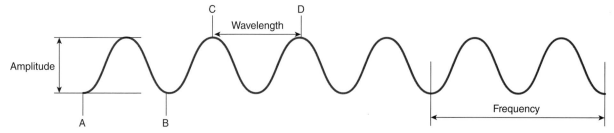

Fig. 1.5 Sine wave demonstrating wavelength, frequency, and amplitude. One wavelength is equal to the distance between two successive troughs (points *A* to *B*) or the distance between two successive crests (points *C* to *D*). Frequency is the number of waves passing a given point per given unit of time (second). Amplitude is the height of the wave.

and frequency are inversely related—that is, as one increases, the other decreases. Higher-energy electromagnetic radiation has high frequencies and low wavelengths.

In a sine wave (see Fig. 1.5), amplitude is a measurement of the height of the wave. For electromagnetic radiations (EMRs), the amplitude or height of the wave does not vary so the most important characteristics of EMR are wavelength and frequency. Amplitude is an important feature of other forms of energy such as electrical current or sound waves.

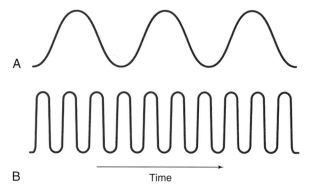

Fig. 1.6 A, Sine wave demonstrating long wavelength and low frequency. **B,** Sine wave demonstrating short wavelength and high frequency; comparison of sine waves. **A** and **B** demonstrate the inverse relationship between wavelength and frequency.

⚡ IMPORTANT RELATIONSHIP

Wavelength and Frequency

> Wavelength and frequency are inversely related. Higher-energy x-rays have decreased wavelength and increased frequency. Lower-energy x-rays have increased wavelength and decreased frequency.

This relationship can be observed in Fig. 1.6 and is demonstrated by the expression $c = \lambda v$, in which c represents the speed of light. In this expression, if wavelength increases, frequency must decrease because the speed of light is a constant velocity (3×10^8 m/s or 186,000 miles/s). Conversely, if wavelength decreases, frequency must increase, again because the speed of light is constant. Mathematically, the formulas are $\lambda = c/v$ to solve for wavelength and $v = c/\lambda$ to solve for frequency. These formulas illustrate the inverse relationship between wavelength and frequency.

X-rays also behave like particles and move as photons or quanta (plural). A photon or quantum (singular) is a small, discrete bundle of energy. For most applications in radiography, x-rays are referred to as *photons*. When x-rays interact with matter, they behave more like particles than waves. The energy of an individual photon is measured in units of electron volts (eV) and the energy of diagnostic x-rays is approximately between 10^4 and 10^5 eV. Decreasing the wavelength and/or increasing the frequency of the x-ray will increase its energy.

Radiation Units of Measurement

It is important to recognize the units of radiation quantity to obtain an accurate understanding of radiation exposure, dose, and biologic effect. There are two systems for quantifying radiation exposure: the Standard (British) System and the International System (SI). SI is the more widely adopted of the two. Radiation exposure can be measured in the following units:

Unit of Measure	Standard	International System (SI)
Exposure in air (a)	Roentgen (R)	coulomb/ kilogram air kerma (Gy$_a$)
Absorbed dose in tissue (t)	radiation absorbed dose (rad)	Gray (Gy$_t$)
Equivalent dose	radiation equivalent in man (rem)	Sievert (Sv)
Effective dose	radiation equivalent in man (rem)	Sievert (Sv)
Radioactivity	Curie (Ci)	Becquerel (Bq)

Exposure

The quantity of radiation exposure expressed in roentgens (R) measures the amount of ionization or electrical charge in a specified amount of air; this is a measure of the *intensity* of radiation exposure. The coulomb/kilogram is equivalent to the roentgen. The coulomb/kilogram is a measure of the number of electrons liberated by ionization per kilogram of air. Ionization is the removal of electrons from atoms. The roentgen or coulomb/kilogram is generally used as a unit of measure for such phenomena as the output intensity of x-ray equipment or intensity in air. The relationship between the two is:

$$1 \text{ C/kg} = 3876 \text{ R}$$

or

$$1 \text{ R} = 2.58 \times 10^{-4} \text{ C/kg}$$

Another radiation quantity used to express exposure or intensity is air kerma (**k**inetic **e**nergy **r**eleased per unit **m**ass). Air kerma is used to describe the quantity of radiation energy delivered to a given point. The quantity of energy released by 1 R of exposure in air is equal to approximately 0.01 air kerma. Air kerma is the amount of energy deposited in a unit mass of air (kg) and expressed in units of joules (J) or J/kg, which is also the radiation unit, the gray (Gy). A unit of 1 R of exposure in air is equal to approximately 0.01 (Gy$_a$) air kerma; however, radiation exposure is typically expressed in smaller units by adding the prefix "milli," in which 1 R = 1000 mR and 1 Gy = 1000 mGy.

Absorbed Dose

The rad and gray are units measuring the transfer of radiation energy into matter (e.g., tissue), known as the absorbed dose. One rad is equal to an energy transfer of 100 ergs per gram of any absorbing matter. One gray (Gy$_t$) is defined as 1 joule of energy absorbed in each kilogram of absorbing material. The joule is the SI unit for the transfer of energy into matter and more commonly used today; 100 ergs per gram is equal to 0.01 joule per kilogram of irradiated matter. One rad is equal to 0.01 gray, and a conversion factor of 0.01 is used to convert a rad into a gray. For example, an absorbed dose of 5 rad = 0.05 Gy$_t$.

Absorbed dose is typically used in referring to patient low-dose medical radiation absorbed exposure and the potential biologic effects and is more commonly expressed as mGy$_t$. The amount of absorbed dose is dependent on the energy of the ionizing radiation and the type of interacting tissues.

Equivalent Dose

The units of equivalent dose (similarly known as dose equivalent) are radiation equivalents in man (rem) and sieverts (Sv). One sievert equals 100 rem or 0.01 Sv equals 1 rem. These units are derived by multiplying a quality factor, radiation weighting factor (W$_r$) for the type of ionizing radiation by the units of absorbed exposure, rads, or grays. The quality factor or W$_r$ takes into consideration the biological effects of different types of ionizing radiation (Table 1.1). Although the quality factor (W$_r$) is not equal for all ionizing radiations, x- and gamma rays have the same quality factor or W$_r$ of 1 and therefore are equal in their biological effect on tissues. Consequently, 1 rad or 0.01 Gy is equal to 1 rem or 0.01 Sv. Differing particulate radiations, such as alpha particles, have differing associated quality factors and

TABLE 1.1 International Commission of Radiologic Protection (ICRP) Radiation Weighting Factors

Type of Radiation	Weighting Factor (Wr)
X-rays, gamma rays, beta particles, and electrons	1
Protons	2
Fast neutrons and alpha particles	20

W_r, resulting in changes in the biologic effects following exposure.

Effective Dose

Effective dose is an expression of the *relative risk to humans* (whole-body exposure) of exposure to ionizing radiation. It is a calculated measure and concept most useful in radiation protection applications. However, effective dose does not consider patient variability such as age, gender, or weight and therefore should be used for populations and not individual patients. It is measured in Sv but is calculated by multiplying the absorbed dose (in Gy [but equal to Sv for x- and gamma rays]), the W_r, and the tissue weighting factor (W_t). W_t is used as a correction factor because not all tissues, organs, or systems have the same level of sensitivity to radiation (radiosensitivity). If more than one tissue, organ, or system is exposed, the effective doses are added together (summed). Table 1.2 is the International Commission of Radiologic Protection (ICRP)–recommended tissue weighting factors.

It is important to note that our knowledge about tissue radiosensitivity and low-dose radiation risk has uncertainties and continues to evolve. There have been variations over the years regarding tissue radiosensitivity because of these inherent uncertainties, and therefore the W_t has varied. Nevertheless, ionizing radiation has the potential to produce biologic harm and should be administered wisely.

Radioactivity

Unstable atoms spontaneously emit particles and energy from the nucleus in an effort to reach stability (radioactivity). This process is called radioactive disintegration or decay. Radioisotopes are the radioactive elements used in nuclear medicine and radiation therapy.

The curie (Ci) and the becquerel (Bq) measure the rate of nuclear disintegration or decay of a material.

Radioactive disintegration or decay refers to the decrease in the activity of a radiation source. Half-life is a term that describes the time it takes for the radiation activity to reduce to 50% of its original activity. For example, radioisotopes used in nuclear medicine typically have half-lives in a number of hours or days.

THE FUNDAMENTALS OF RADIATION PROTECTION

A central message throughout this textbook is that it is the radiographer's responsibility to minimize the radiation dose to the patient, to themselves, and to others in accordance with the **a**s **l**ow **a**s **r**easonably **a**chievable (ALARA) principle. Although the ALARA principle is primarily intended for occupational exposures to imaging professionals, it has also been applied to patient radiation exposure. The concept of *optimization for radiological protection* is currently advocated, meaning the radiation dose should be appropriate to the imaging procedure and avoid unnecessary exposure to the patient while producing quality images for diagnostic interpretation.

> **! RADIATION PROTECTION ALERT**
>
> ### ALARA Principle and Optimization for Radiological Protection
>
> It is the radiographer's responsibility to minimize the radiation dose to the patient, to themselves, and to others in accordance with the as low as reasonably achievable (ALARA) principle. Optimization for radiological protection means the radiation dose should be appropriate to the imaging procedure and avoid unnecessary exposure to the patient while producing quality images for diagnostic interpretation.

TABLE 1.2 International Commission of Radiologic Protection (ICRP)–Recommended Tissue Weighting Factors (ICRP 103)	
Tissue	**Weighting Factor (W_t)**
Breast, adrenals, bone marrow, colon, extrathoracic region, gallbladder, heart, kidneys, lung, lymph nodes, muscle, oral mucosa, pancreas, prostate, small intestine, spleen, stomach, thymus, uterus, cervix	0.12
Gonads	0.08
Bladder, esophagus, liver, thyroid	0.04
Bone surface, brain, salivary glands, skin	0.01

Central to minimizing the radiation dose to oneself and to others are the cardinal principles of shielding, time, and distance. Shielding broadly refers to the use of radiopaque materials (i.e., materials through which x-rays do *not* pass easily) to greatly reduce radiation exposure to radiographers during exams, and to others. Lead-impregnated materials are a common example. Lead aprons must be worn by the radiographer and other health care workers when it is necessary to be in close proximity to the patient during an exposure. In addition, thyroid shields are commonly used in conjunction with lead aprons, especially during fluoroscopic exams by personnel who remain in the room. This collar wraps around the neck and fastens in the back to shield the entire front portion of the neck. Leaded curtains may be draped from the fluoroscopy unit to provide a barrier between the fluoroscopist (one operating the fluoroscope) and the x-ray beam during fluoroscopic exams. The walls of the radiographic suite are permeated with lead or lead equivalent (thicknesses of other materials that provide equivalent radiopaque properties as lead) to limit exposure beyond that intended for the radiological exam. The primary barriers are those to which the x-ray beam is routinely directed, such as the floor beneath the x-ray table and the wall behind the upright Bucky. Secondary barriers are the others, such as the wall separating the control panel from the room and the ceiling to protect those outside the room from scatter radiation. The general rule of thumb is to always maximize shielding (use as much as possible).

Shielding used to reduce radiation exposure to patients' sensitive areas during radiographic imaging has been a standard practice for decades. Recently, regulatory and advisory organizations have recommended discontinuing gonadal shielding during abdominal and pelvic imaging. Digital imaging equipment used today requires significantly reduced radiation exposures, and incorrect placement of shielding devices may obscure visibility of anatomy. In addition, the ICRP tissue weighting factor (W_t) for gonad sensitivity has been lowered from 0.20 to 0.08. These reasons provide support for the decision to discontinue gonadal shielding during abdominal and pelvic imaging. However, knowledge of shielding patient-sensitive areas during radiographic imaging and its practical application will continue to be an important skill set for the radiographer.

Time broadly refers to the duration of exposure to ionizing radiation and the time spent in a health care environment where exposure to ionizing radiation is accumulated. This may include the length of the exposure and number of times the patient is exposed for a radiological exam or the time a radiographer spends in a fluoroscopy suite (or any procedure involving fluoroscopy). Whether one is referring to the patient, to the radiographer, or to other health care workers, the general rule of thumb is to always minimize time (limit duration of exposure to ionizing radiation).

Distance refers to the space between oneself and the source of ionizing radiation. This is an effective means of limiting exposure simply because the intensity (quantity) of radiation diminishes over distance. This is an application of the inverse-square law discussed in detail in Chapter 7. Suffice it to say here that as one increases the distance from an ionizing radiation source, the radiation intensity from that source significantly decreases. This principle is applied mostly to radiographers and others to maintain a safe distance from the source of radiation during exposure. The general rule of thumb is always to maximize distance (maintain a safe distance from the radiation source during exposure).

❗ RADIATION PROTECTION ALERT

Cardinal Principles for Minimizing Radiation Dose

Time: Limit the amount of time exposed to ionizing radiation.
Distance: Maintain a safe distance from the source of ionizing radiation exposure.
Shielding: Maximize the use of shielding from ionizing radiation exposure.

Another important *tool* in radiation protection is the limiting of the field of x-ray exposure, essentially beam restriction, through the use of a collimator. By limiting the area of exposure, this device limits the radiation dose to the patient, that is, the smaller the area of x-ray exposure, the lower the total dose to the patient. When we discuss radiation interactions in the body, we are talking about x-ray photons interacting with atoms of tissue. The greater the volume of tissue we expose, the greater is the opportunity for such interactions to occur. With these interactions, the photon's energy will either be totally absorbed (which contributes to patient dose) or scattered (which may contribute to the dose to radiographers or others if in the immediate area). See Chapter 4 for a full discussion of x-ray interactions with matter.

! RADIATION PROTECTION ALERT

Beam Restriction

Limiting the size of the x-ray exposure field reduces the volume of tissue irradiated and reduces the radiation dose to the patient.

Next among our *tools* of radiation protection are the primary controls of the x-ray beam's kilovoltage peak (kVp), milliamperage (mA), and duration (s), mAs = mA × s. These are the factors selected by the radiographer to produce an x-ray beam of a given quality (penetrating power) controlled by kVp and quantity (number of photons) ultimately controlled by mAs. The combination of kVp and mAs is selected on the basis of a number of considerations, including the anatomic part being examined, patient age, condition, pathology, and so on, and should be ideally suited to the circumstance to minimize radiation dose while producing optimum exposure to the image receptor. See Chapter 7 for a complete discussion of these factors.

! RADIATION PROTECTION ALERT

Primary Exposure Factors

The combination of kVp and mAs is selected based on a number of considerations, including the anatomic part being examined, patient age, condition, and pathology, and should be ideally suited to the circumstance to minimize radiation dose while producing optimum exposure to the image receptor.

Finally, there are a number of daily *workflow* tasks and processes that address radiation protection. A major one, for which the radiographer serves as a frontline advocate for the patient, is the avoidance of unnecessary duplication of exams. This means preventing the patient from having the same exam performed twice owing to an error. With so much computerization, automation, and team approach to patient care, it is easy to duplicate an order (accidentally order the same radiographic

exam more than once) or for two different physicians involved in a patient's care who unknowingly order the same thing. There are instances when a patient's condition rapidly changes, and it is necessary to perform the same exam a number of times in succession, but it is appropriate to double-check an order or to stop and question. The radiographer must recognize and accept this enhanced role as a patient advocate and do what is necessary to avoid unnecessary duplication of exams. Think of each duplicate exam as a doubling of the radiation dose that is otherwise needed (the first exam was a normal dose, and the unnecessary one doubles that dose). Thus, this radiation protection measure alone significantly impacts the radiation dose administered to the patient and to others.

! RADIATION PROTECTION ALERT

Avoid Unnecessary Duplicate Exams

Radiographers must recognize and accept their role as a patient advocate and do what is necessary to avoid unnecessary duplication of exams.

Screening for pregnancy is another important task for minimizing unnecessary exposure to a developing fetus. Departmental protocols for pregnancy screening may vary and should be consistently used. When it is necessary to perform a radiologic exam on a pregnant patient, shielding materials may be used, in special circumstances, along with precise collimation, as discussed previously, to minimize radiation dose administered to the fetus. Be sure to follow the clinical site policy for pregnancy screening.

! RADIATION PROTECTION ALERT

Screening for Pregnancy

Screening for pregnancy is another important task for minimizing unnecessary exposure to a developing fetus. When it is necessary to perform a radiologic exam on a pregnant patient, shielding materials may be used, in special circumstances, along with precise collimation to minimize the radiation dose administered to the fetus.

Last, as a developing radiographer, good work habits and skills have not yet been developed. Use sufficient time and concentration to *get it right the first time.*

BOX 1.2   Summary of Radiation Protection Fundamentals

- Minimize the radiation dose to the patient, to themselves, and to others in accordance with the **as low as reasonably achievable (ALARA)** principle and optimization for radiological protection.
- Limit the amount of *time* exposed to ionizing radiation.
- Maintain a safe *distance* from source of ionizing radiation exposure.
- Maximize the use of *shielding* from ionizing radiation exposure.

- Limit the size of the x-ray exposure field to the area of interest.
- Select a combination of kVp and mAs to produce a diagnostic image while minimizing patient radiation exposure.
- Avoid unnecessary duplicate exams.
- Screen for pregnancy.
- Develop a mental checklist for radiographic procedures and perform consistently.

kVp, Kilovoltage peak; *mAs,* milliamperage-seconds.

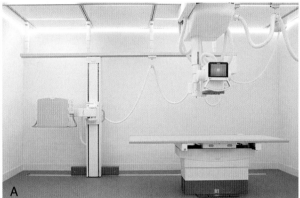
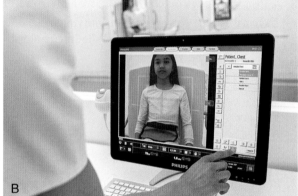

Fig. 1.7 A, Typical radiographic unit showing the x-ray table, overhead x-ray tube with live camera, collimator, and wall stand. **B,** Control panel with touch screen interface. (© 2024 Koninklijke Philips N.V. All rights reserved.)

Develop a mental checklist for radiographic procedures and perform them the same way every time. By doing so, mistakes involving the details of a task can be minimized along with unnecessary radiation dose administered to the patient and to others. See Box 1.2 for a summary of radiation protection fundamentals.

Since the publication of Roentgen's scientific paper, no other properties of x-rays have been discovered. However, the discussion of x-rays has expanded far beyond the early concerns about modesty or even danger. Today, x-rays are accepted as an important diagnostic tool in medicine, and the radiographer is an important member of the health care team. The radiologic imaging professional is responsible for the care of the patient in the radiology department, the production and control of x-rays, and the formation of a quality radiographic image. Fig. 1.7 shows a standard radiographic room that includes an x-ray table, an overhead x-ray tube and collimator, and a control panel for the selection of exposure technique factors. The subsequent chapters of this book uncover the intricate and fascinating details of the art and science of medical radiography.

CHAPTER SUMMARY

- X-rays were discovered on November 8, 1895, by Dr. Wilhelm Conrad Roentgen, a German physicist, mathematician, and recipient of the first Nobel Prize for physics.

- The discovery of x-rays was met with skepticism and curiosity and subsequently by acceptance of its medical benefit.

- X-rays have several important characteristics. They are invisible and electrically neutral, have no mass, travel at the speed of light, penetrate matter, and can cause chemical and biologic changes.
- X-rays are a type of electromagnetic radiation with both electrical and magnetic properties.
- Electromagnetic radiation is a form of energy that moves in waves with wavelength and frequency.
- Wavelength and frequency are inversely related. Higher-energy x-rays have decreased wavelength and increased frequency.
- X-rays act like both waves and particles and have a higher energy than other types of electromagnetic radiation, such as visible light.
- There have been two systems of quantifying radiation exposure: the standard system and the International System (SI). The International System (SI) is the more widely adopted today. Exposure in air: coulomb/kilogram, roentgen (R), and air kerma (Gy_a); absorbed dose: radiation absorbed dose (rad) and gray (Gy_t); equivalent dose: radiation equivalent in man (rem) and sievert (Sv); effective dose: an expression of the relative risk to humans of exposure to ionizing radiation; radioactivity: curie (Ci) and becquerel (Bq).
- The fundamentals of radiation protection include adhering to the ALARA principle, optimization of radiological protection, time, distance, shielding, beam restriction, careful selection of exposure technique factors, avoidance of duplicate exams, and screening for pregnancy.

REVIEW QUESTIONS

1. In what year were x-rays discovered?
   A. 1892
   B. 1895
   C. 1898
   D. 1901
2. In what year were some of the biologically damaging effects of x-rays discovered?
   A. 1892
   B. 1895
   C. 1898
   D. 1901
3. X-rays were discovered in experiments dealing with electricity and _____.
   A. ionization
   B. magnetism
   C. atomic structure
   D. vacuum tubes
4. X-rays were discovered when they caused a barium platinocyanide–coated plate to _____.
   A. fluoresce
   B. phosphoresce
   C. vibrate
   D. burn and redden
5. X-radiation is classified in which spectrum?
   A. Radiation
   B. Energy
   C. Atomic
   D. Electromagnetic
6. X-rays have a dual nature, which means that they behave like both _____.
   A. atoms and molecules
   B. photons and quanta
   C. waves and particles
   D. charged and uncharged particles
7. The wavelength and frequency of x-rays are _____ related.
   A. directly
   B. inversely
   C. partially
   D. not
8. X-rays have _____ electrical charge.
   A. a positive
   B. a negative
   C. an alternately positive and negative
   D. no
9. X-rays have _____.
   A. no mass
   B. the same mass as electrons
   C. the same mass as protons
   D. the same mass as neutrons
10. The x-ray beam used in diagnostic radiography can be described as being _____.
   A. homogeneous
   B. monoenergetic
   C. polyenergetic
   D. scattered

11. The unit that measures the transfer of radiation energy into tissues is known as the _____.
    A. roentgen
    B. kerma
    C. gray
    D. sievert

12. What is defined as the measure of the intensity of radiation exposure?
    A. Absorbed dose
    B. Exposure
    C. Equivalent dose
    D. Effective dose

13. What is the radiation weighting factor (W_r) for x- and gamma rays?
    A. 1
    B. 2
    C. 10
    D. 20

14. Which of the following will minimize radiation exposure to the patient?
    A. Limiting the x-ray exposure field
    B. Controlling quality and quantity of the x-ray beam
    C. Avoiding unnecessary duplicate exams
    D. All of the above

Fundamentals of Radiation Production

CHAPTER OUTLINE

X-ray Production
  Cathode
  Anode
  X-ray Tube Housing
The X-ray Circuit
  Transformers

Resistors
Current Rectification
Current Waveforms
High-Frequency Generators

OBJECTIVES

After completing this chapter, the reader will be able to perform the following:
1. Define all the key terms in this chapter.
2. State all the important relationships in this chapter.
3. Describe the construction of an x-ray tube.
4. Differentiate between the functions of the cathode and anode.
5. Describe the process to produce x-rays.
6. State the purpose of the x-ray circuit.

7. Identify the major components found in the high- and low-voltage sides of the x-ray circuit.
8. Explain the process of obtaining the high voltage required for x-ray production.
9. Define the role of resistors in regulating current during x-ray exposure.
10. Explain the need for an autotransformer and both step-up and step-down transformers during x-ray production.
11. State the advantages of high-frequency generators.

KEY TERMS

anode	focusing cup	step-down transformers
autotransformer	leakage radiation	step-up transformers
capacitors	mutual induction	stator
cathode	off-focus radiation	target
circuit	rectification	thermionic emission
dielectric	resistance	transformers
diode	resistors	
filament	rotor	

The x-ray tube is the most important part of the x-ray machine because the tube is where the x-rays are produced. Radiographers must understand the construction and operation of an x-ray tube and its basic circuit design features. The radiographer controls many actions that

occur within the tube. Kilovoltage peak (kVp), milliamperage (mA), exposure time, and focal spot size all are factors that the radiographer adjusts on the control panel to produce a quality image. There are additional controls such as distance (source-image-receptor distance [SID]) that can be selected to optimize image quality at safe radiation dosages. The radiographer also needs to be aware of the amount of heat produced during x-ray production because excessive heat can damage the tube.

X-RAY PRODUCTION

As an essential electrical component in the x-ray system, the x-ray tube is considered a diode in that it has polarity with a positively charged anode and negatively charged cathode. The x-ray tube performs two functions: x-ray production and circuit continuity. If the x-ray tube fails, electron flow through the circuit stops and the system is inoperable.

The production of x-rays requires a rapidly moving stream of electrons that are suddenly decelerated or stopped. The source of electrons is a cathode, or negative electrode. The negative electrode is heated, and electrons are emitted. The electrons are attracted to the positively charged anode (positive electrode) and move rapidly toward the anode, where they are stopped or decelerated. When the kinetic energy (energy of motion) of the electrons is transferred to the anode, x-rays and heat are produced (Fig. 2.1). Unfortunately, it is a very inefficient process with most electron kinetic energy converted to heat.

Cathode

The cathode of an x-ray tube is a negatively charged electrode. It comprises a coiled, tungsten wire filament that is precisely positioned in a concave focusing cup (Fig. 2.2).

Most x-ray tubes are referred to as *dual-focus tubes* because they have two filaments: one large and one small. Only one filament is energized at any one time during x-ray production. If the radiographer selects a large focal spot when setting the control panel, the large filament is energized. If a small focal spot is chosen, the

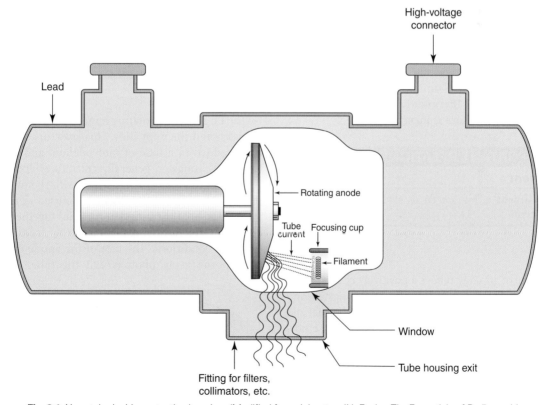

Lead

High-voltage connector

Rotating anode

Tube current   Focusing cup

Filament

Window

Tube housing exit

Fitting for filters, collimators, etc.

Fig. 2.1 X-ray tube inside protective housing. (Modified from Johnston JN, Fauber TL. *Essentials of Radiographic Physics and Imaging*. 2nd ed. St. Louis: Mosby; 2016.)

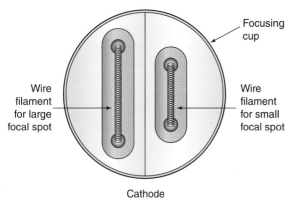

Fig. 2.2 Frontal view of cathode small and large filaments recessed into the concave contour of the focusing cup design.

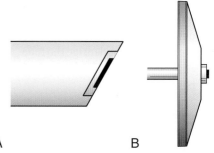

Fig. 2.3 **A,** Side views of a stationary anode. **B,** A rotating anode.

small filament is energized. The **focusing cup** is made of nickel and nearly surrounds the filament. It is open at one end to allow electrons to flow freely across the tube from the cathode to the anode. It has a negative charge, which keeps the cloud of electrons emitted from the filament from spreading apart. The purpose of the focusing cup is to electrically focus the stream of electrons from the filament toward the anode target.

Just prior to the actual exposure, the cathode filament heats up to extreme temperatures and liberates or "boils off" electrons as a "cloud" around the filament wire. This process is known as **thermionic emission** and occurs when the x-ray exposure sequence is initiated.

IMPORTANT RELATIONSHIP

Filament

The **filament** is the source of electrons during x-ray production.

Anode

The **anode** of an x-ray tube is a positively charged electrode composed of molybdenum, copper, tungsten, and graphite. These materials are used for their thermal and electrical conductive properties. The anode assembly consists of a target and, in rotating anode tubes, a stator and rotor. The **target** is made of a metal that abruptly decelerates and stops electrons in the tube current, allowing the production of x-rays. The target can be either rotating or stationary. Tubes with rotating targets are more common than tubes with stationary ones,

which are popular in the dental industry. Rotating anodes are manufactured to rotate at a set speed ranging from 3000 to 10,000 revolutions per minute (rpm). Fig. 2.3 shows how a rotating anode and stationary anode differ in appearance.

IMPORTANT RELATIONSHIP

Target

The target is the part of the anode that is struck by the focused stream of electrons coming from the cathode. The target stops the electrons and creates the opportunity for the production of x-rays.

The target of the rotating anode tubes is made of a tungsten and rhenium alloy. This layer, or focal track, is embedded in a base of molybdenum and graphite (Fig. 2.4). Tungsten generally constitutes 90% of the composition of the rotating target, with rhenium constituting the other 10%. Rhenium is used as an alloy material to hold the tungsten particles together under high heat and centrifugal force (away from axis of rotation) conditions. The face of the anode is angled to help the x-ray photons exit the tube. Rotating

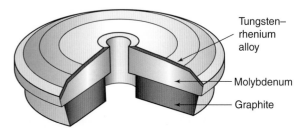

Fig. 2.4 Typical construction of a rotating anode.

targets generally have a target angle ranging from 5 to 20 degrees. Tungsten is used for both rotating and stationary targets because it has a high atomic number of 74 for effective x-ray production and a high melting point of 3400°C (6152°F). Most of the energy produced by an x-ray tube is heat; thus melting of the target can sometimes become a problem, especially with high exposures.

IMPORTANT RELATIONSHIP
Tungsten

> Because tungsten has a high atomic number (74) and a high melting point (3400°C [6152°F]), it effectively produces x-rays.

To turn the anode during x-ray production, a rotating anode tube requires a stator and rotor (Fig. 2.5). The **stator** is an electric motor that turns the rotor at very high speed. The **rotor** (made of copper) is rigidly connected to the target through the anode stem (made of molybdenum), causing the target to rapidly rotate during x-ray production. High-strength ball bearings in the rotor allow it to smoothly rotate at high speeds.

During x-ray production, most of the energy produced at the anode is heat, with a very small percentage being x-ray energy. Heat can pose a problem if allowed to build up; hence, it is transferred to the envelope and then to the **dielectric** (nonconducting material and considered an insulator since it does not conduct electricity) oil surrounding the tube. Moreover, many tube

assemblies have a fan that blows air over the tube to help dissipate heat. X-ray tube manufacturers have developed creative methods to help dissipate x-ray tube heat such as liquid-bearing rotors, larger diameter anodes, and water-cooled tubes.

IMPORTANT RELATIONSHIP
Dissipating Heat

> The heat produced when the x-ray exposure is activated is transferred to the electrical insulating, dielectric oil that surrounds the x-ray tube.

Rotating anodes can withstand high heat loads; this ability relates to the actual focal spot, which is the physical area of the target that is bombarded by electrons during x-ray production. With stationary targets, the focal spot is a fixed area on the surface of the target. With rotating targets, this area is represented by a focal track. Fig. 2.6 shows the stationary anode's focal spot and the rotating anode with its focal track. The size of the focal spot is not altered with a rotating anode, but the actual physical area of the target bombarded by electrons is constantly moving, causing a greater area of the *focal track* to be exposed to electrons. Because of the

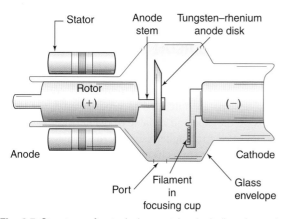

Fig. 2.5 Structure of a typical x-ray tube, including the major operational parts.

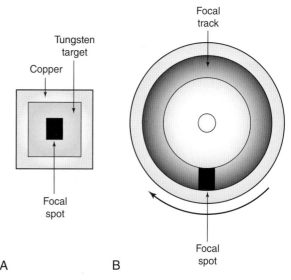

Fig. 2.6 A, Front view of a stationary anode. **B,** The target area of the rotating anode turns during exposure along with an increased physical area—a focal track—that is exposed to electrons.

larger area of the target being bombarded during an exposure, the rotating anode is able to withstand higher heat loads produced by greater exposure factors. Rotating anode x-ray tubes are used in all applications in radiography, whereas stationary anode tubes are limited to studies of small anatomic structures such as teeth.

 IMPORTANT RELATIONSHIP

Rotating Anodes

Rotating anodes can withstand higher heat loads than stationary anodes because the rotation causes a greater physical area, or focal track, to be exposed to electrons.

X-ray Tube Housing

The components necessary for x-ray production are housed in a glass or metal envelope. Fig. 2.7 shows the appearance of a glass x-ray tube. Metal envelopes are more commonly used because of their superior electrical properties.

A disadvantage of a glass envelope x-ray tube is that tungsten evaporated from the filament and anode surface during exposure can be deposited upon the inside of the glass, especially in the middle portion of the envelope. This buildup of tungsten particles can affect the flow of electrons by arcing and cause the tube to fail. Replacing this section of glass with metal (metal window tube) prevents these problems and extends the tube life.

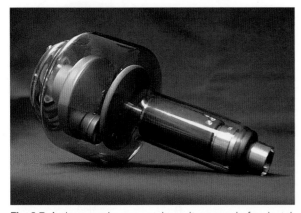

Fig. 2.7 A glass envelope x-ray tube as it appears before installation in a tube housing. (From Johnston JN and Fauber TL. *Essentials of Radiographic Physics and Imaging*. 3rd ed. St. Louis: Mosby; 2020.)

An additional advantage of a metal envelope is the reduction of off-focus radiation. Off-focus radiation occurs when projectile electrons from the cathode strike areas of the anode surface other than the actual focal spot area such as the anode stem and anode edge. This x-ray production is undesirable and diminishes image quality. The metal tube envelope can collect these electrons and conduct them away from the anode.

The envelope allows air to be completely evacuated from the x-ray tube, which in turn allows an efficient flow of electrons from cathode to anode. The envelope serves two additional functions: it provides some insulation from electrical shock that may occur because the cathode and anode contain electrical charges, and it dissipates heat in the tube by conducting it to the insulating oil surrounding the envelope. The purpose of insulating oil is to provide more insulation from electrical shock and to help dissipate heat away from the tube. All of these components are surrounded by the metal tube housing on all sides except for a port, or window, which allows the primary beam to exit the tube. It is the metal tube housing that the radiographer observes and handles when moving the x-ray tube. The tube housing has an inside lining of lead to provide additional shielding from leakage radiation. Leakage radiation refers to any x-rays, other than the primary beam, that escape the tube housing. The tube housing is required to allow a leakage radiation of no more than 1 mGy$_a$/h (100 mR/h) to escape when measured at 1 m from the source while the tube operates at maximum output. Electrical current is supplied to the x-ray tube housing assembly. X-ray production is a high-voltage process and because of this, the spacing between the anode and cathode electrodes is important and is typically 1 to 2 cm.

THE X-RAY CIRCUIT

As you might expect, the sophistication of x-ray systems involves complex electronic circuits and components. These designs are intended to produce an x-ray beam that is predictable and capable of delivering the correct amount of electromagnetic energy to an image receptor. Generally, the x-ray circuit is intended to raise the incoming voltage to very high levels momentarily at precise milliamperage levels for x-ray exposure. At the same time, circuit safety features ensure that exposure parameters are within allowable limits and that circuit components are protected from damage.

A circuit is a fixed path that electricity flows through, and its purpose is to precisely control the flow and intensity of electrons as they travel through the circuit pathways and components. Electrons only work for us when they flow through circuits in electrical devices to create energy, and the x-ray tube is an example of this process. Electrons can flow in a water-based (aqueous) solution, gaseous environment, vacuum, and solid conductor. The x-ray tube is an example of electron flow in a vacuum and electrical circuits using copper wires as conductors illustrate electron flow in a solid material. Many of the x-ray circuits are contained in layered, circuit boards with components positioned to ensure that the output from the board is precise in terms of amperage and voltage.

 IMPORTANT RELATIONSHIP

Circuits

> Circuits precisely control the flow and intensity of electrons as they travel through the circuit pathways and components. Electrons only work for us when they flow through circuits in electrical devices to create energy, and the x-ray tube is an example of this process.

All electrical devices behave according to the electrical power formula. Power is expressed in Watts (W) and is the product of amperage and voltage.

$$\text{Power (W)} = \text{Amps (I)} \times \text{Volts (V)}$$

X-ray production is a high-voltage process and can range from 50,000 to 150,000 Volts (50–150 kV), and because of this, the amperage necessarily must drop to milliamperage (mA) values. One mA equals 1/1000 amps. X-ray machine power is expressed in kilowatts (kW) and typically ranges from 30 to 100 kW. Higher kW systems naturally offer more power and therefore higher mA and kilovoltage peak (kVp) values. As a practical matter for radiographers, this means shorter exposure times at higher mA and kVp values.

 IMPORTANT RELATIONSHIP

High Voltage

> X-ray production is a high-voltage process and can range from 50,000 to 150,000 Volts (50–150 kV), and because of this, the amperage necessarily must drop to milliamperage (mA) values. Higher kW systems naturally offer more power and therefore higher mA and kVp values.

Electrical power entering the system on the primary side must equal the output power delivered on the secondary side, according to the power formula.

$$P_{input} = P_{output}$$

The x-ray circuit is divided into two major divisions: a high-voltage side and a low-voltage filament side (see Fig. 2.8). The primary (main) circuit is considered the high-voltage side and its design takes the incoming voltage (220 V/480 V) and increases it to kilovoltage peak (kVp) values during x-ray exposure. Most units use 440 to 480 V since this is a more reliable voltage value that can be provided by the power utility. See Box 2.1 for x-ray circuit terminology.

Transformers

Regulating voltage in an x-ray system generally employs the use of transformers, which are devices that consist of copper wire coils wound around a central core material of laminated, steel plates. All transformers have an input and output side. The input side contains a primary coil, and the output side contains the secondary coil. The ratio of wire windings between the primary and secondary sides determines whether the transformer is a step-up or step-down transformer. The transformer law determines the amount of induced voltage according to this formula:

$$V_s/V_p = N_s/N_p$$

Vs = Voltage induced on secondary coil; Ns = Number of turns on secondary coil

Vp = Voltage coming into primary coil; Np = Number of turns on primary coil

Kilovoltage peak (kVp) values required for x-ray exposure are obtained using high-voltage transformers operating on the principle of mutual induction. The principle of electromagnetic induction was discovered by the English scientist, Michael Faraday (1791–1867) and with this discovery he began to understand the relationship between electricity and magnetic fields. Conducting materials carrying electrical current have a magnetic field surrounding this conductor and the orientation of this magnetic field is related to the direction of electrical flow. Additionally, if you place a varying magnetic field in close proximity to a closed-circuit conducting material (copper), an electrical current will be induced. This is what happens in a transformer. An electrical current coming into a set of coils on the input side (primary side) will create an electrical current and voltage in the secondary coil windings, the

X-ray circuit

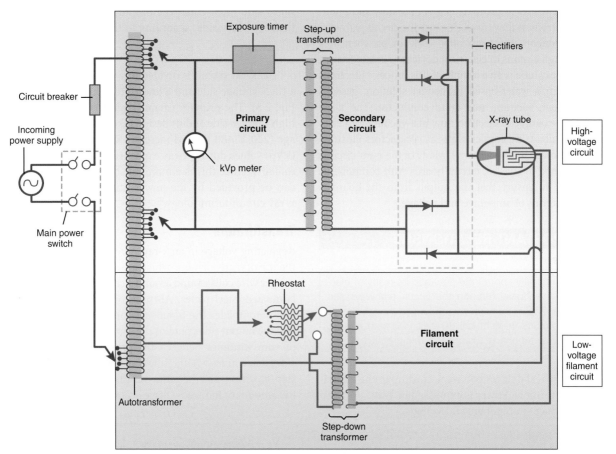

Fig. 2.8 Typical x-ray circuit demonstrating two main divisions. (Modified from Johnston JN and Fauber TL. *Essentials of Radiographic Physics and Imaging.* 3rd ed. St. Louis: Mosby; 2020.)

output side. This is termed mutual induction as both coils (primary and secondary) work together in a mutual magnetic-electrical fashion to create varying magnetic fields around the primary side of the transformer coil windings, and alternating electrical current (AC) is required for the efficient operation of all transformers.

⏩ IMPORTANT RELATIONSHIP

Transformers and Mutual Induction

Transformers regulate voltage on the principle of mutual induction. All transformers have an input side, the primary coil, and an output side, the secondary coil. An electrical current coming into a set of coils on the input side (primary side) will create an electrical current and voltage in the secondary coil windings, the output side. The ratio of wire windings between the primary and secondary sides determines whether the transformer is a step-up or step-down transformer.

Kilovoltage selection occurs through an **autotransformer**, which determines the induced voltage going to the primary side of the high-tension transformer. These voltage changes happen momentarily, only during the actual x-ray exposure.

X-ray production is considered an ultra-high-voltage electrical process. This is different than the simple operation of electrical devices such as electric ranges, clothes dryers, or air conditioners, which operate at

BOX 2.1 X-ray Circuit Terminology

Autotransformer determines the induced voltage going to the primary side of the high-tension transformer.

Capacitors are charge storage components and when placed in the circuit with the inverter, the stored charges are released in a sequential fashion that result in a current waveform with a very small voltage fluctuation, known as ripple.

Circuit— a fixed path that electricity flows through and its purpose is to precisely control the flow and intensity of electrons as they travel through the circuit pathways and components.

Diodes use solid-state, semiconductor materials that permit current flow in only one direction.

Mutual induction—the process of an electrical current coming into a set of coils on the input side (primary side) will create an electrical current and voltage in the secondary coil windings, the output side.

Rectification—changing alternating current (AC) to direct current (DC).

Resistance—electric friction that inherently impedes the flow of electrons along its pathway.

Resistors regulate the amount of current passing through the cathode filament during exposure and are used to control amperage.

Step-down transformers have more core windings on the primary side than on the secondary side and reduce the incoming voltage to a lower value.

Step-up transformers have fewer core windings on the primary side than on the secondary side and increase the incoming voltage to a higher value.

Transformer regulates voltage in an x-ray system. The ratio of wire windings between the primary and secondary sides determines whether the transformer is a step-up or step-down transformer.

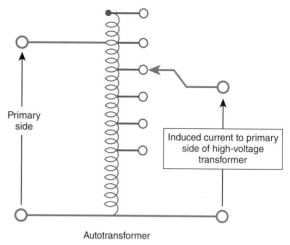

Fig. 2.9 Electrical symbol for an autotransformer. (Source: 1200px-Tapped_autotransformer.svg.png [1200 × 960] [wikimedia.org].)

240 to 480 Volts. X-ray systems use large transformers to create very high voltages for the momentary production of x-ray energies. These transformers generally are used to control voltage values on the secondary side and are constructed with a set of primary copper wire windings that are electrically insulated and wrapped around a larger set of secondary windings. Referred to as step-up transformers, these devices have no moving parts, produce a small amount of heat, and are considered very efficient as electrical components. They are encased in a metal container that is filled with a dielectric oil to absorb the heat they produce and to prevent electrical shock when the high voltages are produced during x-ray production. The high-voltage transformer is in the x-ray system's electronics cabinet and produces the characteristic soft "humming" sound that is heard in most rooms.

Working in conjunction with the high-tension, step-up transformer, the autotransformer consists of a single coil winding that acts as both a primary and secondary coil. It supplies an induced voltage to the primary windings of the step-up transformer and permits the selection of kilovoltage peak (kVp) values by the operator. It also works on the principle of mutual induction, and the degree of induced voltage created by the autotransformer is dependent upon the number of coiled windings that are electrically contacted or "tapped" as contact points (Fig. 2.9).

Generally, transformers are used to create and regulate voltage values in circuits and in doing so effectively produce an inverse change in current (amperes). If voltage is increased, the current is decreased proportionally. Since x-ray production is a high-voltage production process, the amperage values used necessarily drop to milliamperage (mA) levels.

Resistors

By design, electrical circuits take advantage of moving electron charges as they travel along circuit pathways, known as "traces." Conducting pathways inherently impede the flow of electrons along its pathway, primarily due to electron friction. This results in a resistance to the flow of electrical current and all circuit paths put up a degree of resistance to the flow of these negative electron charges. Controlling these resistive values is very precise in circuits and often a function of the length, temperature, and type of conducting material. Electronic engineers purposely design circuits to be as short as possible, using a low-resistance conducting material such as copper, silver, or even gold, and at safe temperatures. Often, circuits in an x-ray system are cooled using whisper fans and ventilation panels in spacious electronic cabinets. Circuits that get too warm do not perform as designed and create system malfunctions.

Milliamperage selection occurs using precise resistors that regulate the amount of current passing through the cathode filament during exposure. Resistors are designed to impede the flow of current flowing through them as a circuit component. The internal structure of a resistor controls electron flow by conductor material type and thickness and they come in a wide variety of resistive values, with a color-coded striping on their surface to indicate their resistive value as well as tolerance or accuracy (see Fig. 2.10). Generally, they are used to control amperage and it is this resistor technology that allows for the specific selection of mA values such as 100, 200, or even 1000 mA. With sensitive, modern digital receptors for image formation, the exposure requirements for quality images are much lower than in years past. Low mAs levels typically use very short exposure times in the milliseconds and these very short times can cause a degree of cathode filament instability. Circuit components, such as resistors, help correct for filament variations to ensure consistent x-ray output.

 IMPORTANT RELATIONSHIP

Resistors

Negative electron charges moving along circuit pathways inherently impede the flow of electrons, known as resistance, primarily due to electron friction. Resistors regulate the amount of current passing through the cathode filament during exposure and are used to control amperage. Resistors allow for the specific selection of mA values such as 100, 200, or even 1000 mA.

The cathode filament is controlled by the low-voltage side of the circuit, which operates like the filament wire seen in an incandescent light bulb. When not making an x-ray exposure, typical filament amperages range from 3 to 6 amps. During exposure, however, high voltage flows through the x-ray tube at low milliamperages. The power maintenance formula (P input = P output) necessarily requires that as voltage increases, amperage decreases proportionally. Because of this, the filament circuit uses low-voltage, step-down transformers. These transformers have more core windings on the primary

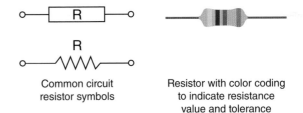

Fig. 2.10 Resistor symbols. (From Zizou7. Fixed resistor symbol on white background [photograph 1661117008]. https://www.shutterstock.com/image-vector/fixed-resistor-symbol-on-white-background-1661117008) and color coding of a resistor component (from Spacefem. 47K Ohm resistor PNG icon [photograph #93147]. March 16, 2018.)

side than on the secondary side and reduce the incoming voltage to a lower value. The x-ray tube cathode filament transformer is step-down and keeps the filament in a standby state with a voltage of 5 to 15 V and 3 to 5 amperes. These current values keep the filament warm in preparation for high-voltage x-ray production. When an exposure is made, the voltage increases dramatically to kilovoltage peak values, and the x-ray tube current drops to milliamperage (mA) levels.

 MIND IMAGE

Incandescence

An incandescent light bulb has a tungsten filament inside and when the electrical current heats the tungsten filament, light is produced by heat (incandescence). Similar to an x-ray tube, there is more heat produced in an incandescent bulb than light.

 IMPORTANT RELATIONSHIP

Step-up and Step-down Transformers

Transformers operate on the principle of mutual induction, are used to control voltage values on the secondary side, and are constructed with a set of primary copper wire windings that are electrically insulated and wrapped around a larger set of secondary windings, referred to as step-up transformers. Working in conjunction with the high-tension, step-up transformer, the autotransformer consists of a single coil winding that acts as both a primary and secondary coil. It supplies an induced voltage to the primary windings of the step-up transformer and permits the selection of kilovoltage peak (kVp) values by the operator.

The cathode filament is controlled by the low-voltage side of the circuit. During exposure, high voltage flows through the x-ray tube at low milliamperages. Because the filament circuit uses low voltage, step-down transformers have more core windings on the primary side than on the secondary side and reduce the incoming voltage to a lower value.

Current Rectification

X-ray tubes perform most efficiently with direct current (DC) passing through from cathode to anode. Transformers necessarily require alternating current (AC) and this AC must be changed to DC prior to the current entering the x-ray tube. This process is known as rectification and employs sophisticated rectification diodes that permit current flow in only one direction. Diodes use solid-state, semiconductor materials that, when positioned correctly in a "stack," allow electrons to travel across in only one direction.

Rectifiers are precisely placed in the circuit and contained within the high-tension transformer cabinet and immersed in a dielectric oil. With the correct number of rectifiers in the circuit, the AC current waveform is now rectified to DC and sent to the x-ray tube.

 IMPORTANT RELATIONSHIP

Rectification

Electrical power supplied by the power utility to a modern x-ray system is typically three-phase, alternating current (AC). Because x-ray tubes perform most efficiently with direct current (DC), rectification is the process of changing alternating current (AC) to direct current (DC). Rectification diodes permit current flow in only one direction.

Current Waveforms

Electrical power supplied by the power utility to a modern x-ray system is typically three-phase, alternating current (AC). X-ray generators will convert this three-phase energy to a higher frequency using electrical waveform "choppers" and capacitors through inverter circuits. Capacitors are charge storage components and when placed in the circuit with the inverter, the stored charges are released in a sequential fashion according to a phase-timing controller. The result is a current waveform that has a very small voltage fluctuation, known as ripple. Without this inverter step, the voltage level could

vary as much as 13% from its peak value. Inverters take the DC current and modify this waveform, so the ripple is approximately 1%. The result is a current waveform that is nearly flat, at the desired high-voltage level. This yields a very efficient, high-quality x-ray beam with a higher average energy that minimizes patient x-ray exposure without negatively affecting image quality.

 IMPORTANT RELATIONSHIP

Capacitors

Capacitors are charge storage components and when placed in the circuit with the inverters result in a current waveform that has a very small voltage fluctuation, known as ripple. This provides a very efficient, high-quality x-ray beam with a higher average energy that minimizes patient x-ray exposure without negatively affecting image quality.

 IMPORTANT RELATIONSHIP

X-ray System Circuits

X-ray system circuits, by design, take incoming alternating current (AC) at voltage levels supplied by the power utility and increase it to kilovoltage peak (kVp) levels, and convert the AC to a direct current (DC) waveform with a voltage fluctuation (ripple) that is minimal.

HIGH-FREQUENCY GENERATORS

Most all modern x-ray systems now use high-frequency (HF) generator technology. The advantages are many. These systems can use a single-phase or three-phase power supply and convert it to a high-frequency waveform expressed in Hertz (Hz) ranging from 100 Hz to 400 kHz. Additionally, because of HF efficiencies, the circuit components can be minimized resulting in smaller electronics cabinets. Older systems were much larger, and the high-tension transformer was often in its own large cabinet.

HF technology has downsized the transformers to the point that they can now be encased in a single, electronic cabinet with all the other circuit components. HF technology permits more accurate kVp regulation and easier calibration for service engineers. Computer microprocessors are now integral to HF circuit designs that monitor all electrical conditions of exposure in real time and provide feedback on exposure variances and errors to service personnel. The addition of microprocessor computer chips has produced x-ray systems that are more precise, easier to operate and repair, and with a user-friendly operator interface and control.

The current flow through the x-ray tube is difficult to precisely control as it is a function of the kVp selected for the exposure. During exposure, the high voltage places an electrical load on the x-ray tube, which affects the current flowing through the cathode filament. Many x-ray generators use filament regulators known as stabilizers to help provide a constant supply of voltage to the filament circuits. With today's high-frequency generators, the current is more stable and monitored by frequency sensors to help stabilize it during exposure.

Additionally, circuit designers have incorporated various components that make up a "safe circuit" to protect all the critical elements. This is particularly necessary because the x-ray circuit operates momentarily at very high-voltage levels during the x-ray exposure. Safe circuit components are part of the entire system circuit and work to protect the x-ray tube and circuits during the high-voltage conditions that occur during exposure. Safe circuits control anode rotation speeds, allowable exposure factor combinations, x-ray tube anode heat load calculations, and anode stator and rotor controls.

All circuit conditions necessary for successful exposure must be in place to enable the actual x-ray exposure. Generator consoles typically provide a "ready light" as part of the exposure preparation sequence. When that does not occur, x-ray exposure will be prohibited to protect the patient and expensive x-ray circuitry. Modern systems now provide microprocessor intelligence to determine the presence of incorrect exposure sequencing and often display an error message. This information needs to be noted and passed along to trained x-ray service engineers. Without these safe circuit designs, damage could occur to the system and successful operation. It is important to understand that when you select exposure conditions and prepare to make an exposure, seeing the "ready light" ensures that the safe circuit is working as designed.

As we can see, the complexities and sophistication of x-ray-generating equipment require particular attention to electronic circuit designs and components. The designs have evolved over many decades of research and product development. Operating these systems may seem easy and trouble-free, but the intent is still to produce a reliable electron flow through the x-ray tube, at very high voltages and low milliamperages, with an electrical waveform that has negligible ripple. This yields the most energetic and quality x-ray beam possible for safe radiation dosages to patients and personnel.

CHAPTER SUMMARY

- The production of x-rays requires a rapidly moving stream of electrons that are suddenly decelerated or stopped.
- X-rays are produced when electrons are boiled off (thermionic emission) the cathode filament, accelerated across to the anode target, and suddenly stopped. Heat is also produced.
- The cathode of an x-ray tube is a negatively charged electrode. It comprises a filament and a focusing cup.
- The filament is a coiled tungsten wire, which is the source of electrons during x-ray production.
- The purpose of the focusing cup is to focus the stream of electrons from the filament toward the anode target.
- The anode target is made of a metal with a high atomic number and melting point that abruptly decelerates and stops electrons in the tube current, allowing the production of x-rays.

- During x-ray production, most of the energy produced at the anode is heat, with a very small percentage being x-ray energy.
- Rotating anodes can withstand higher heat loads than stationary anodes because the rotation causes a greater physical area, or focal track, to be exposed to electrons.
- All the x-ray tube components are surrounded by a metal tube housing envelope on all sides except for a port, or window, which allows the primary beam to exit the tube.
- The envelope allows air to be completely evacuated from the x-ray tube, which in turn allows an efficient flow of electrons from cathode to anode.
- Complex electronic circuits and components are intended to produce an x-ray beam that is predictable and capable of delivering the correct amount of electromagnetic energy to an image receptor.

- By design, circuit components raise the incoming voltage to very high levels at precise milliamperage levels for x-ray exposure.
- All electrical devices behave according to the electrical power formula. Power is expressed in Watts (W) and is the product of amperage and voltage.
- The x-ray circuit is divided into two major divisions: a high-voltage side and a low-voltage side which keeps the cathode filament ready for thermionic emission.
- The primary (main) circuit is considered the high-voltage side and its design takes the incoming voltage (220 V/480 V) and increases it to kilovoltage peak (kVp) values during x-ray exposure.
- The cathode filament is controlled by the low-voltage side of the circuit. The power maintenance formula requires that as voltage increases, amperage decreases, proportionally. When an exposure is made, the voltage across the x-ray tube circuit increases dramatically to kilovoltage peak (kVp) values, and the amperage drops to milliamperage levels.

- Transformers require alternating current (AC) and this AC must be changed to direct current (DC) prior to the current entering the x-ray tube. This process is known as rectification and employs sophisticated rectification diodes that permit current flow in only one direction.
- Capacitors using inverter circuits take the direct current and modify this waveform, so the ripple is approximately 1%. The result is a very efficient, high-quality x-ray beam with a higher average energy that minimizes patient x-ray exposure without negatively affecting image quality.
- The addition of microprocessor computer chips in high-frequency generators produces x-ray systems that are more precise, easier to operate and repair, and with a user-friendly operator interface and control.
- It is important to understand that when you select exposure conditions and prepare to make an exposure, seeing the "ready light" ensures that the safe circuit is working as designed.

REVIEW QUESTIONS

1. Which x-ray tube component serves as a source of electrons for x-ray production?
   A. Focusing cup
   B. Filament
   C. Stator
   D. Target

2. What precisely controls the flow and intensity of electrons in the x-ray tube?
   A. Cathode
   B. Capacitor
   C. Transformer
   D. Circuit

3. The burning or boiling-off of electrons at the cathode is referred to as _____.
   A. thermionic emission
   B. space charge
   C. space charge effect
   D. tube current

4. Electrons interact with the _____ to produce x-rays and heat.
   A. focusing cup
   B. filament
   C. stator
   D. target

5. Rotating anodes withstand greater heat loads than stationary anodes because:
   A. their increased weight
   B. off-focus radiation
   C. greater number of electrons bombarding
   D. greater physical area

6. Most of the energy produced during x-ray production is _____.
   A. x-rays
   B. scatter x-rays
   C. heat
   D. leakage radiation

7. Electrical power is measured in _____.
   A. Kilovolts
   B. Milliamperes
   C. Watts
   D. Coulombs

8. In electric circuits, resistors are used to primarily regulate _____.
   A. heat
   B. voltage
   C. amperage
   D. capacitance

9. The electrical process of _____converts alternating current to direct current.
   A. capacitance
   B. mutual induction
   C. self-induction
   D. rectification

10. The autotransformer in an x-ray circuit creates an induced voltage that is supplied to the_____ of the high-tension transformer.
   A. secondary side
   B. primary side
   C. rectifiers
   D. capacitors

11. With modern high-frequency radiographic generators using inverter technology, the voltage ripple is typically _____.
   A. 1%
   B. 5%
   C. 13%
   D. 50%

12. _____ regulates the x-ray tube voltage.
   A. Transformers
   B. Capacitors
   C. Resistors
   D. Rectifiers

13. The element _____is used to stabilize the rotating anode materials during high heat and rotational speed conditions.
   A. nickel
   B. molybdenum
   C. copper
   D. rhenium

14. _____ is more stable with the use of high-frequency generators.
   A. Current
   B. Heat
   C. Vibration
   D. Noise

The X-ray Beam

CHAPTER OUTLINE

OBJECTIVES

After completing this chapter, the reader will be able to perform the following:

1. Define all the key terms in this chapter.
2. State all the important relationships in this chapter.
3. Describe how x-rays are produced.
4. Explain the role of the primary exposure factors in determining the quality and quantity of x-rays.
5. Explain the line-focus principle.
6. State how the anode heel effect can be used in radiography.
7. Differentiate among the types of filtration and explain their purpose.
8. Explain the purpose of measuring the x-ray beam's half-value layer.
9. Calculate heat units.
10. Recognize how changing generator output, kVp, mA, and filtration affect the x-ray emission spectrum.
11. Analyze a typical x-ray beam graphical emission spectrum.
12. List the guidelines followed to extend the life of an x-ray tube.

KEY TERMS

actual focal spot size
added filtration
anode heel effect
bremsstrahlung interactions
characteristic interactions
compensating filters
dosimeter
effective focal spot size
electron transition

exposure time
filament current
half-value layer (HVL)
heat unit (HU)
inherent filtration
kilovoltage
line-focus principle
milliamperage (mA)
space charge

space charge effect
thermionic emission
total filtration
trough filter
tube current
voltage ripple
wedge filter
x-ray emission spectrum

As discussed in Chapter 2, x-rays are produced from a specially designed x-ray tube. The purpose of the x-ray circuit is to produce a reliable electron flow through the x-ray tube, at very high voltages and low milliamperages with a voltage waveform that has negligible ripple. This chapter will discuss the production of radiation inside the x-ray tube and factors that affect the safe operation of the x-ray tube and image quality.

PRODUCING X-RAYS

The production of x-rays requires a rapidly moving stream of electrons that are suddenly decelerated or stopped. The source of electrons is a cathode, or negative electrode. The negative electrode is heated, and electrons are emitted through the process of thermionic emission. The electrons are attracted to the positively charged anode (positive electrode) and move rapidly toward the anode, where they are stopped or decelerated. When the kinetic energy (energy of motion) of the

electrons is transferred to the anode, x-rays and heat are produced (Fig. 3.1).

TARGET INTERACTIONS

The electrons that move from the cathode to the anode travel extremely fast, approximately at half the speed of light. The moving electrons, which have high kinetic energy, strike the target and interact with the tungsten atoms in the anode to produce x-rays. These interactions occur within the top 0.5 mm of the anode surface. Two types of interactions produce x-ray photons: bremsstrahlung interactions and characteristic interactions.

📼 IMPORTANT RELATIONSHIP
Production of X-rays

As electrons strike the target, their kinetic energy is transferred to the tungsten atoms in the anode to produce x-rays. Bremsstrahlung interactions and characteristic interactions both produce x-ray photons.

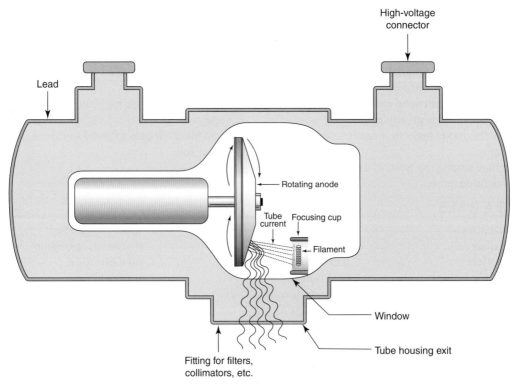

Fig. 3.1 X-ray tube inside protective housing. (Modified from Johnston JN, Fauber TL. *Essentials of Radiographic Physics and Imaging.* 2nd ed. St. Louis: Mosby; 2016.)

Bremsstrahlung Interactions

Bremsstrahlung is a German word meaning *braking* or *slowing down radiation*. Bremsstrahlung interactions occur when a projectile (incident) electron completely avoids the orbital electrons of a tungsten atom and travels very close to its nucleus. The very strong negative electrostatic force surrounding the positively charged nucleus causes the incident electron to suddenly *slow down*. As the electron loses energy, it suddenly changes its direction, and the energy loss then reappears as an x-ray photon (Fig. 3.2). The closer the projectile electron travels to the nucleus, the stronger the attraction.

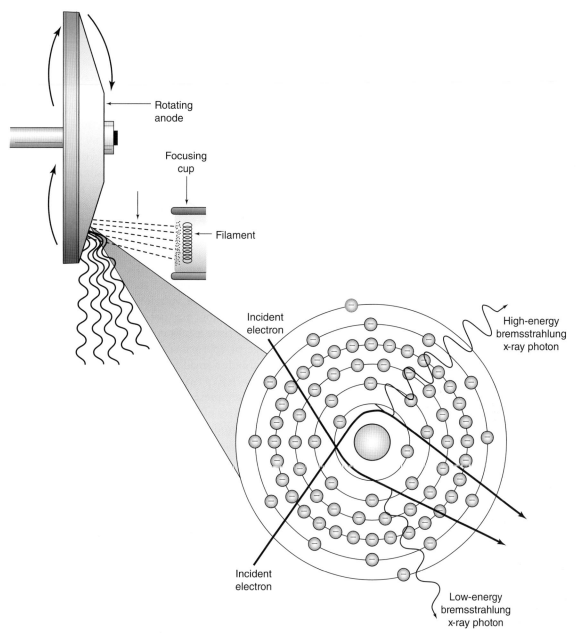

Rotating anode

Focusing cup

Filament

Incident electron

High-energy bremsstrahlung x-ray photon

Incident electron

Low-energy bremsstrahlung x-ray photon

Fig. 3.2 Bremsstrahlung interaction. X-ray photons are created when the incident (projectile) electrons travel close to the atom's nucleus of the rotating tungsten anode.

The stronger this attraction, the more energy the projectile electron loses and the stronger the resultant x-ray photon (higher energy). The continuous deceleration of the projectile electron produces this "braking" or bremsstrahlung radiation. Projectile electrons that travel farther from the nucleus create x-ray photons with less energy.

X-ray energy is measured in kiloelectron volts (keV [1 keV = 1000 electron volts]). The energy of a bremsstrahlung x-ray photon can be found by subtracting the energy that the projectile electron exits the atom with from the energy it had upon entering. For example, a projectile electron enters an atom with 120 keV of energy, passes very close to the nucleus, and exits with 40 keV of energy. The x-ray photon produced is 80 keV (120 keV − 40 keV = 80 keV). If that same projectile electron traveled farther from the nucleus and exited with 90 keV of energy, the x-ray photon produced would be 30 keV (120 keV − 90 keV = 30 keV).

In the diagnostic energy range from 30 to 150 keV, most x-ray interactions are bremsstrahlung. Below 70 kVp (with a tungsten target), 100% of the x-ray beam results from bremsstrahlung interactions. Above 70 kVp, approximately 85% of the beam results from bremsstrahlung interactions.

 IMPORTANT RELATIONSHIP

Bremsstrahlung Interactions

Bremsstrahlung interactions occur when a projectile (incident) electron completely avoids the orbital electrons of a tungsten atom and travels very close to its nucleus. The closer the projectile electron travels to the nucleus, the stronger the attraction. The stronger this attraction, the more energy the projectile electron loses and the stronger the resultant x-ray photon (higher energy). Projectile electrons that travel farther from the nucleus create x-ray photons with less energy. Most x-ray interactions in the diagnostic energy range are bremsstrahlung.

Characteristic Interactions

Characteristic interactions are produced when a projectile (incident) electron interacts with an electron from the inner shell (K-shell) of a tungsten atom. The projectile electron must have enough energy to eject the K-shell electron of a tungsten atom from its orbit.

TABLE 3.1 Binding Energies for Tungsten	
Electron Shell	**Binding Energy (keV)**
K-shell	69.5
L-shell	12.1
M-shell	2.82
N-shell	0.6
O-shell	0.08
P-shell	0.008

The electron shells of each element have specific binding energies (Table 3.1). K-shell electrons in tungsten have the strongest binding energy at 69.5 keV. For a projectile electron to remove this orbital electron, it must possess energy equal to or greater than 69.5 keV. When the K-shell electron is ejected from its orbit, an outer-shell electron drops into the open position and creates an energy difference. This is referred to as an electron transition and generally consists of an M to K or L to K transition. The energy difference is emitted as an x-ray photon (Fig. 3.3). Electrons from the L-, M-, O-, and P-shells of the tungsten atom are also ejected from their orbits, as they are attracted to the open positions nearer to the nucleus. However, the photons created from these interactions have very low energy and, depending on beam filtration, may not even reach the patient. K-shell characteristic x-rays in the x-ray beam have an energy range of approximately 57 to 69 keV; therefore they contribute a small percentage to the useful x-ray beams. Below 70 kVp (with a tungsten target), no characteristic x-rays are present in the beam; above 70 kVp, approximately 15% of the beam consists of characteristic x-rays. X-rays produced through these interactions are termed *characteristic x-rays* because their energies are characteristic of the tungsten target element and its binding energy values.

 IMPORTANT RELATIONSHIP

Characteristic Interactions

Characteristic interactions are produced when a projectile (incident) electron interacts with an electron from the inner shell (K-shell) of a tungsten atom. Characteristic x-rays can be produced in a tungsten target only when the kVp is set at 70 or greater because the binding energy of the K-shell electron is 69.5 keV.

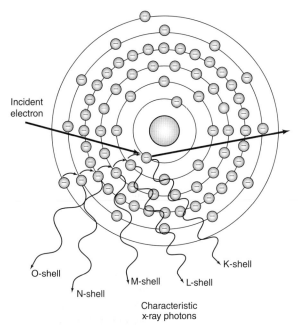

Incident
electron

O-shell

N-shell

M-shell

L-shell

K-shell

Characteristic
x-ray photons

Fig. 3.3 Characteristic interaction. X-ray photons are created when the incident electrons interact with inner-shell electrons within the atoms of the rotating tungsten anode.

⯈ **MATHEMATICAL APPLICATION**

Characteristic X-ray Photons

To find the energy of a characteristic x-ray photon, one must know the shell-binding energies of the element and the shells involved. The projectile electron must possess kinetic energy equal to or greater than the shell-binding energy to remove it from orbit. The photon energy is then equal to the difference in the binding energy of the shells involved.

Example:
A projectile electron removes a K-shell electron, and an
    L-shell electron fills the vacancy:
K-shell binding energy = 69.5 keV
L-shell binding energy = 12.1 keV
69.5 − 12.1 = 57.4 keV
The energy of the K-shell characteristic x-ray photon
    produced is 57.4 keV.

To summarize, when comparing bremsstrahlung and characteristic interactions, most x-ray interactions produced in diagnostic radiology result from bremsstrahlung interactions. There is no difference between a bremsstrahlung x-ray and a characteristic x-ray at the same energy level; they are simply produced by different processes.

X-RAY EMISSION SPECTRUM

The x-ray beam is polyenergetic (has many energies) and consists of a wide range of energies known as the x-ray emission spectrum. The lowest energies are always approximately 15 to 20 keV, and the highest energies cannot exceed the kVp set on the control panel. For example, an 80 kVp x-ray exposure technique produces x-ray energies ranging from 15 to 80 keV (Fig. 3.4). The smallest number of x-rays occurs at the extreme low and high ends of the spectrum. The greatest number of x-ray energies (peak of the curve) occurs between 30 and 40 keV for an 80 kVp exposure (about one-third of the kVp selected). The x-ray emission spectrum, or the range and intensity of x-rays emitted, changes with different exposure technique settings on the control panel. The graphic illustration of the spectrum (Fig. 3.4) demonstrates a large bremsstrahlung portion and a characteristic "spike" at the specific energy level of approximately 69 keV. This characteristic energy level is particularly important when contrast media is used to visualize specific anatomical structures.

❓ **MIND IMAGE**

Visible Light

Visible light is polyenergetic and like x-rays include electromagnetic energy that varies in wavelength. These wavelengths of visible light, ranging from 380 to 700 nanometers (10^{-6} m), can be seen in a rainbow as colors from red to violet.

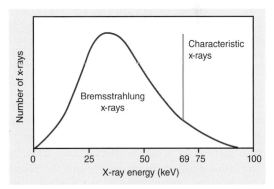

Fig. 3.4 An 80 kVp x-ray emission spectrum from a tungsten target. Most x-rays occur between 30 and 40 keV. Characteristic x-ray energies are discrete and are represented by the line at 69 keV. (From Johnston JN, Fauber TL. *Essentials of Radiographic Physics and Imaging.* 2nd ed. St. Louis: Mosby; 2016.)

X-RAY EXPOSURE

A radiographic exposure is produced by a radiographer using two switches located on the control panel of the x-ray unit. These are sometimes combined into a single switching device that has two levels of operation corresponding to rotor preparation and x-ray exposure. In either case, the switches that are used to make an x-ray exposure are called *deadman switches*. Deadman switches require positive pressure to be applied during the entire x-ray exposure process. If the radiographer lets off either switch, thus releasing positive pressure, the exposure process is immediately terminated.

The first switch is usually called the *rotor*, or *prep button*, and the second switch is usually called the *exposure*, or *x-ray button*. The activation of the exposure switch by the radiographer produces specific reactions inside the x-ray tube. The rotor must be activated before the x-ray exposure to properly produce an x-ray exposure.

Pushing the rotor, or prep button, causes an electrical current to be induced across the filament in the cathode. This filament current is approximately 3 to 5 A and operates at approximately 10 V. The amount of current flowing through the filament depends on the mA set at the control panel. The filament current heats the tungsten filament. This heating of the filament causes thermionic emission to occur. Thermionic emission refers to the boiling off of electrons from the filament.

 IMPORTANT RELATIONSHIP

Thermionic Emission

When the tungsten filament gains enough heat (therm), the outer-shell electrons of the filament atoms are boiled off, or emitted, from the filament, which creates free electrons as ions.

The electrons liberated from the filament during thermionic emission form a thermionic cloud around the filament called space charge. This term is descriptive because there is an actual negative charge from these electrons that exists in the space around the filament. The space charge effect refers to the tendency of the space charge to prevent more electrons to be boiled off of the filament. The focusing cup, with its own negative charge, forces the electrons in the space charge to remain together.

By pushing the rotor, or prep button, the radiographer also activates the stator that drives the rotor and rotating target (Box 3.1). While thermionic emission is occurring and the space charge is forming, the stator starts to turn the anode, accelerating it to top speed in preparation for x-ray production. If an exposure were to be made before the target was up to speed, the heat produced would be too great for the slowly rotating target, causing serious damage to the anode surface. The machine, through its safe-circuit components, does not allow such an exposure to occur until the target is up to full speed, even when the exposure switch is activated. The radiographer can press the rotor and exposure switches one after the other, and the machine makes the exposure as soon as it is ready, with no damage to the tube. It takes only a few seconds for the space charge to be produced and for the rotating target to reach its top speed (Fig. 3.5).

When the radiographer pushes the exposure, or x-ray button, the x-ray exposure begins (Box 3.2). The kVp level, which depends on the actual kVp value set on the control panel by the radiographer, is applied across the tube from cathode to anode. This creates a potential difference in charge between the anode and cathode, and the cathode becomes highly negatively charged and the anode has a strong positive charge which attracts the electrons.

Electrons that comprised the space charge now flow quickly from the cathode to the anode in a current. Tube current refers to the flow of electrons from cathode to anode and is measured in units called *milliamperes*. Note that electrons flow only in one direction in the x-ray tube—from cathode to anode.

BOX 3.1   Preparing the Tube for Exposure

When the rotor, or prep button, is activated:

On the Cathode Side of the X-ray Tube
1. The filament current heats up the filament.
2. This heat boils electrons off the filament (thermionic emission).
3. These electrons gather in a cloud around the filament (space charge).
4. The negatively charged focusing cup keeps the electron cloud focused together.
5. The number of electrons in the space charge is limited (space charge effect).

On the Anode Side of the X-ray Tube
1. The rotating target begins to turn rapidly, quickly reaching top speed.

As these electrons strike the anode target, their kinetic energy is converted into either electromagnetic energy (x-rays) or thermal energy (heat); in other words, an energy conversion occurs. Most of the electron kinetic energy in the tube current (>99%) is converted to heat, whereas less than 1% of it is converted to x-rays. These events are illustrated in Fig. 3.6.

IMPORTANT RELATIONSHIP

Energy Conversion in the X-ray Tube

As electrons strike the anode target, more than 99% of their kinetic energy is converted to heat, whereas less than 1% of their energy is converted to x-rays.

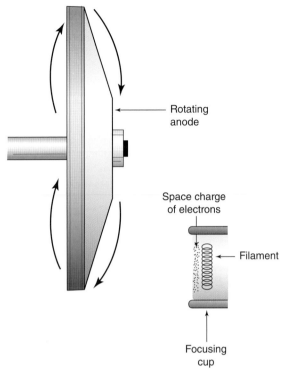

Fig. 3.5 When the radiographer activates the rotor, or prep button, a filament current is induced across the filament, causing electrons to be burned off and gather in a cloud around the filament. Simultaneously, the rotating anode begins to turn.

BOX 3.2 Making an X-ray Exposure

After activation of the rotor and the exposure is initiated:

On the Cathode Side of the X-ray Tube
1. High negative charge strongly repels electrons.
2. These electrons stream away from the cathode and toward the anode (tube current).

On the Anode Side of the X-ray Tube
1. High positive charge strongly attracts electrons in the tube current.
2. These electrons strike the anode.
3. X-rays and heat are produced.

IMPORTANT RELATIONSHIP

Tube Current

Electrons flow only in one direction in the x-ray tube—from cathode to anode. This flow of electrons is called the *tube current* and is measured in mA.

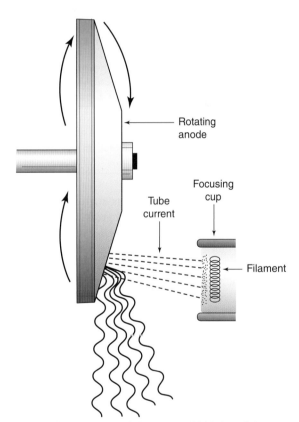

Fig. 3.6 After activation of the rotor and initiation of the exposure, a high voltage, or kilovoltage, is applied across the tube, making the cathode highly negative and the anode highly positive. Electrons are repelled from the cathode side and attracted to the anode side. The negatively charged focusing cup focuses the electrons into a stream, and they quickly cross the tube gap in a tube current. The kinetic energy of electrons interacting with the target is converted into x-rays and heat.

X-RAY QUALITY AND QUANTITY

The radiographer initiates and controls the production of x-rays. Manipulating the prime exposure factors on the control panel (kVp, mA, and exposure time) allows both the quantity and the quality of the x-ray beam to be altered. The quantity of the x-ray beam indicates the number of x-ray photons in the primary beam, and the quality of the x-ray beam indicates its penetrating power. Knowledge of the prime exposure factors and their effect on the production of x-rays assists the radiographer in producing quality radiographic images.

Kilovoltage

The kilovoltage that is set by the radiographer and applied across the x-ray tube at the time the exposure is initiated determines the speed at which the electrons in the tube current move. It is a direct relationship, but not proportional.

 IMPORTANT RELATIONSHIP

Kilovoltage and the Speed of Electrons

> The speed of the electrons traveling from the cathode to the anode increases as the kilovoltage applied across the x-ray tube increases. It is a direct relationship, but not proportional.

Selecting a higher voltage results in greater repulsion of electrons from the cathode and greater attraction of electrons toward the anode. The speed at which the electrons in the tube current move determines the quality or energy of the x-rays that are produced. The higher the energy of the x-ray photons, the greater their penetrability, or ease with which they move through tissue. It is important to note that changing kVp directly affects the energy or quality of the x-rays produced but it is not a proportional relationship. Whether addressing the x-ray photons themselves or the primary beam, *quality* refers to the energy level of the radiation produced (Box 3.3).

 IMPORTANT RELATIONSHIP

Speed of Electrons and Quality of X-rays

> The speed of the electrons in the tube current directly affects the quality or energy of the x-rays that are produced but it is not a proportional relationship. The quality or energy of the x-rays in turn determines the penetrability of the primary beam (ease with which it moves through tissue).

BOX 3.3   kVp and X-ray Quality

1. Higher kVp results in electrons that move faster in the tube current from the cathode to the anode.
2. The faster the movement of the electrons in the tube current, the greater the energy of the x-rays produced.
3. Changing kVp directly affects the energy or quality of the x-rays produced but it is not a proportional relationship.
4. The greater the energy of the x-rays produced, the greater the penetrability of the primary beam.
5. The quality of the x-ray beam refers to its energy level; hence, adjusting kVp affects the quality of the x-ray beam.

kVp, Kilovoltage peak.

 IMPORTANT RELATIONSHIP

kVp and Beam Penetrability

> As kVp increases, beam penetrability increases; as kVp decreases, beam penetrability decreases.

In addition to kVp affecting the quality of x-ray photons produced, it affects the quantity or number of x-ray photons produced since higher kVps produce more bremsstrahlung interactions (Fig. 3.7). Increased kVp results in more x-rays being produced because it increases the efficiency of x-ray production. (Box 3.4 describes quality control methods for evaluating kilovoltage accuracy.)

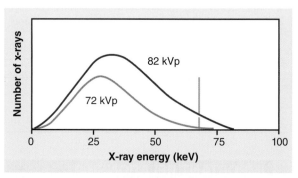

Fig. 3.7 Increasing the kVp from 72 to 82 shows an increase in the quantity of x-rays (amplitude), and the x-ray emission shifts toward the right, indicating an increase in the energy or quality of the beam. *kVp,* Kilovoltage peak. (From Johnston JN, Fauber TL. *Essentials of Radiographic Physics and Imaging.* 2nd ed. St. Louis: Mosby; 2016.)

To provide a sufficient potential difference (kVp) to allow x-ray production, a generator is required to convert low voltage (volts) to high voltage (kilovolts), 1 kilovolt = 1000 volts. Three basic types of x-ray generators are available: single-phase, three-phase, and high-frequency. Modern generators are high-frequency but each type of generator produces a different voltage waveform (Fig. 3.8). These waveforms are a reflection of the consistency of the voltage supplied to the x-ray tube during an x-ray exposure. The term voltage ripple describes voltage waveforms in terms of how much the voltage varies during x-ray production. Fig. 3.8 shows that for single-phase generators, voltage varies from the peak to a value of zero. The voltage ripple for single-phase generators is said to be 100% because there is total variation in the voltage waveform, from peak voltage to zero voltage. The most efficient x-ray production happens when the voltage is at the top 1/3 of peak value. For three-phase generators, the voltage ripple is 13% for the 6-pulse mode and 4% for the

12-pulse mode. High-frequency generators produce a voltage ripple of less than 1%. Voltage used in the x-ray tube is most consistent with high-frequency generators. The more consistent the voltage applied to the x-ray tube throughout the exposure, the greater the quantity and energy level (quality) of the x-ray beam. Fig. 3.9 shows x-ray emissions for different types of generators.

Milliamperage

Milliamperage (mA) is selected on the x-ray control panel to operate the tube current. Tube current is the number of electrons flowing per unit time between the cathode and the anode. For example, at 200 mA, there is a specific amount of current applied to the filament, causing a certain amount of thermionic emission. Based on the amount of thermionic emission, there is a space charge consisting of a certain number of electrons; 200 mA indicates the number of electrons (based on the space charge) flowing in the tube per second. Generally, changing to the 400 mA station on the control panel causes twice as much thermionic emission, twice as big a space charge, and twice as many electrons to flow per second. The mA set by the radiographer determines the number of electrons flowing in the tube and the quantity of x-rays produced (Box 3.5). The quantity of electrons in the tube current is directly proportional to the mA. If the mA increases, the quantity of electrons and x-rays proportionally increases, and if it decreases,

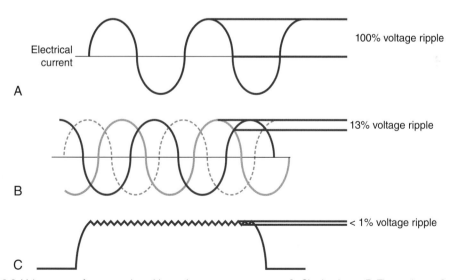

Fig. 3.8 Voltage waveforms produced by various x-ray generators. **A,** Single-phase. **B,** Three-phase. **C,** High-frequency.

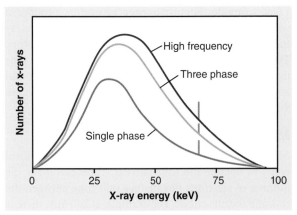

Fig. 3.9 The quantity (amplitude) and the quality (shift to the right) of the x-ray beam are increased when using high-frequency and three-phase generators because they are more efficient in x-ray production. (From Johnston JN, Fauber TL. *Essentials of Radiographic Physics and Imaging*. 2nd ed. St. Louis: Mosby; 2016.)

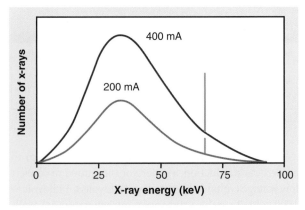

Fig. 3.10 Changing the mA results in a proportional change in the quantity (amplitude) of x-rays produced. *mA*, Milliamperage. (From Johnston JN, Fauber TL. *Essentials of Radiographic Physics and Imaging*. 2nd ed. St. Louis: Mosby; 2016.)

BOX 3.5 mA and X-ray Quantity

1. Higher mA results in more electrons moving in the tube current from the cathode to the anode.
2. The more electrons in the tube current, the more x-rays produced.
3. The number of x-rays produced is directly proportional to mA.

, Milliamperage.

---

the quantity of electrons and x-rays proportionally decreases. The mA does not affect the quality or energy of the x-rays produced (Fig. 3.10).

⬛ IMPORTANT RELATIONSHIP

mA, Tube Current, and X-ray Quantity

The quantity of electrons in the tube current and quantity of x-rays produced are directly proportional to the mA.

Exposure Time

Exposure time determines the length of time over which the x-ray tube produces x-rays. The exposure time set by the radiographer can be expressed in seconds or milliseconds (ms) as either a fraction (older units) or a decimal (1 s = 1000 ms). This exposure time determines the length of time for which the tube current is allowed to flow from cathode to anode. The longer the exposure

time, the greater the quantity of electrons that flow from the cathode to the anode and the greater the quantity of x-rays produced (Box 3.6). For example, if an exposure time of 0.25 s at 400 mA hypothetically produces 5000 x-rays, then doubling the exposure time to 0.50 s at 400 mA would produce 10,000 x-rays. Changes in exposure time produce the same effect on the number of x-rays produced as do changes in mA. (Box 3.7 describes quality control methods for evaluating exposure timer accuracy.)

BOX 3.6 Exposure Time and X-ray Quantity

1. A longer exposure time results in more electrons moving in the tube current from the cathode to the anode.
2. The more electrons in the tube current, the more x-rays produced.
3. The number of x-rays produced is directly proportional to the exposure time.

BOX 3.7 Quality Control Check: Exposure Timer Accuracy

- X-ray quantity can be affected if the actual exposure time used is inaccurate. A digital timer device measures the actual exposure time. This is generally measured by a qualified medical physicist or service engineer.
- The maximum variability of the exposure timer is ±5% for times >10 ms and ±10% for times <10 ms.

MIND IMAGE

Quantity of X-rays Produced

Producing x-rays is like plumbing in your household. Water coming out of a faucet into your sink has both pressure or velocity and volume or quantity. When you turn on the faucet, water flows in gallons (liters) per minute. For example, if you close the sink drain and turn on the faucet, 6 gallons (23 liters) of water will flow per minute. Turning the faucet off after 30 seconds or 0.5 minutes would result in approximately half the amount of water at 3 gallons (11.5 liters) in your sink. If you kept the water running for a total of 45 seconds or 0.75 minutes, you would have approximately 4.5 gallons (17 liters) of water in your sink. In the x-ray tube, selecting mA and time is similar. If you select 100 mA (100 milliamperage flowing per second) for 0.5 s, you will have half the x-rays produced.

IMPORTANT RELATIONSHIP

Exposure Time, Tube Current, and X-ray Quantity

The quantity of electrons flowing from the cathode to the anode and the quantity of x-rays produced are directly proportional to the exposure time.

Milliamperage and Time

When mA is multiplied by exposure time, the result is known as mAs (milliamperage-seconds), which the radiographer can set at the control panel. Mathematically, mAs is simply expressed as follows: $mA \times s = mAs$, where s represents the exposure time in fractions of a second (as actual fractions or in decimal form) or in seconds. Milliseconds (ms) of time must be converted to seconds to calculate $mA \times s = mAs$.

 MATHEMATICAL APPLICATION

Calculating mAs

$mAs = mA \times seconds$ (1 second = 1000 ms)

Examples: $200\ mA \times 0.25\ s\ (250\ ms) = 50\ mAs$

$500\ mA \times 2/5\ s = 200\ mAs$

$800\ mA \times 100\ ms\ (0.1\ s) = 80\ mAs$

The quantity of electrons flowing from the cathode to the anode is directly proportional to mAs (Box 3.8). The quantity of x-ray photons produced is directly proportional to this quantity of electrons. An increase or decrease in mA, exposure time, or mAs directly affects the quantity of x-rays produced; mAs has no effect on the quality of the x-rays produced. (Box 3.9 describes quality control methods for evaluating radiation output.)

BOX 3.8 mAs and X-ray Quantity

1. Higher mAs results in more electrons moving within the tube current from the cathode to the anode.
2. The more electrons in the tube current, the more x-rays produced.
3. The number of x-rays produced is directly proportional to the mAs.
4. mAs affects only the quantity of x-rays produced; it has no effect on the quality of the x-rays.

mAs, Milliamperage-seconds.

BOX 3.9 Quality Control Check: Radiation Output

- Variations in the generator or x-ray tube performance may cause inconsistent exposures and affect the x-ray quantity. Three quality control tests are typically performed with a dosimeter (a device that measures x-ray exposure) to evaluate the radiation output by measuring the radiation intensity: reproducibility of exposure, mAs reciprocity, and mA and exposure time linearity.
- **Reproducibility of exposure** verifies the consistency of the radiation output for a given set of exposure factors. The maximum variability of the reproducibility of radiation exposures is ±5%.
- **mAs reciprocity** verifies the consistency of radiation intensity for changes in mA and exposure time with constant mAs. The maximum variability of reciprocity is ±10%.
- **mA and exposure time linearity** verifies that proportional changes in mA or exposure time or both likewise change the radiation intensity. Doubling the mA or exposure time should double the radiation intensity. The maximum variability of linearity is ±10%.

mAs, Milliamperage-seconds.

IMPORTANT RELATIONSHIP

Quantity of Electrons, X-rays, and mAs

The quantity of electrons flowing from the cathode to the anode and the quantity of x-rays produced are directly proportional to mAs.

LINE-FOCUS PRINCIPLE

The line-focus principle describes the relationship between the actual and the effective focal spots in an x-ray tube.

 IMPORTANT RELATIONSHIP

Line-Focus Principle

The line-focus principle describes the relationship between the actual focal spot, where the electrons in the tube current bombard the target, and the effective focal spot, which is the same area as seen from directly below the tube.

The actual focal spot size refers to the size of the area on the anode target that is exposed to electrons from the tube current. It depends on the size of the filament producing the electron stream. The effective focal spot size refers to the projected focal spot size as measured directly under the anode target (Fig. 3.11).

A tube's focal spot is an important factor because a large focal spot can withstand the heat produced by large exposures, whereas a small one produces better image quality. The line-focus principle demonstrates how, by angling the face of the anode target, the actual focal spot can remain relatively large while the effective focal spot is reduced in size. Greater heat capacity can be achieved while maintaining good image quality. A smaller effective focal spot yields better spatial resolution on the image.

When manufactured, every tube has a specific anode target angle, typically ranging from 5 to 20 degrees. Based on the line-focus principle, the amount of the target angle determines the size of the effective focal spot. It should be noted that the anode target angle is determined on the basis of the intended use of the tube and is not something the radiographer *selects* at the operating console.

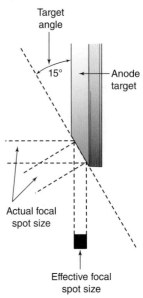

Fig. 3.11 The line-focus principle addresses the relationship between the size of the actual focal spot (where the electrons actually bombard the target) and the effective focal spot (the same area as viewed and measured directly below the target).

A larger target angle produces a larger effective focal spot, and a smaller target angle produces a smaller one. The relationship among target angle, effective focal spot size, and actual focal spot size is illustrated in Fig. 3.12.

 IMPORTANT RELATIONSHIP

Anode Angle and Effective Focal Spot Size

Based on the line-focus principle, the smaller the anode target angle, the smaller the effective focal spot size.

ANODE HEEL EFFECT

A phenomenon known as the anode heel effect occurs because of the angle of the target. The heel effect describes how the x-ray beam has greater intensity (number of x-rays) on the cathode side of the tube but a lower intensity toward the anode side (Fig. 3.13).

 IMPORTANT RELATIONSHIP

Anode Heel Effect

X-rays are more intense on the cathode side of the tube; their intensity decreases toward the anode side.

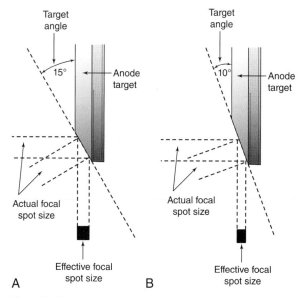

Fig. 3.12 **A,** Based on the line-focus principle, a large target angle produces a large effective focal spot size. **B,** A small target angle produces a small one. Both actual focal spot sizes are the same, meaning that they can withstand the same heat loading. The smaller effective focal spot results in improved image quality.

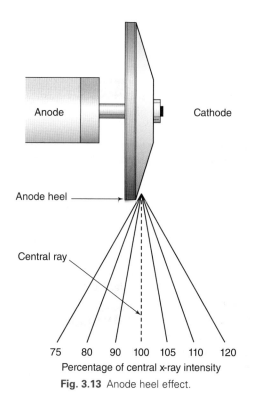

Fig. 3.13 Anode heel effect.

As x-rays are produced, they leave the anode in all directions. The x-rays that are emitted toward the anode side of the tube have farther to travel, and some are absorbed by the anode itself (anode heel), reducing them in number compared with the photons that are emitted in the direction of the cathode. The difference in the intensities between the two ends can be as much as 45%. The heel effect can be used to advantage in radiography because the cathode end of the tube can be placed over a thicker body part, resulting in a more even exposure to the image receptor.

The anode heel effect can be used in imaging the thoracic spine, which has small vertebrae at the top and large vertebrae at the bottom. By placing the patient's head under the anode end of the tube, more intense radiation is directed toward the lower, larger portion of the spine, and the upper, smaller vertebrae are exposed to less intense radiation exposure.

BEAM FILTRATION

The x-ray beam produced at the anode exits the tube housing to become the primary beam. The remnant (exit) beam is the x-ray beam that eventually records the body part onto the image receptor. The x-rays that exit the tube are polyenergetic; they consist of low-energy, medium-energy, and high-energy photons. The low-energy photons cannot penetrate parts of the anatomy and do not contribute to image formation. They contribute only to patient dose and are undesirable.

IMPORTANT RELATIONSHIP
Low-Energy Photons, Patient Dose, and Image Formation

Low-energy photons serve only to increase patient dose and do not contribute to image formation.

Reduction of the low-energy photons requires that filtration be added to the x-ray beam to attenuate or absorb these photons. Added filtration describes the filtration that is added anywhere below the port of the x-ray tube. Aluminum is the material primarily used for this purpose because it absorbs more low-energy photons while the useful higher-energy photons can penetrate the aluminum and exit (Fig. 3.14).

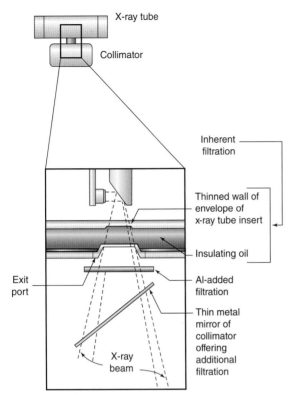

Fig. 3.14 Aluminum *(Al)*-added filtration is shown at the port, or window, of the x-ray tube and the collimator mirror. The inherent filtration of the envelope and the oil are shown.

🔍 MIND IMAGE

X-ray Beam Filtration

Think of an x-ray beam like a pot of coffee. Brewed coffee is a heterogeneous mixture, not unlike the x-ray beam. Coffee filters remove the undesirable parts of the coffee brew to improve its taste and purity. X-ray beam filtration removes the low-energy photons to improve the primary beam.

Various components within the x-ray tube assembly also contribute to the attenuation of low-energy x-rays. Inherent filtration refers to the filtration that is permanently in the path of the x-ray beam. Three components contribute to inherent filtration: (1) the envelope of the tube, (2) the oil that surrounds the tube, and (3) the window in the tube housing. The mirror inside the collimator (beam restrictor located just below the x-ray tube) is considered added filtration since it is not part

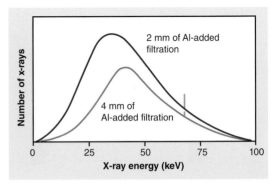

Fig. 3.15 Increasing beam filtration decreases the quantity (amplitude) and increases the quality (shift to the right) of the x-ray beam. *Al,* Aluminum. (From Johnston JN, Fauber TL. *Essentials of Radiographic Physics and Imaging.* 2nd ed. St. Louis: Mosby; 2016.)

of the x-ray tube/housing construction (see Fig. 3.14). The total filtration in the x-ray beam is the sum of the added and inherent filtration. The US government sets standards for total filtration to ensure that patients receive minimal doses of radiation. The current guidelines state that x-ray tubes operating at or above 70 kVp must have a minimum total filtration of 2.5 mm of aluminum or its equivalent. Increasing the amount of tube filtration increases the x-ray beam quality because there is a greater percentage of x-rays that have high energy rather than low energy. In addition, increasing tube filtration decreases the quantity of x-rays or x-ray emission (Fig. 3.15). (Box 3.10 describes quality control methods for evaluating filtration.)

❗ RADIATION PROTECTION ALERT

Beam Filtration

Low-energy photons, created during x-ray production, are unable to penetrate the patient. Patients are protected from unnecessary exposure to this low-energy radiation by the placement of inherent and added filtration in the path of the x-ray beam.

Half-Value Layer

Because the x-ray beam is polyenergetic it is difficult to express the quality of the beam with a single value such as kVp or keV. This heterogeneous makeup of the beam requires a method that takes into account all of the x-ray beam energies as they penetrate a selected material.

BOX 3.10   Quality Control Check: Beam Filtration

- Half-value layer (HVL), the amount of filtration that reduces the intensity of the x-ray beam to half of its original value, is considered the best method for describing x-ray quality.
- The HVL can be used as an indirect measure of the total filtration in the path of the x-ray beam. It is expressed in millimeters of aluminum (mm-Al).
- During the HVL test, a radiation-measuring device, such as a dosimeter, is used to measure both the radiation intensity of the original exposure and that following the addition of increasing mm-Al filtration in the path of the primary beam. The radiation intensity can be graphed for the increasing levels of aluminum filtration to determine the HVL.
- According to the NCRP Report #102, for equipment operated at or above 70 kVp, the required minimum total filtration should be at least 2.5 mm, which indicates the total filtration in the x-ray tube is adequate to protect patients from unnecessary low-energy radiation.
- Normal HVL of general diagnostic beams is 3 to 5 mm-Al.

Aluminum is the chosen material, and the original x-ray beam intensity is measured with a dosimeter. Using the identical exposure conditions, a series of exposures are made, each with added aluminum to the beam, usually in mm thicknesses. When the x-ray beam intensity is half its original intensity, we have measured the total x-ray beam and express it as its half-value layer (HVL). This method naturally takes into account the entire beam and its exposure conditions.

The amount of added filtration to the beam (usually in mm of aluminum) that reduces the beam intensity to half its original intensity is called the beam half-value layer (HVL). One HVL reduces beam intensity by 50% and two HVLs reduce the beam again by 50% and so on.

 IMPORTANT RELATIONSHIP

Half-Value Layer (HVL)

Half-value layer is the amount of added filtration to the beam (usually in mm of aluminum) that reduces the beam intensity to half its original intensity. HVL is an effective and relatively convenient method for tracking x-ray system output over time as a function of usage.

The practical value of this comes into play when the overall output of an x-ray system, including the x-ray tube, is in question. Over time, x-ray machine output can decrease, particularly with x-ray tube aging. When the system is new, the HVL is measured and recorded and reassessed on an annual basis by a qualified medical physicist.

As systems age, subsequent HVL measurements are compared to the original HVL, and when the output reaches an unacceptable level based upon its HVL, the x-ray tube is replaced after inspection by a qualified medical physicist.

Using HVL is an effective and relatively convenient method for tracking x-ray system output over time as a function of usage. It accounts for the entire x-ray beam makeup as well as x-ray exposure parameters. Over time, it takes less added aluminum filtration to the beam to reduce it by 50% and generally this is because metallic tungsten particles have adhered to the inside of the x-ray tube glass envelope and increased the tube's inherent filtration component. At a certain point, a poor HVL will require a new tube.

COMPENSATING FILTERS

Compensating filters can be added to the primary beam to alter its intensity. These types of filters are used to image anatomic areas that are nonuniform in makeup and assist in producing more consistent exposure to the image receptor.

The most common type of compensating filter is a simple wedge filter (Fig. 3.16A). The thicker part of the wedge filter is lined up with the thinner portion of the anatomic part being imaged, allowing fewer x-ray photons to reach that end of the part. A wedge filter may be used for an anteroposterior (AP) projection of the femur, where the hip end is considerably larger than the knee end. A trough filter performs a function similar to a wedge filter; however, it is differently designed (Fig. 3.16B). In particular, the trough filter has a double wedge. A trough filter may be used for an AP projection of the thorax to compensate for the easily penetrated air-filled lungs.

HEAT UNITS

During x-ray production, most of the kinetic energy of the electrons is converted to heat. This heat can damage the x-ray tube and the anode target. The amount of heat

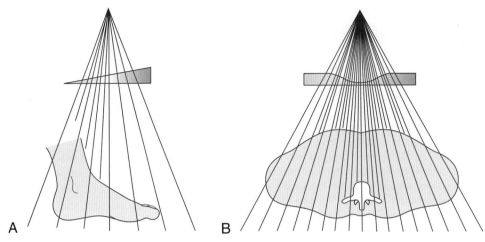

Fig. 3.16 A, Wedge filter. **B,** Trough filter.

produced from any given exposure is expressed by the **heat unit (HU)**. The number of HUs produced depends on the type of x-ray generator being used and the exposure factors selected for a particular exposure and can be mathematically expressed as follows:

$$HU = mA \times Time \times kVp \times Generator\ Factor$$

The generator factor (Table 3.2) accounts for the fact that the use of more consistent x-ray generators results in more heat.

 MATHEMATICAL APPLICATION

Calculating Heat Units

An exposure is made with a three-phase x-ray unit at 600 mA and 75 kVp over 0.05 s. How many heat units are produced from this exposure?

$$HU = mA \times Time \times kVp \times Generator\ Factor$$

$$HU = 600 \times 0.05 \times 75 \times 1.35$$

$$3037.5\ HU$$

TABLE 3.2 Generator Factor

Generator Type	Factor
Single-phase	1.00
Three-phase	1.35
High-frequency	1.40

Different models of x-ray tubes vary in their ability to withstand the heat produced by x-ray exposures. Prior to modern x-ray tubes, radiographers were responsible for evaluating their exposure technique selection to avoid excessive heat load. Box 3.11 and Fig. 3.17 explain the use of tube-rating charts to avoid heat damage. Manufacturers of current x-ray units build their equipment so that tube-damaging exposures cannot be made. In general, if an inappropriate technique is set, the radiographer sees a message such as *Technique Overload*, or the machine may simply not expose after the button is activated. The routine use of high-exposure techniques, although within the x-ray tube's limit, can potentially damage the x-ray tube.

EXTENDING X-RAY TUBE LIFE

X-ray tubes are expensive devices that can fail because of radiographer errors or carelessness. Not only do failed tubes result in an expense for purchasing a new tube, but there is also a downtime for a radiographic room when a failed tube is being replaced, thus decreasing the room's productivity. A few simple but important guidelines for x-ray tube operation should be consistently adhered to by the radiographer to extend tube life:

- If applicable, warm up the tube according to the manufacturer's specifications, especially if it has not been energized for 2 hours or more.
- Avoid excessive heat unit generation. Repeatedly using exposure techniques near an x-ray tube's limit

BOX 3.11 Tube-Rating Charts

Before the development of today's x-ray tubes, manufacturers used instantaneous-load tube-rating charts, also called *single-exposure rating charts*, to describe the exposure limits of x-ray tubes. An instantaneous-load tube-rating chart is used to determine whether a particular exposure would be safe to make and to determine what limits on kVp, mA, and exposure time must be made for safe exposure. Violation of these limits, as indicated by the tube-rating chart, would almost certainly result in permanent and irreparable damage to the x-ray tube. Fig. 3.17 shows a typical instantaneous-load tube-rating chart. For example, the maximum kVp that can be used with 700 mA and 0.3 s exposure time is 90 kVp. The maximum mA that can be used with 105 kVp and 0.2 s exposure time is 600 mA. The

maximum exposure time that can be used with 85 kVp and 900 mA is 0.05 s. Although 130 kVp, 500 mA, and 0.1 s would produce a safe exposure, 130 kVp, 500 mA, and 0.2 s would not.

In addition to tube-rating charts, manufacturers provided anode and housing cooling charts. Based on the quantity of heat units, these charts provided radiographers with information regarding the amount of time that must elapse before initiating another exposure. Modern generators with their microprocessor controls have x-tube rating and anode cooling charts programmed into their computer memories to prevent unacceptable exposure conditions and x-ray tube damage.

kVp, Kilovoltage peak; *mA,* milliamperage.

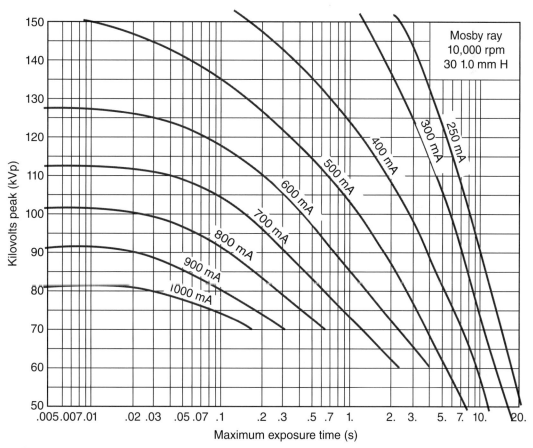

Fig. 3.17 Typical instantaneous-load tube-rating chart that can be used to determine safe and unsafe exposures.

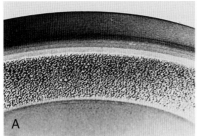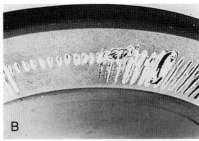

A   B

Fig. 3.18 Two heat-damaged anode targets. **A,** Target shows pitting of the anode track caused by consistent overloading of exposure factors. **B,** Target shows melting of the focal track caused by failure of the rotor to rotate the anode. This failure is usually due to heat damage to the rotor bearings from overloading the exposure factors. (Courtesy Varian Medical Systems, North Charleston, SC.)

increases the total number of heat units. Fig. 3.18 shows anode targets that have been damaged as a result of excessive heat loading.

- Do not hold down the rotor button without making an exposure. Unnecessarily holding down the rotor button causes excessive wear on both the filament and the rotor.
- Use lower tube currents with longer exposure times when possible to minimize wear on the filament.
- Do not move the tube while it is energized. This movement can cause damage to the anode and anode stem as a result of torque (a twisting or rotation force).
- If the rotor makes noticeable noise, stop using the tube until it has been inspected by a qualified service personnel. Noises can be indicative of a potentially serious problem.

Radiographers create diagnostic images by producing an x-ray beam to visualize anatomic structures. The x-rays produced by the radiographer affect not only the quality of the image but also the life of the x-ray tube. Understanding the prime exposure factors and their effect on the x-ray beam and knowing what happens inside the x-ray tube are important considerations in radiography. The basic design and operation of x-ray tubes has not changed significantly over the past few years as we still deal with x-ray tube heat loading and filament characteristics. The most dramatic innovations in the medical imaging process have been on the side of the image receptor and its technologies. We will study this at greater depth in upcoming chapters.

CHAPTER SUMMARY

- X-rays are produced when electrons are boiled off (thermionic emission) the cathode filament, accelerated across to the anode target, and suddenly stopped. Heat is also produced.
- The anode, containing a tungsten-rhenium alloy target, typically rotates, allowing for larger exposures.
- X-rays are produced by bremsstrahlung (primarily) and characteristic interactions that occur as the electrons interact with the tungsten atoms in the target.
- Manipulation of the primary factors affects the quality and quantity of radiation. kVp affects both the quality (energy and penetrability) and the quantity of x-rays, whereas mA and exposure time (or mAs when combined) affect only quantity.

- The line-focus principle describes the relationship between the anode angle and the effective focal spot. Smaller focal spots yield better spatial resolution. The anode heel effect results in more intense radiation exiting the tube toward the cathode side.
- Added and inherent beam filtration ensures that a minimal amount of low-energy x-ray photons reach the patient. The half-value layer (HVL) is an indirect measure of total filtration and is used to describe x-ray beam quality.
- There are numerous methods for extending tube life, including attending to the amount of heat produced during x-ray production. Heat units are the measure of the amount of heat produced using specific exposure factors.

REVIEW QUESTIONS

1. Which x-ray tube component serves as a source of electrons for x-ray production?
   A. Focusing cup
   B. Filament
   C. Stator
   D. Target

2. Electrons interact with the _____ to produce x-rays and heat.
   A. focusing cup
   B. filament
   C. stator
   D. target

3. The cloud of electrons that forms before x-ray production is referred to as _____.
   A. thermionic emission
   B. space charge
   C. space charge effect
   D. tube current

4. The burning or boiling off of electrons at the cathode is referred to as _____.
   A. thermionic emission
   B. space charge
   C. space charge effect
   D. tube current

5. Which primary exposure factor influences both the quantity and the quality of x-ray photons?
   A. mA
   B. mAs
   C. kVp
   D. Exposure time

6. The unit used to express tube current is _____.
   A. mA
   B. mAs
   C. kVp
   D. s

7. What percentage of the kinetic energy is converted to heat when moving electrons strike the anode target?
   A. 1%
   B. 25%
   C. 59%
   D. 99%

8. The intensity of the x-ray beam is greater on the _____.
   A. cathode side of the tube
   B. anode side of the tube
   C. short axis of the beam
   D. long axis of the beam

9. According to the line-focus principle, as the target angle decreases, the _____.
   A. actual focal spot size decreases
   B. actual focal spot size increases
   C. effective focal spot size decreases
   D. effective focal spot size increases

10. _____ extends x-ray tube life.
    A. Selecting higher tube currents
    B. Using small focal spots when possible
    C. Producing exposures with a wide range of kVp values
    D. Warming up the tube after 2 hours of non-use

11. Which type of target interaction is responsible for most of the x-rays in the diagnostic beam?
    A. Characteristic interaction
    B. Thermionic emission
    C. Bremsstrahlung interaction
    D. None of the above

12. What value of mAs is produced when the radiographer sets a kVp of 70, an mA of 600, and an exposure time of 50 ms?
    A. 3.5 mAs
    B. 30 mAs
    C. 300 mAs
    D. 350 mAs

13. Increasing the kVp results in _____.
    A. x-rays with higher energy
    B. x-rays with lower energy
    C. more x-rays
    D. A and C
    E. B and C

14. Total filtration in the x-ray beam includes _____.
    A. compensating filters
    B. inherent filtration
    C. added filtration
    D. B and C
    E. A and C

15. How many heat units result from an exposure made on a single-phase x-ray unit using a beam current of 400 mA, an exposure time of 0.2 s, and a kVp of 70?
    A. 5600 HU
    B. 7560 HU
    C. 7896 HU
    D. 8120 HU

16. On a typical x-ray beam emission spectral graph, the increase in x-ray output due to characteristic radiation from tungsten occurs at approximately:
    A. 12 keV
    B. 37 keV
    C. 69 keV
    D. 81 keV

17. As x-ray systems age due to usage, the HVL:
    A. decreases
    B. increases
    C. remains unaffected
    D. requires longer exposure times

Image Formation and Radiographic Quality

CHAPTER OUTLINE

OBJECTIVES

After completing this chapter, the reader will be able to perform the following:

1. Define all the key terms in this chapter.
2. State all the important relationships in this chapter.
3. Describe the overall process of radiographic image formation.
4. Explain the process of beam attenuation.
5. Identify the factors that affect beam attenuation.
6. Describe the x-ray interactions termed photoelectric effect and Compton effect.
7. Define the term ionization.
8. State the composition of exit radiation.
9. Describe the process of creating the raw image data in the image receptor.
10. Identify the attributes of a quality radiographic image.
11. Explain the importance of the displayed brightness and contrast to image quality.
12. Differentiate between displayed high-contrast and low-contrast images.
13. Explain the importance of temporal and spatial resolution, size, and shape distortion to displayed image quality.
14. State the effects of quantum noise, scatter, and image artifacts on displayed image quality.
15. Explain the importance of radiographic opacities and contrast to image interpretation.
16. Differentiate radiographic imaging from dynamic imaging.

KEY TERMS

absorption
artifact
attenuation
brightness
coherent scattering
Compton effect
Compton electron
contrast resolution
differential absorption
distortion

dynamic range
electronic data set
elongation
exit radiation
fluoroscopy
fog
foreshortening
grayscale
high-contrast images
image receptor (IR)

ionization
low-contrast images
magnification
orthogonal
photoelectric effect
photoelectron
quantum noise
remnant radiation
saturation
scattering

To produce a radiographic image, x-ray photons must pass through tissue and interact with an image receptor (IR), a device that receives the radiation leaving the patient. As discussed in Chapter 3, the radiographer manipulates and controls the radiation exposure exiting the x-ray tube (primary x-ray beam). Both the quantity and the quality of the primary x-ray beam affect its interactions within the various tissues that make up anatomic parts. In addition, the composition of the anatomic tissues affects the x-ray beam interaction. The absorption characteristics of the anatomic part are determined by its thickness, atomic number of the atoms contained within it, and tissue density or compactness of the cellular structures. Finally, the radiation that exits the patient (remnant beam) is composed of varying energies and interacts with the IR to create the raw image data which then must be computer processed. Because digital images are created electronically, the raw image data are considered an electronic data set, which are electronic signal values created by the ionization energies when the exit radiation interacts with an image receptor.

The quality of the digital image is primarily dependent on computer processing the electronic signal values and manipulating the image displayed on the monitor. However, it is important for the radiographer to comprehend the attributes of a quality digital image, and therefore these attributes will be briefly discussed in this chapter. Digital image receptors, computer processing, and displayed image manipulation will be discussed in detail in subsequent chapters.

IMAGE FORMATION

Differential Absorption

The process of image formation is a result of differential absorption of the x-ray beam as it interacts with anatomic tissue. Differential absorption is a process whereby some amount of the x-ray beam is absorbed in the tissue, and some passes through (transmits) the anatomic part. The term *differential* is used because varying anatomic parts do not *absorb* the primary beam to the same degree. Anatomic parts composed of substances such as bone absorb more x-ray photons than parts filled with air. Differential absorption of the primary x-ray beam creates an image that structurally represents the anatomic area of interest (Fig. 4.1).

IMPORTANT RELATIONSHIP
Differential Absorption and Image Formation

A radiographic image is created when an x-ray beam passes through a patient and then interacts with an IR, such as a digital image receptor. The variations in the absorption and transmission of the exiting x-ray beam structurally represent the anatomic area of interest.

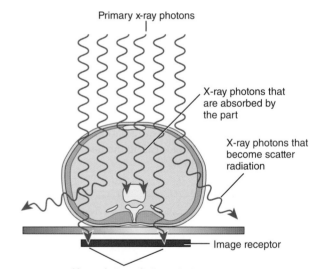

Primary x-ray photons

X-ray photons that are absorbed by the part

X-ray photons that become scatter radiation

Image receptor

X-ray photons that penetrate the part to help form the image

Fig. 4.1 As the primary x-ray beam interacts with an anatomic part, photons are absorbed, scattered, and transmitted. The differences in the absorption characteristics of the anatomic part create an image that structurally represents the part. (From Johnston JN, Fauber TL. *Essentials of Radiographic Physics and Imaging*, 3rd ed. St. Louis: Mosby; 2020.)

Creating a radiographic image by differential absorption requires several processes to occur: beam attenuation (absorption and scattering) and transmission.

Beam Attenuation

As the primary x-ray beam passes through anatomic tissue, it loses some of its energy (intensity). Fewer x-ray photons remain in the beam after it interacts with anatomic tissue. This reduction in the intensity or number of photons in the primary x-ray beam is known as attenuation. Beam attenuation occurs because of the photon interactions with the atomic structures that comprise the tissues. Two distinct processes occur during beam attenuation: absorption and scattering.

Absorption. As the energy of the primary x-ray beam is deposited within the atoms comprising the tissue, some x-ray photons are completely absorbed. Complete absorption of the incoming x-ray photon occurs when it has enough energy to remove (eject) an inner-shell electron. The ejected electron is called a photoelectron, and it quickly loses energy by interacting with nearby tissues. The ability to remove (eject) electrons, known as ionization, is a characteristic of x-rays. In the diagnostic range, this x-ray interaction with matter is known as the photoelectric effect.

With the photoelectric effect, an ionized atom has a vacancy, or electron hole, in its inner shell. An electron from an outer shell drops down to fill this vacancy. Because of the difference in binding energies between the two electron shells, a secondary x-ray photon is emitted (Fig. 4.2). This secondary x-ray photon typically has a very low energy and is unlikely to exit the patient.

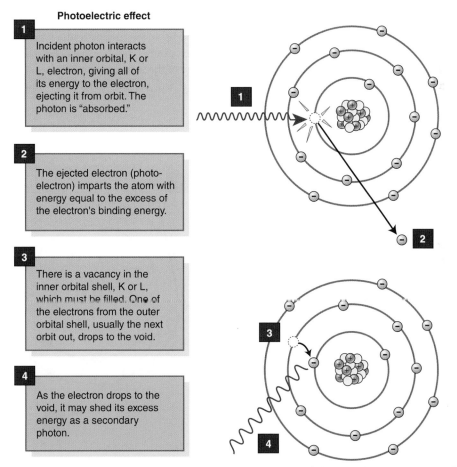

Photoelectric effect

1 Incident photon interacts with an inner orbital, K or L, electron, giving all of its energy to the electron, ejecting it from orbit. The photon is "absorbed."

2 The ejected electron (photoelectron) imparts the atom with energy equal to the excess of the electron's binding energy.

3 There is a vacancy in the inner orbital shell, K or L, which must be filled. One of the electrons from the outer orbital shell, usually the next orbit out, drops to the void.

4 As the electron drops to the void, it may shed its excess energy as a secondary photon.

Fig. 4.2 The photoelectric effect is responsible for total absorption of the incoming x-ray photon. (From Johnston JN, Fauber TL. *Essentials of Radiographic Physics and Imaging*, 3rd ed. St. Louis: Mosby; 2020.)

IMPORTANT RELATIONSHIP

X-ray Photon Absorption

During attenuation of the x-ray beam, the photoelectric effect is responsible for the total absorption of the incoming x-ray photon.

The probability of total photon absorption by the photoelectric effect depends on the energy of the incoming x-ray photon and the atomic number of the anatomic tissue. The energy of the incoming x-ray photon must be at least equal to the binding energy of the inner-shell electron. After absorption of a portion of x-ray photons, the overall quantity of the primary beam decreases as it passes through the anatomic part.

Scattering. Some incoming photons are not absorbed but lose energy and change direction during interactions with the atoms comprising the tissue. This process is called scattering. It results from an interaction between diagnostic x-rays and matter, known as the Compton effect. The loss of energy of the incoming photon occurs when it ejects an outer-shell electron from a tissue atom. The ejected electron is called a Compton electron or secondary electron. The remaining lower-energy x-ray photon changes direction and may leave the anatomic part and interact with the IR (Fig. 4.3).

 IMPORTANT RELATIONSHIP

X-ray Beam Scattering

During attenuation of the x-ray beam, the incoming x-ray photon may lose energy and change direction as a result of the Compton effect.

Compton interactions can occur at any diagnostic x-ray energy and are an important interaction in radiography. The probability of a Compton interaction occurring depends on the energy of the incoming photon. It does not depend on the atomic number of the anatomic tissue. For example, a Compton interaction is just as likely to occur in soft tissue as in tissue composed of bone; however, if the tissue has more complex atoms, there are more opportunities for interaction. With higher atomic number particles, such as bone, if the energy of the incoming photon is sufficiently high, more scatter will occur; otherwise, more absorption will

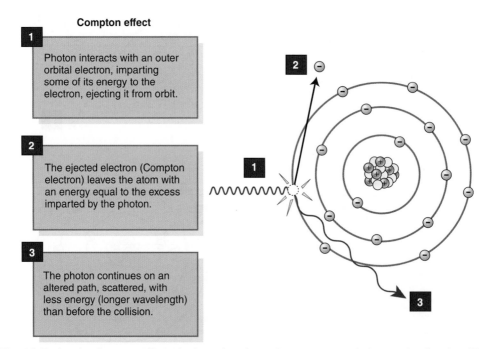

Compton effect

1 Photon interacts with an outer orbital electron, imparting some of its energy to the electron, ejecting it from orbit.

2 The ejected electron (Compton electron) leaves the atom with an energy equal to the excess imparted by the photon.

3 The photon continues on an altered path, scattered, with less energy (longer wavelength) than before the collision.

Fig. 4.3 During the Compton effect, the incoming photon loses energy and changes its direction. (From Johnston JN, Fauber TL. *Essentials of Radiographic Physics and Imaging*, 3rd ed. St. Louis: Mosby; 2020.)

occur. For Compton interactions to occur, the energy of the photon is more important, whereas the atomic number of elements in the tissue is only related to the opportunity for x-ray interactions. When a higher kilovoltage peak (kVp) within the diagnostic range is used, the overall number of x-ray interactions within matter decreases because of increased photon transmission; however, the percentage of Compton interactions increase and photoelectric interactions decrease. Box 4.1 compares photoelectric and Compton interactions. Scattered and secondary radiations provide no useful clinical information and must be controlled during radiographic imaging.

Coherent scattering is an interaction that occurs with low-energy x-rays, typically below the diagnostic range, also known as classical scattering. The incoming photon interacts with the atom as a whole and does not invade the electron cloud surrounding the nucleus, causing it to become excited. The x-ray does not lose energy, but it changes direction (Fig. 4.4). Coherent scattering could occur within the diagnostic range of the x-rays and may interact with the IR, but it is not considered an important interaction in radiography.

If a scattered photon strikes the IR, it does not contribute any useful information about the anatomic area of interest. If scattered photons are absorbed within the anatomic tissue, they contribute to radiation exposure to the patient. In addition, if the scattered photon leaves the patient and does not strike the IR, it could contribute to radiation exposure of anyone near the patient.

BOX 4.1 Comparing the Photoelectric and Compton Effects

Photoelectric Effect
- An incoming photon has sufficient energy to eject an inner-shell electron and be completely absorbed.
- An electron from an upper-level shell fills the electron hole or vacancy.
- A secondary photon is created equal to the difference in the electrons' binding energies.
- The probability of this effect depends on the energy of the incoming x-ray photon and the composition of the anatomic tissue.
- Fewer photon interactions occur at a higher kilovoltage peak (kVp), but of those interactions, a smaller percentage are photoelectric interactions.

Compton Effect
- An incoming photon loses energy when it ejects an outer-shell electron and changes direction.
- The scattered photon may be absorbed within the patient tissues, leave the anatomic part, interact with the image receptor (IR), or expose anyone near the patient.
- Scattered photons that strike the IR provide no useful information.
- The probability of this effect depends on the energy of the incoming x-ray photon but not on the composition of the anatomic tissue.
- Fewer photon interactions occur at a higher kVp, but a greater percentage of those interactions are Compton interactions.

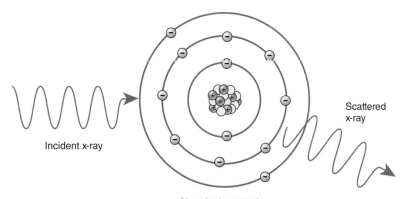

Classical scattering

Fig. 4.4 Coherent (classical) scattering. The incoming photon interacts with the atom, causing it to become excited. The x-ray does not lose energy, but it changes direction. (From Johnston JN, Fauber TL. *Essentials of Radiographic Physics and Imaging*, 3rd ed. St. Louis: Mosby; 2020.)

The preceding discussion focused on photon interactions that occur in radiography when using x-ray energies within the moderate range. X-rays with energies above the diagnostic range result in other interactions, namely, pair production and photodisintegration. X-ray interactions above the diagnostic range are important in positron emission tomography (PET) and radiation therapy.

Factors Affecting Beam Attenuation

The amount of x-ray beam attenuation is affected by the thickness of the anatomic part, the atomic number of the atoms contained within it, its tissue density, and the energy of the x-ray beam.

Tissue Thickness. Increasing the thickness of a given anatomic tissue increases beam attenuation by either absorption or scattering (Fig. 4.5). X-rays are exponentially attenuated and are generally reduced by approximately 50% for each 4 to 5 cm (1.6–2 inches) of tissue thickness (Fig. 4.6). More x-rays are needed to produce a radiographic image for a thicker anatomic part. Fewer x-rays are needed to produce a radiographic image for a thinner anatomic part.

Type of Tissue. Tissues composed of substances with a higher effective atomic number, such as bone (which has an effective atomic number of 13.8), attenuate the x-ray beam more than tissue composed of substances with a lower effective atomic number, such as fat (which has an effective atomic number of 6.3). The higher atomic number indicates that there are more atomic particles with higher electron binding energies, for

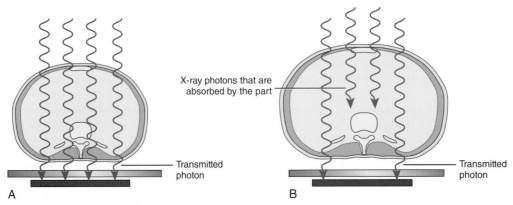

Fig. 4.5 A, A thinner patient transmits more radiation than a thicker patient. **B,** A thicker patient absorbs more radiation than a thinner patient. (From Johnston JN, Fauber TL. *Essentials of Radiographic Physics and Imaging,* 3rd ed. St. Louis: Mosby; 2020.)

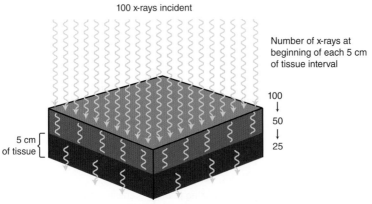

Fig. 4.6 X-rays are exponentially attenuated and generally reduced by approximately 50% for each 4 to 5 cm (1.6–2 inches) of tissue thickness. (From Johnston JN, Fauber TL. *Essentials of Radiographic Physics and Imaging,* 3rd ed. St. Louis: Mosby; 2020.)

interactions with x-ray photons. X-ray absorption is more likely to occur in tissues with a higher effective atomic number than in those with a lower effective atomic number (Fig. 4.7).

Tissue density (matter per unit volume), or the compactness of atomic particles composing the anatomic part, also affects the amount of beam attenuation. For example, muscle (effective atomic number 7.4) and fat (effective atomic number 6.3) tissue are similar in effective atomic number; however, their atomic particles differ

in compactness, and their tissue densities vary. Muscle tissue has atomic particles that are more densely packed or compact and therefore attenuate the x-ray beam more than fat cells. Bone is composed of tissue with a higher effective atomic number, and the atomic particles are more compacted or densely packed. Anatomic tissues are typically ranked based on their attenuation properties. Five substances account for most of the beam attenuation in the human body: mineral such as bone, water such as muscle, fat (adipose), air (gas), and foreign substances, such as metal. Bone attenuates the x-ray beam more than muscle, muscle attenuates the x-ray beam more than fat, and fat attenuates the x-ray beam more than air. The effective atomic number of the anatomic part and its tissue density affect x-ray beam attenuation.

X-ray Beam Quality. The quality of the x-ray beam or its penetrating ability affects its interaction with anatomic tissue. Higher-penetrating x-rays (shorter wavelength with higher frequency) are more likely to be transmitted through anatomic tissue without interacting with the tissues' atomic structures. Lower-penetrating x-rays (longer wavelength with lower frequency) are more likely to interact with the atomic structures and be absorbed. The kilovoltage selected during x-ray production determines the energy or penetrability of the x-ray photon, and this affects its attenuation in anatomic tissue (Fig. 4.8). Beam attenuation decreases with a higher-energy x-ray beam and increases with a lower-energy x-ray beam. See Table 4.1 for factors affecting beam attenuation.

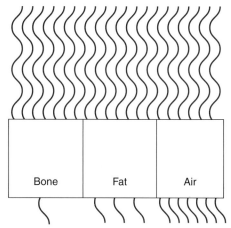

Fig. 4.7 Bone absorbs more radiation than fat and air. Air transmits more radiation than fat and bone. (From Johnston JN, Fauber TL. *Essentials of Radiographic Physics and Imaging*, 3rd ed. St. Louis: Mosby; 2020.)

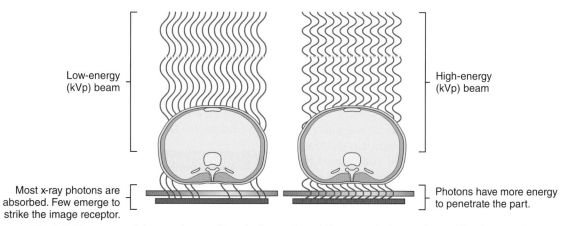

Fig. 4.8 The energy of the x-ray beam affects its interaction within anatomic tissues. Lower kilovoltage peak (*kVp*) results in more absorption in the tissue; higher kVp results in more transmission through the tissue. (From Johnston JN, Fauber TL. *Essentials of Radiographic Physics and Imaging*, 3rd ed. St. Louis: Mosby; 2020.)

Factor	Beam Attenuation	Absorption	Transmission
TABLE 4.1 Factors Affecting Beam Attenuation			
Tissue Thickness			
• Increasing thickness	↑	↑	↓
• Decreasing thickness	↓	↓	↑
Tissue Atomic Number			
• Increasing atomic number	↑	↑	↓
• Decreasing atomic number	↓	↓	↑
Tissue Density			
• Increasing tissue density	↑	↑	↓
• Decreasing tissue density	↓	↓	↑
X-Ray Beam Quality			
• Increasing beam quality	↓	↓	↑
• Decreasing beam quality	↑	↑	↓

IMPORTANT RELATIONSHIP
Factors Affecting Beam Attenuation

Increasing tissue thickness, higher effective atomic number, and tissue density increases x-ray beam attenuation because more x-rays are absorbed by the tissue. Increasing the quality of the x-ray beam decreases beam attenuation because the higher-energy x-rays penetrate the tissue.

Transmission. If the incoming x-ray photon passes through the anatomic part without any interaction with the atomic structures, it is called transmission (Fig. 4.9). The combination of absorption and transmission of the x-ray beam provides an image that structurally represents the anatomic part. Because scatter radiation is also a process that occurs during interaction of the x-ray beam and the anatomic part, the quality of the image created is compromised if scattered photons strike the IR.

Exit Radiation

When the attenuated x-ray beam leaves the patient, the remaining x-ray beam, referred to as exit radiation or remnant radiation, is composed of both transmitted and scattered radiation (Fig. 4.10). This remnant radiation will ultimately produce an electronic data set in a digital image receptor. The varying amounts of transmitted and absorbed radiation (differential absorption) create an image that structurally represents the anatomic

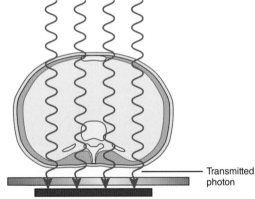

Fig. 4.9 Some incoming x-ray photons pass through the anatomic part without any interactions. (From Johnston JN, Fauber TL. *Essentials of Radiographic Physics and Imaging*, 3rd ed. St. Louis: Mosby; 2020.)

area of interest. Scatter exit radiation (Compton interactions) that reaches the IR does not provide any diagnostic information about the anatomic area. Scatter radiation creates unwanted exposure on the image called fog. Methods used to decrease the amount of scatter radiation reaching the IR are discussed in Chapter 8.

IMPORTANT RELATIONSHIP
X-ray Interaction With Matter

When the diagnostic primary x-ray beam interacts with anatomic tissues, three processes occur: absorption, scattering, and transmission.

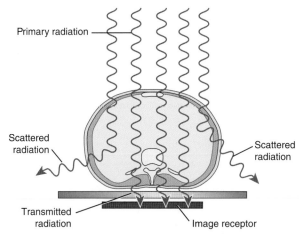

Fig. 4.10 Radiation that exits the anatomic part comprises transmitted and scattered radiation. (From Johnston JN, Fauber TL. *Essentials of Radiographic Physics and Imaging*, 3rd ed. St. Louis: Mosby; 2020.)

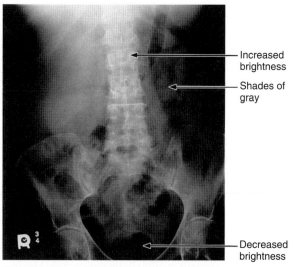

Fig. 4.11 Anatomic tissues vary in their absorption and transmission of x-ray photons to create the range of gray levels that structurally represent the anatomic area of interest. Radiopaque tissues display increased brightness from absorbed radiation, whereas radiolucent tissues display decreased brightness from transmitted radiation. (From Johnston JN, Fauber TL. *Essentials of Radiographic Physics and Imaging*, 3rd ed. St. Louis: Mosby; 2020.)

The areas within the anatomic tissue that absorb incoming x-ray photons (photoelectric effect) are considered radiopaque and create the light areas (increased brightness) on the displayed image. The areas within the anatomic tissues that transmit the incoming photons are considered radiolucent and create dark areas (decreased brightness) on the displayed image. Anatomic tissues that vary in absorption and transmission range between radiopaque and radiolucent to create a range of dark and light areas (shades of gray) (Fig. 4.11). The various shades of gray displayed in the radiographic image make anatomic tissues visible. Skeletal bones are differentiated from the air-filled lungs because of their differences in absorption and transmission.

 IMPORTANT RELATIONSHIP

Displayed Image Gray Levels

Anatomic tissues that vary in absorption and transmission range between radiopaque and radiolucent to create a range of dark and light areas (shades of gray).

Less than 5% of the primary x-ray beam interacting with the anatomic part reaches the IR, and an even lower percentage is used to create the radiographic image. When the exit or remnant radiation interacts with the digital IR, it is converted to the electronic signal values. The strength (intensity) of the signal value and the differences in adjacent signal values are a result

of x-ray beam attenuation with the varying anatomic tissues. The electronic data set is computer processed to produce a visible image displayed on a monitor. IRs, acquisition, processing, and display are discussed in Chapters 5 and 6.

 IMPORTANT RELATIONSHIP

Electronic Signal Values

When the exit or remnant radiation interacts with the digital IR, it is converted to the electronic signal values. The strength (intensity) of the signal value and the differences in adjacent signal values are a result of x-ray beam attenuation with the varying anatomic tissues.

RADIOGRAPHIC QUALITY

A quality radiographic image accurately represents the anatomic area of interest, and information is well visualized for diagnosis. It is important to identify the attributes of a quality radiographic image before comprehending all the factors that affect its quality.

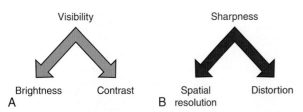

Fig. 4.12 Factors affecting radiographic image quality. **A,** Visibility factors. **B,** Sharpness factors. (From Johnston JN, Fauber TL. *Essentials of Radiographic Physics and Imaging*, 3rd ed. St. Louis: Mosby; 2020.)

The *visibility* of the anatomic structures and the *accuracy* of their recorded structural lines (sharpness) determine the overall quality of the radiographic image. The visibility of the anatomic detail refers to the *brightness* and *contrast* of the displayed image, and the accuracy of the structural lines is achieved by maximizing the amount of *spatial resolution* and minimizing the amount of *distortion* (Fig. 4.12). Visibility of the anatomic structures is achieved by the proper balance of image brightness and contrast.

Displayed Image Brightness

Because the digital image is composed of electronic data, the brightness level displayed on the computer monitor can be easily altered to visualize the range of anatomic structures recorded. Brightness is the amount of luminance (light emission) of a display monitor.

A digital image must have sufficient brightness displayed to visualize the anatomic structures of interest (Fig. 4.13). A digital image that is too light has too much brightness to visualize the structures of the anatomic part (Fig. 4.14). Conversely, a digital image that is too dark has insufficient brightness, and the anatomic part cannot be well visualized (Fig. 4.15). The radiographer must evaluate the overall brightness in the displayed image to determine whether it is sufficient to visualize the anatomic area of interest. The radiographer then decides whether the digital image is diagnostic or unacceptable.

> ### ◆ IMPORTANT RELATIONSHIP
> #### *Displayed Brightness and Digital Image Quality*
> A digital image must have sufficient brightness to visualize the anatomic structures of interest.

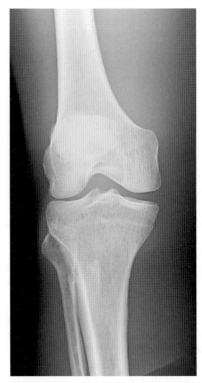

Fig. 4.13 Displayed brightness. Digital image with sufficient brightness. (From Johnston JN, Fauber TL. *Essentials of Radiographic Physics and Imaging*, 3rd ed. St. Louis: Mosby; 2020.)

The x-ray beam that exits the patient contains a wide range of x-ray intensities (often varying by more than 1000-fold). To adequately capture these intensity extremes, a receptor with a wide dynamic range (the range of exposure intensities an IR can accurately detect) is required. Because digital imaging provides a wide dynamic range and the computer can adjust for exposure errors, a greater margin of error in exposure exists to produce a diagnostic image.

Because digital image processing can compensate for exposure errors, the image may display the appropriate level of brightness yet also have been over- or underexposed. As a result, the radiographer may be unaware of the exposure error. However, extreme exposure errors can affect image quality and be visible to the radiographer. When exposure to the digital IR is too low for the anatomic area, excessive quantum noise (discussed later in this chapter) may be visible. When the IR is extremely overexposed, saturation of IR elements may occur where the image cannot be properly processed, and the quality is severely degraded (Fig. 4.16).

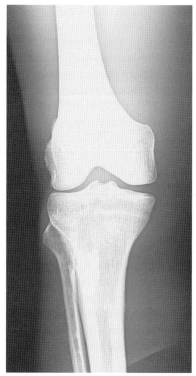

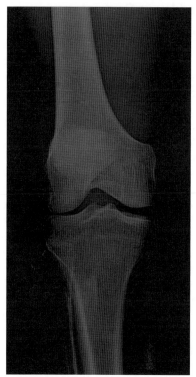

Fig. 4.14 Displayed brightness. Digital image with excessive brightness. Brightness altered at the display monitor. (From Johnston JN, Fauber TL. *Essentials of Radiographic Physics and Imaging*, 3rd ed. St. Louis: Mosby; 2020.)

Fig. 4.15 Displayed brightness. Digital image with insufficient brightness. Brightness altered at the display monitor. (From Johnston JN, Fauber TL. *Essentials of Radiographic Physics and Imaging*, 3rd ed. St. Louis: Mosby; 2020.)

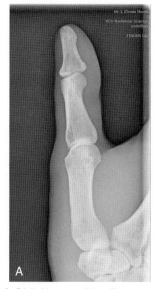

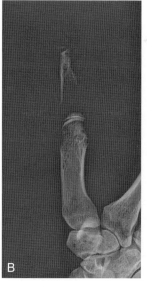

Fig. 4.16 Saturation. **A,** Digital image with sufficient exposure. **B,** Digital image with extreme overexposure; the quality is severely degraded. (From Johnston JN, Fauber TL. *Essentials of Radiographic Physics and Imaging*, 3rd ed. St. Louis: Mosby; 2020.)

Displayed Image Contrast

In addition to sufficient brightness, the digital image must exhibit variations in the brightness levels (image contrast) to differentiate among anatomic tissues. The range of brightness levels displayed is, in part, a result of the tissues' differential absorption of the x-ray photons. An image that has sufficient brightness but no differences appears as a homogeneous object (Fig. 4.17). This appearance indicates that the absorption characteristics of the object are equal. When the absorption characteristics of an object differ, the image has varying levels of brightness displayed (Fig. 4.18). The anatomic tissues are easily differentiated because of these variations in brightness levels (i.e., contrast). Tissues that attenuate the x-ray beam equally are more difficult to visualize because the brightness levels are too similar to differentiate.

Displayed image contrast is the combined result of multiple factors associated with the anatomic structure, radiation quality, image-receptor characteristics, computer processing, and display monitor. Subject contrast refers to the absorption characteristics of the anatomic tissue imaged and the quality of the x-ray beam. Differences in tissue thickness, density, and effective atomic number contribute to subject contrast (Fig. 4.19). For example, the chest is composed of tissues that vary greatly in x-ray lucency, such as the air-filled lungs, the heart, and the bony thorax. This anatomic region creates high subject contrast because the tissues attenuate the x-ray beam very differently compared with the abdomen for the same beam quality. When the thorax is imaged, great differences in brightness levels are displayed for the varying tissues (Fig. 4.20). The abdomen is composed of tissues that attenuate the x-ray beam similarly and is a region of low subject contrast. The brightness levels representing the organs in the abdomen are more similar (Fig. 4.21). Therefore it is difficult to distinguish the liver from the kidneys. As previously discussed, the quality of the x-ray beam also affects its attenuation in tissues, which alters subject contrast. Increasing the penetrating power of the x-ray beam decreases attenuation, reduces absorption, and increases x-ray transmission, resulting in fewer differences in the brightness levels recorded in the radiographic image (lower contrast).

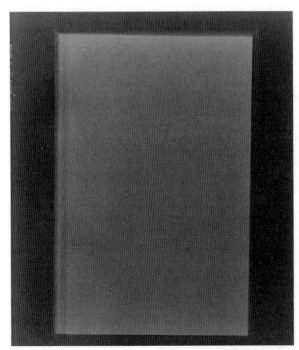

Fig. 4.17 Radiographic image of a homogeneous object having no differences in brightness levels.

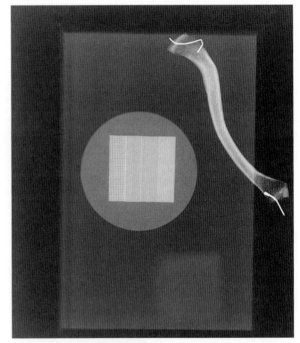

Fig. 4.18 An object with different absorption characteristics produces an image with varying brightness levels.

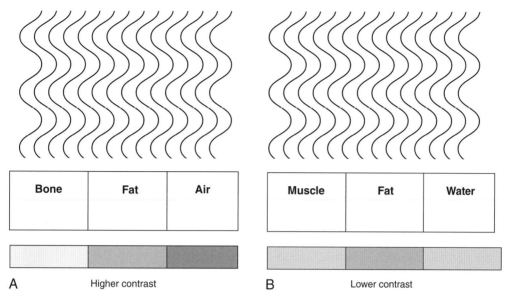

Bone	Fat	Air

A   Higher contrast

Muscle	Fat	Water

B   Lower contrast

Fig. 4.19 A, Higher subject contrast resulting from great differences in radiation absorption between tissues that vary greatly in composition. **B,** Lower subject contrast resulting from fewer differences in the radiation absorption for tissues that are more similarly composed.

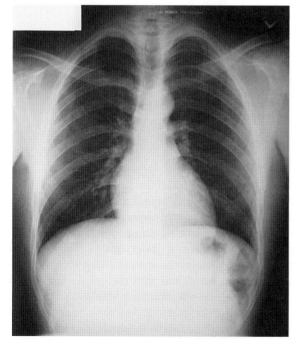

Fig. 4.20 The thorax is an anatomic area of high subject contrast because there is great variation in tissue composition.

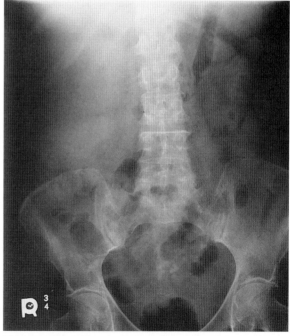

Fig. 4.21 The abdomen is an anatomic area of low subject contrast because it is composed of similar tissue types.

Differentiating Among Anatomic Tissues

The ability to distinguish among types of tissues is determined by the differences in brightness levels in the displayed image, or contrast. Anatomic tissues that attenuate the beam similarly have low subject contrast. Anatomic tissues that attenuate the beam very differently have high subject contrast.

Brightness is easily measurable; however, contrast is a more complex attribute. Evaluating digital image quality in terms of displayed contrast is more subjective. (It is affected by individual preferences.) The level of displayed contrast desired in an image is determined by the composition of the anatomic tissue to be imaged and the amount of information needed to visualize the tissue for an accurate diagnosis. For example, the level of contrast desired in a chest image is different from that required in an extremity image.

Radiographic or *image contrast* is a term used to describe variations in displayed brightness levels. In digital imaging, the number of different shades of gray that can be stored and displayed by a computer system is termed grayscale. Because the digital image is processed and reconstructed in the computer as electronic data, its grayscale or contrast can be altered. Digital images can be displayed to show a range of gray levels from high to low contrast. High-contrast images display fewer shades of gray but greater differences between them (Fig. 4.22). Low-contrast images display a greater number of gray shades but smaller differences between them (Fig. 4.23).

Contrast resolution is used to describe the ability of the digital imaging system to distinguish between small objects that attenuate the x-ray beam similarly. The contrast resolution of the imaging system determines the level of visibility of small objects having similar brightness levels or shades of gray. Increasing the number of shades of gray available for display increases the contrast resolution within the image. An image with increased contrast resolution increases the visibility of anatomic structures and the ability to distinguish among small anatomic areas of interest. The ability to detect anatomic substances having low contrast is important in radiography, such as visualization of soft tissue anatomy. Displayed image contrast is a product of both the subject contrast and the contrast resolution of the digital image receptor. In

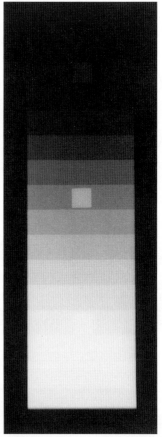

Fig. 4.22 High-contrast image showing fewer gray levels and greater differences between them.

addition, contrast can be altered with computer processing before and after the image is displayed.

Spatial Resolution

The quality of a digital image depends on both the visibility and the accuracy of the anatomic structural lines (sharpness) displayed. Adequate visualization of the anatomic area of interest (brightness and contrast) is just one component of image quality. To produce a quality digital image, the anatomic structures must be accurately displayed and with the greatest amount of sharpness. Spatial resolution is a term used to evaluate the accuracy of the anatomic structural lines displayed. Spatial resolution refers to the smallest object that can be detected in an image.

The ability of a digital image to demonstrate sharp lines determines the quality of the spatial resolution.

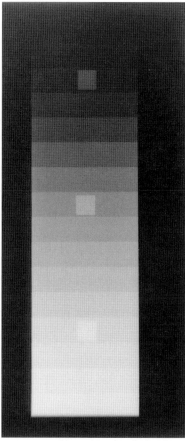

Fig. 4.23 Low-contrast image showing many gray levels and few differences between them.

The imaging process makes it impossible to produce a digital image without a certain degree of unsharpness. A digital image that has greater spatial resolution minimizes the unsharpness of the anatomic structural lines.

IMPORTANT RELATIONSHIP

Sharpness of Anatomic Detail

> The accuracy of the anatomic structural lines displayed in the digital image is determined by its spatial resolution.

Temporal Resolution

There is some motion unsharpness on all images due to the uncontrolled motion of anatomy such as the heart-beat, bowel contractions, and pulsating major blood vessels. To minimize this type of motion unsharpness,

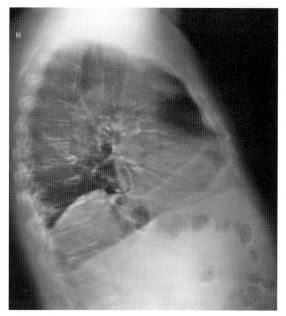

Fig. 4.24 Image showing motion unsharpness. (From *Mosby's Instructional Radiographic Series: Radiographic Imaging.* St. Louis: Mosby; 1998.)

exposures are taken using the shortest exposure time possible, typically in milliseconds (ms). Temporal resolution is the inherent resolution on an image as a function of image acquisition time. Increasing the time of exposure during image acquisition can increase motion unsharpness and therefore decrease temporal resolution, even if it is not visible on the displayed image.

A radiographic image cannot be an exact reconstruction of the anatomic structure. Some information is always lost during the process of image formation. In addition, factors such as patient motion increase the amount of unsharpness recorded in the image (Fig. 4.24). Eliminating motion unsharpness is an important skill required of the radiographer. Voluntary motion, under the control of the patient, is best alleviated by effective communication. However, in some situations such as with children and older adults, patients may have difficulty controlling voluntary motion. Reducing the exposure time and using immobilization devices may be needed in addition to effective communication. Reducing the exposure time is the best method to eliminate motion unsharpness for involuntary motion (temporal resolution), not under the control of the patient. A less common type of motion unsharpness is a result of equipment malfunction and is more difficult to identify.

It is the radiographer's responsibility to minimize the amount of information lost by manipulating the factors that affect the sharpness of the displayed image. Diagnostic quality is achieved by maximizing the amount of spatial resolution and minimizing the amount of image distortion.

The sharpness and visibility of the anatomic structural details have typically been discussed as two separate qualities of a radiographic image. Generally, this separation remains true except when imaging small anatomic structures. A small anatomic structure is best visualized when its displayed brightness varies significantly from the background. If unsharpness is increased, the visibility of small anatomic details is compromised. An increase in the amount of unsharpness displayed in the image decreases the displayed contrast of small anatomic structures, reducing the overall visibility of the structural lines. The spreading of the structural lines with increased unsharpness decreases the differences in displayed brightness levels between the structural lines of the area of interest and the background. As a result, the difference in brightness levels between the area of interest and the background lessens (low contrast) and the visibility of the anatomic structure is reduced (Fig. 4.25).

Distortion

Distortion results from the radiographic misrepresentation of either the size (magnification) or the shape of the anatomic part. When an image is distorted, spatial resolution is also reduced.

Size Distortion (Magnification)

The term size distortion (or magnification) refers to an increase in the image size of an object compared with its true or actual size. Radiographic images of objects are always magnified in terms of the true object size. The source-to-image receptor distance (SID) and object-to-image receptor distance (OID) have a geometric relationship and play an important role in minimizing the amount of size distortion of the radiographic image.

Because radiographers produce radiographs of three-dimensional objects, some size distortion always occurs because of OID. The parts of the object that are farther away from the IR are radiographically represented with greater size distortion than the parts of the object that are closer to the IR. Even if the object is in close contact with the IR, some part of the object is farther away than other parts of the object. SID also influences the total amount of magnification of the image. As SID increases,

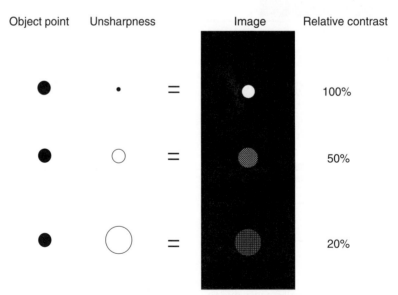

Object point	Unsharpness		Image	Relative contrast
●	·	=	○	100%
●	○	=	◉	50%
●	○	=	◉	20%

Fig. 4.25 Unsharpness and image contrast. Increasing the amount of unsharpness decreases the brightness between the area of interest and its surrounding background. (Modified from Sprawls P. *Physical Principles of Medical Imaging Online*, 2nd ed. http://www.sprawls.org/ppmi2.)

size distortion (magnification) decreases; as SID decreases, size distortion (magnification) increases.

Size Distortion

> Radiographic images of objects are always magnified in terms of the true object size. The SID and OID have a geometric relationship and play an important role in minimizing the amount of size distortion of the radiographic image.

Shape Distortion

In addition to size distortion, objects that are being imaged can be radiographically misrepresented by distortion of their shape. Shape distortion can radiographically appear in two different ways: elongation or foreshortening. Elongation refers to images of objects that appear longer than the true objects. Foreshortening refers to images that appear shorter than the true objects. Examples of elongation and foreshortening can be seen in Fig. 4.26.

Shape distortion can arise from inaccurate central ray (CR) alignment of the tube, the part being radiographed, or the IR. Any misalignment of the CR among these three factors—tube, part, or IR—alters the shape of the part recorded in the image.

Shape Distortion

> Shape distortion can occur from inaccurate CR alignment of the tube, the part being radiographed, or the IR. Elongation refers to images of objects that appear longer than the true objects. Foreshortening refers to images that appear shorter than the true objects.

Sometimes shape distortion is advantageous in projections or positions. For example, CR angulation is sometimes required to elongate a part so that a particular anatomic structure can be visualized better. Also, rotating the part (and therefore creating shape distortion) is sometimes required to eliminate superimposition of objects that normally obstruct visualization of

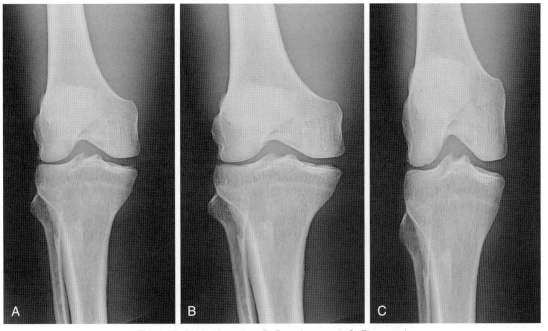

Fig. 4.26 A, No distortion. **B,** Foreshortened. **C,** Elongated.

the area of interest. In general, shape distortion is not a necessary or desirable characteristic of radiographic images and an orthogonal or right-angle relationship between the CR and the image receptor is preferred.

Both SID and OID determine the amount of magnification of the anatomic structures on the image. In addition, improper alignment of the CR, anatomic part, IR, or a combination of these components distorts the shape of the image.

Scatter

Scatter radiation, as previously described, can add unwanted exposure to the radiographic image because of Compton interactions. Unwanted exposure or fog on the image does not provide information about the anatomic area of interest. Scatter degrades or decreases the visibility of the anatomic structures. The scatter or unwanted exposure displayed in the image has the effect of decreasing the contrast by masking the desired brightness of the image and changing the adjacent brightness levels (Fig. 4.27).

Fog produced because of scatter reaching the IR can be visualized on a digital image as noise. Even though the computer can change the contrast or gray levels

displayed in a digital image, scatter radiation reaching the IR does not provide any information about the area of interest. Because digital IRs can detect low levels of radiation intensity, they are more sensitive to scatter radiation.

Quantum Noise

Image noise contributes no useful diagnostic information and serves only to detract from the quality of an image. Quantum noise (mottle) is a concern in digital imaging and is photon dependent. Quantum noise is visible as brightness fluctuations and graininess in the image. The fewer the photons reaching the IR to form the image, the greater the visibility of quantum noise on the digital image.

Quantum noise negatively affects the visibility of structural details on an image and is related to exposure.

IMPORTANT RELATIONSHIP
Number of Photons and Quantum Noise

Decreasing the number of photons reaching the IR may increase the amount of quantum noise within the radiographic image; increasing the number of photons reaching the IR may decrease the amount of quantum noise within the radiographic image.

As previously mentioned, the digital computer system can adjust for low or high x-ray exposures during image acquisition. When the x-ray exposure to the IR is too low (i.e., when there are fewer photons), computer processing alters the appearance of the digital image to make the brightness acceptable, but the image displays increased quantum noise (Fig. 4.28). Certain postprocessing options can be used to enhance image quality by decreasing the visibility of image noise.

The exposure technique should be selected based on the requirements of the type of imaging procedure being performed. Although the computer can adjust for both low- and high-exposure technique errors, the radiographer is still responsible for selecting exposure techniques that produce diagnostic-quality images while avoiding unnecessary exposure to the patient. Exposures that are too low adversely affect the quantum noise of an image even though the computer can adjust the brightness. Exposures that are too high result in excessive radiation exposure to the patient and may impact image quality.

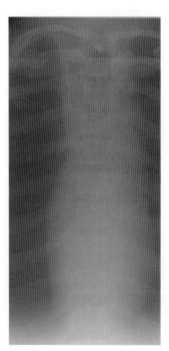

Fig. 4.27 Scatter and fog.

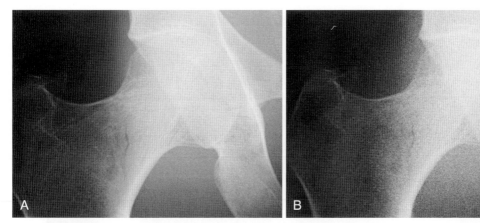

Fig. 4.28 A, Image created using an appropriate x-ray exposure technique. **B,** Image shows increased quantum noise because of insufficient x-ray exposure to the image receptor. (From Johnston JN, Fauber TL. *Essentials of Radiographic Physics and Imaging*, 3rd ed. St. Louis: Mosby; 2020.)

Image Artifacts

The goal with all medical imaging is to produce images that accurately reflect the true nature of a patient's structure and function. An artifact is any unwanted brightness level on a radiographic image that is not part of the patient's anatomy. Artifacts are detrimental to images because they can impede the visibility of anatomy or pathologic conditions. They decrease the overall quality of the radiographic image.

Errors such as double exposing a computed radiography IR or the improper use of equipment can result in image artifacts and must be avoided. Foreign bodies are a class of artifacts imaged within a patient's body. Variation in exposure techniques may be necessary when imaging for a suspected foreign body.

Artifacts from patient clothing and items imaged that are not a part of the area of interest are the same regardless of the type of imaging systems. The radiographer must be diligent in removing clothing or items that could obstruct visibility of the anatomic area of interest (Fig. 4.29). Scatter radiation or fog and image noise have also been classified as radiographic artifacts because they add unwanted information on the displayed image.

Digital image artifacts can be a result of errors during extraction of the electronic data set from the IR, inadequate computed radiography imaging plate erasure, or performance of the electronic detectors and will be discussed in subsequent chapters.

RADIOGRAPHIC IMAGE INTERPRETATION

Knowing that image production is a function of differential absorption of the variations in tissue thickness and composition, radiologists use their deep understanding of human anatomy and structure to understand what they view on medical images.

To the radiologist, there are five basic radiographic substances, and they understand that human anatomy is a combination of these radiographic substances, and they look for these opacities when interpreting images (Fig. 4.30). Anatomy such as muscle, liver tissue, lymph nodes, and blood vessels are water-based tissues that are lower in subject contrast because they attenuate the x-ray beam similarly. Fat (adipose) is scattered throughout our anatomy and is used diagnostically to help in interpretation, as it can be an indicator of an underlying pathology. Our skeletal system represents mineral substances as do blood vessel calcifications, gallstones, kidney stones, etc., and illustrates higher subject contrast because they absorb more of the x-rays through photoelectric interactions. Air in the lungs as well as bowel gas illustrates the role of a radiolucent substance that is visualized as higher contrast with its surrounding tissues.

Visualizing Anatomy on Radiographic Images

Visualizing anatomy depends upon these five substances (air [gas], fat [adipose], water, mineral, and metal), being in anatomical, physical contact (adjacent) to each other.

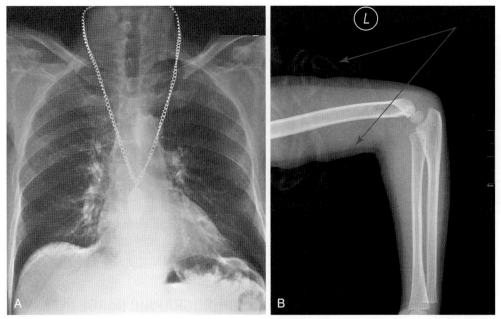

Fig. 4.29 Image artifacts. **A,** Jewelry. **B,** Clothing. (**A,** From Long B, Rollins J, Smith B. *Merrill's Atlas of Radiographic Positioning and Procedures*, 13th ed. St. Louis: Mosby; 2016. **B,** Modified from © Nevit Dilmen [CC BY-SA 3.0 (https://creativecommons.org/licenses/by-sa/3.0)]).

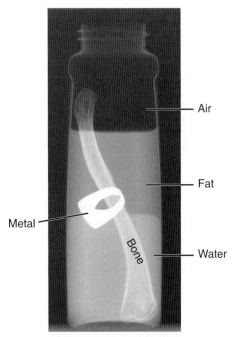

Fig. 4.30 Image of the five radiographic substances. (From Marchiori, DM. *Clinical Imaging: With Skeletal, Chest and Abdomen Pattern Differentials*. 3rd ed. St. Louis: Elsevier Inc.; 2014.)

Simply stated, anatomy of different radiographic substances that are adjacent to each other will contrast each other (higher subject contrast). The heart, which is muscle as a water-based tissue, is positioned between the two lungs, which are gas. Water against gas will attenuate the x-ray beam differently, so subject contrast is increased. Bones of the leg are surrounded by muscle bundles, nerves, connective tissues, and blood vessels and because of the adjacent contact between bone and water-based tissues, the bony anatomy is well visualized. We cannot differentiate between the adjacent muscle fibers, nerves, blood vessels, and so on because they are all water-based and attenuate the x-ray beam similarly. Water against water displays very low subject contrast. This is because substances of similar radiographic opacities adjacent to each other will display decreased subject contrast.

Radiologists clearly understand this principle of radiographic opacities and image contrast and use it as a principle of radiographic image interpretation. They also understand that there are limitations to the visualization of anatomy that attenuate the x-ray beam similarly and use contrast medium such as iodine and barium to help visualize anatomical structures. For example, we know the heart has four internal chambers with valves as well as coronary arteries and veins on the surface of heart myocardium. These tissues are all water-based substances and adjacent to each other. With the injection of an iodine contrast medium into the heart and coronary arteries, the blood vessel and internal heart anatomy are better visualized during an angiographic heart study. Iodine (atomic number 53) is a mineral substance and attenuates (absorbs) the x-ray beam more than the adjacent water-based heart tissues, therefore increasing subject contrast. This same principle is true with the use of barium (atomic number 56) as a contrast medium when used to visualize the digestive system.

Adipose tissue (fat) is significant as a radiolucency, particularly with studies of extremities such as the elbow, ankle, knee, and wrist. Because of its low effective atomic number (6.3) and its contact with surrounding tissues, which are water based (7.4), the x-ray beam attenuation between water and adipose is evident, but more subtle. Visualizing changes in the adipose tissue surrounding extremities may indicate injury or pathology and is important to the radiologist (see Fig. 4.31).

In reviewing the radiographic images you create, practice identifying the five basic radiographic substances (Fig. 4.32). Optimizing image quality through proper exposure selection (as discussed in Chapter 7) is a key responsibility of radiographers for radiologists to interpret radiographic images accurately.

DYNAMIC IMAGING: FLUOROSCOPY

Fluoroscopy (Fig. 4.33) differs from static imaging by its use of a continuous beam of x-rays to create images of moving internal anatomic structures that can be viewed on a display monitor. Internal structures, such as the vascular or gastrointestinal systems, can be visualized in their normal state of motion with the aid of special liquid or gas substances (contrast media) that are either injected or instilled (i.e., ingested). The equipment used in fluoroscopy has undergone major changes over the past few years. Image-intensified fluoroscopy is being replaced with flat-panel detector fluoroscopy. Regardless of the type of fluoroscopic equipment, the x-ray tube is

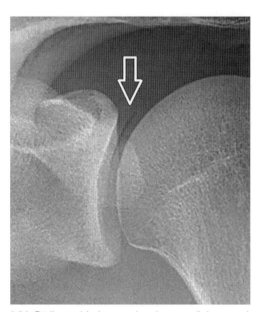

Fig. 4.31 Radiographic image showing a radiolucency in the shoulder joint following an injury. The gas transmits more x-rays than the surrounding soft tissues and therefore demonstrates higher contrast with the adjacent soft tissues. (From https://upload.wikimedia.org/wikipedia/commons/7/74/X-ray_of_shoulder_with_vacuum_sign_-_annotated.jpg.)

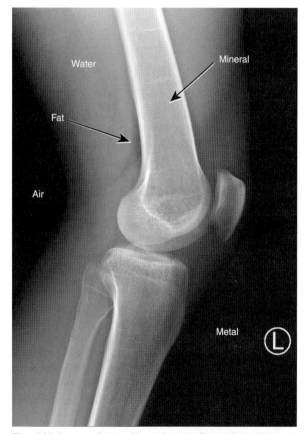

Fig. 4.32 Image of knee illustrating the five radiographic substances. (Netter, FH. Netter *Atlas of Human Anatomy: Classic Regional Approach*. 8th ed. St. Louis: Elsevier; 2023.)

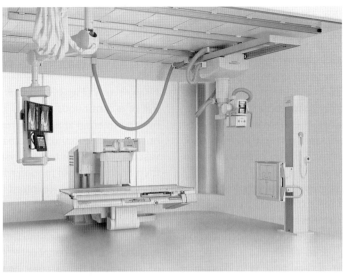

Fig. 4.33 Digital fluoroscopy using flat-panel detector technology. (Courtesy Siemens Healthcare, Malvern, PA.)

still the functional component of the equipment and may be positioned above or below the patient depending upon equipment design. The x-ray beam passes through the patient, and remnant x-ray energy strikes a solid-state, digital flat-panel detector. This x-ray energy is quickly converted to light and electrons as an analog signal and then to a digital signal data set. The data set is then processed at high speeds to yield a fluoroscopic image that displays patient anatomy and movement in real time to the observer.

 IMPORTANT RELATIONSHIP

Fluoroscopy

Dynamic imaging of internal anatomic structures can be visualized with the use of a flat-panel detector. The exit radiation interacts with the acquisition device, is processed, and is then transmitted to the display monitor for viewing.

Fluoroscopy is discussed in detail in Chapter 10.

Regardless of the type of imaging system (radiographic or fluoroscopic), the process of differential absorption for image formation remains the same. The varying x-ray intensities exiting the patient structurally represent the area of interest in the displayed image.

 IMPORTANT RELATIONSHIP

Image Formation

The process of differential absorption for image formation remains the same regardless of the type of imaging system, radiographic or fluoroscopic. The varying x-ray intensities exiting the patient structurally represent the area of interest in the displayed image.

CHAPTER SUMMARY

- A radiographic image is a result of the differential absorption of the primary x-rays that interact with tissues of varying composition within the anatomic area of interest.
- Beam attenuation occurs when the primary x-ray beam loses energy as it interacts with anatomic tissues.

- X-rays have the ability to eject electrons (ionization) from atoms within anatomic tissue.
- Three primary processes occur during x-ray interaction with anatomic tissues: absorption, scattering, and transmission.
- Total absorption of the incoming x-ray photon is a result of the photoelectric effect.

- Scattering of the incoming x-ray photon is a result of the Compton effect.
- Scatter radiation reaching the IR provides no useful information and creates unwanted exposure or fog on the radiographic image.
- The process of differential absorption remains the same for image formation regardless of the type of IR.
- A radiographic image is composed of varying brightness levels that structurally represent the anatomic area of interest.
- The visibility and accuracy of the recorded anatomic structural lines determine the overall quality of the radiographic image.
- Visibility of the anatomic structures is achieved by the proper balance of image brightness and contrast.
- Image contrast provides the ability to distinguish among the types of irradiated tissues.
- Grayscale is the number of different shades of gray that can be stored and displayed in a digital image.

- Spatial resolution refers to the accuracy of the anatomic structural lines displayed.
- Image sharpness is a function of geometric and temporal factors of image formation.
- Distortion describes the magnification or misrepresentation in shape of the anatomic structures.
- Scatter radiation produces unwanted exposure on the image, known as fog.
- Quantum noise is a result of too few photons reaching the IR and is a concern in digital imaging.
- An artifact is any unwanted brightness level on a radiographic image that does not accurately portray patient anatomy.
- The visualization of anatomic tissues is due to the physical relationship among five attenuating substances: gas, fat, water, mineral, and metal.
- Fluoroscopy differs from static imaging by its use of a continuous beam of x-rays to create images of moving internal structures (dynamic imaging) that can be viewed on a display monitor.

REVIEW QUESTIONS

1. The process whereby a radiographic image is created by variations in absorption and transmission of the exiting x-ray beam is known as _____.
   A. attenuation
   B. the photoelectric effect
   C. the Compton effect
   D. differential absorption

2. Which of the following processes occur during the x-ray beam interaction with tissue?
   A. Absorption and photon transmission
   B. Absorption and scattering
   C. Photon transmission and scattering
   D. Absorption, photon transmission, and scattering

3. The ability of an x-ray photon to remove an atom's electron is a characteristic known as _____.
   A. attenuation
   B. scattering
   C. ionization
   D. absorption

4. The x-ray interaction responsible for absorption is _____.
   A. differential
   B. photoelectric
   C. attenuation
   D. Compton

5. The x-ray interaction responsible for scattering is _____.
   A. differential
   B. photoelectric
   C. attenuation
   D. Compton

6. What interaction causes unwanted exposure to the image, known as fog?
   A. Compton
   B. Transmitted
   C. Photoelectric
   D. Absorption

7. Which of the following factors would affect beam attenuation?
   A. Tissue atomic number
   B. Beam quality
   C. Fog
   D. Tissue atomic number and beam quality

8. The high brightness areas on a displayed digital image are created by _____.
   A. transmitted radiation
   B. scattered radiation
   C. absorbed radiation
   D. primary radiation

9. An anatomic part that transmits the incoming x-ray photon with low absorption would create an area of _____ on the radiographic image.
   A. fog
   B. high brightness
   C. low brightness
   D. noise

10. The process of creating a radiographic image by differential absorption varies for fluoroscopy and static radiographic imaging.
   A. True
   B. False

11. Which attribute(s) of a radiographic image affect(s) the visibility of sharpness?
   A. Distortion
   B. Contrast
   C. Brightness
   D. B and C

12. A radiographic image with many shades of gray but few differences between them is said to have _____.
   A. high contrast
   B. low contrast
   C. saturation
   D. excessive noise

13. Which of the following is defined as the range of exposure intensities that an image receptor can accurately detect?
   A. Saturation
   B. Spatial resolution
   C. Quantum noise
   D. Dynamic range

14. Fluoroscopy uses a continuous beam of x-rays to create images of moving internal anatomic structures.
   A. True
   B. False

15. Which of the anatomic tissues below would not represent water as a radiographic substance?
   A. Liver
   B. Sternal sutures
   C. Abdominal aorta
   D. Kidney

16. Radiographic images that demonstrate motion distortion generally demonstrate poor _____.
   A. temporal resolution
   B. contrast resolution
   C. spatial resolution
   D. A and C

17. Anatomic substances are best visualized when they _____.
   A. transmit more x-rays.
   B. attenuate the x-rays differently from their adjacent tissues.
   C. create more quantum noise.
   D. attenuate the x-rays similarly from their adjacent tissues.

18. Which of the following substances absorb more of the x-ray beam?
   A. Muscle
   B. Fat
   C. Water
   D. Contrast medium

Digital Image Characteristics, Receptors, and Image Acquisition

CHAPTER OUTLINE

Digital Image Characteristics
Spatial Frequency and Spatial Resolution
Dynamic Range
Dose Monitoring
Modulation Transfer Function
Detective Quantum Efficiency

Signal-to-Noise Ratio
Contrast-to-Noise Ratio
Digital Image Receptors and Image Acquisition
Computed Radiography
Digital Radiography
Quality Control

OBJECTIVES

After completing this chapter, the reader will be able to perform the following:

1. Define all the key terms in this chapter.
2. State all the important relationships in this chapter.
3. Compare and contrast the attributes of a digital image.
4. Explain the digital characteristics of matrix and pixels.
5. Recognize the relationship among pixel size, display field of view, and matrix size.
6. State the relationship between spatial frequency and spatial resolution.
7. Explain the importance of dynamic range and exposure latitude in exposure technique selection, image quality, and patient exposure.
8. Define *modulation transfer function* and *detective quantum efficiency* and explain their relationship to digital image quality.

9. Define *signal-to-noise ratio* and explain its importance to digital image quality.
10. Define *contrast-to-noise ratio* and explain its importance to digital image quality.
11. Differentiate between computed radiography (CR) and digital radiography (DR) image receptors (IRs) in acquiring the image.
12. Explain the importance of sampling frequency in reproducing a quality digital image.
13. Describe how the size of a CR imaging plate can affect spatial resolution.
14. Recognize the differences between indirect and direct conversion digital IRs.
15. State the importance of proper DR handling and how it is prepared for x-ray exposure.
16. List quality control checks the radiographer can do to evaluate digital equipment performance.

KEY TERMS

air kerma
bit
bit depth
byte
cassette
charge-coupled device (CCD)
complementary metal oxide
    semiconductor (CMOS)

contrast-to-noise ratio (CNR)
CR fading
detective quantum efficiency
    (DQE)
detector elements (DELs)
dose area product (DAP)
dynamic range
exposure latitude

field of view (FOV)
fill factor
flat-panel detectors (FPDs)
grayscale
imaging plate (IP)
kerma area product (KAP)
luminescence
matrix

During radiographic imaging, the radiation exiting a patient (remnant radiation) is composed of a range of intensities that reflect the absorption and transmission characteristics of the anatomic tissues. The image receptor (IR) receives the exit radiation and creates the invisible raw image data. The raw image data are differently acquired depending on the type of IR. This chapter describes the digital image characteristics, common types of digital IRs used in radiography, and how the image is acquired.

DIGITAL IMAGE CHARACTERISTICS

In digital imaging, the raw image data are stored as an electronic data set and must be processed by a computer for viewing on a display monitor. Digital imaging can be accomplished using a specialized IR that can produce a computerized radiographic image. Two types of digital radiographic systems are in common use today: computed radiography (CR) and digital radiography (DR). Regardless of whether the imaging system is CR or DR, the computer can manipulate the radiographic image in various ways after the image has been digitally created.

Digital images are composed of electronic data that can be easily manipulated by a computer. When displayed on a computer monitor, there is tremendous flexibility in terms of altering the brightness and contrast of a digital image. The practical advantage of such capability is that regardless of the original exposure technique factors (within reason), any anatomic structure can be independently and well visualized. Computers can also perform various pre- and postprocessing image manipulations to further improve the visibility of the anatomic region.

A digital image is recorded as a matrix or combination of rows and columns (array) of small, usually square, "picture elements" called pixels. The size of a pixel is measured in microns (100 microns = 0.1 mm).

Each pixel is recorded as a single numerical value, which is represented as a single brightness and shade of gray on a display monitor. The location of the pixel within the image matrix corresponds to an area within the patient or volume of tissue (Fig. 5.1). This is known as the spatial domain of the data set. Each data point has an "address" and when reconstructed, the data point is placed in its precise spatial position, representing patient anatomy.

Given the dimensions of an anatomic area of interest, or exposure field of view (FOV), a matrix size of 1024 × 1024 has 1,048,576 individual pixels; a matrix size of 2048 × 2048 has 4,194,304 pixels. Digital image quality is improved with a larger matrix size that includes a greater number of smaller pixels (Fig. 5.2 and Box 5.1). Although image quality is improved for

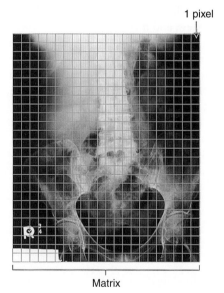

Fig. 5.1 Location of the pixel within the image matrix corresponds to an area within the patient or volume of tissue. Note: Pixel size is not to scale and is used for illustration only.

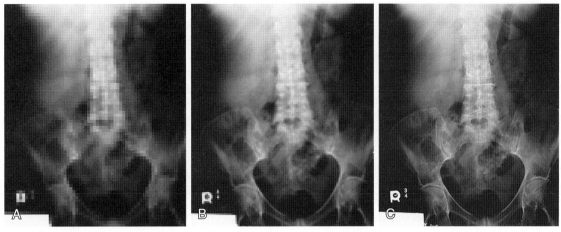

Fig. 5.2 For a given exposure field of view (FOV), the larger the matrix size, the greater the number of smaller individual pixels. Increasing the number of pixels improves the spatial resolution of the image. **A,** Matrix size is 64 × 64. **B,** Matrix size is 215 × 215. **C,** Matrix size is 2048 × 2048.

BOX 5.1 Digital Imaging Terminology

Matrix—image displayed as a combination of rows and columns (array); a larger matrix size improves spatial resolution for a given exposure field of view (FOV).

Pixel—smallest component of the matrix; a greater number of smaller pixels improves spatial resolution.

Pixel bit depth—number of bits that determines the precision with which the exit radiation is recorded and controls the exact pixel brightness that can be displayed.

---

a larger matrix size and smaller pixels, computer processing time, network transmission time, and digital storage space increase as the matrix size increases.

There is a relationship among pixel size, displayed FOV (the dimensions of an anatomic area displayed on the computer monitor), and matrix size, as demonstrated in the following formula:

$$\text{Pixel size} = \frac{\text{FOV}}{\text{Matrix size}}$$

This relationship demonstrates that if the FOV displayed on the monitor is increased for a fixed matrix size, then the pixel size is also increased (direct relationship). However, if the matrix size is increased for a fixed FOV, then the pixel size is decreased (inverse relationship).

▶▶ MATHEMATICAL APPLICATION

Pixel Size and Displayed FOV

FOV = 17 inches (431.8 mm) and matrix size = 1024:

$$\frac{431.8}{1024} = 0.42 \text{ mm pixel size}$$

If the FOV displayed was decreased to 12 inches (304.8 mm) for the same matrix size of 1024:

$$\frac{304.8}{1024} = 0.30 \text{ mm pixel size}$$

Decreasing the FOV displayed for a given matrix size will decrease the size of the pixels and increase spatial resolution.

▶▶ MATHEMATICAL APPLICATION

Pixel Size and Matrix Size

Displayed FOV = 17 inches (431.8 mm) and matrix size = 1024:

$$\frac{431.8}{1024} = 0.42 \text{ mm pixel size}$$

If the matrix size was increased to 2048 for the same FOV displayed:

$$\frac{431.8}{2048} = 0.21 \text{ mm pixel size}$$

Increasing the matrix size for a given FOV displayed will decrease the size of the pixels and increase spatial resolution.

IMPORTANT RELATIONSHIP

Pixel Size, Displayed FOV, and Matrix Size

The pixel size is directly related to the FOV displayed and inversely related to the matrix size. Increasing the FOV displayed for the same matrix size will increase the size of the pixel and decrease spatial resolution, whereas increasing the matrix size for the same FOV displayed will decrease the pixel size and increase spatial resolution.

The numerical value assigned to each pixel is determined by the relative attenuation of x-rays passing through the corresponding volume of tissue. Pixels representing highly attenuating tissues (increased absorption) such as bone are assigned a different numerical value for higher brightness than pixels representing tissues of low x-ray attenuation (decreased absorption) (Fig. 5.3). Each pixel also has a bit depth, or number of bits (Box 5.2), that determines the amount of precision in digitizing the analog signal and therefore the number of shades of gray that can be displayed in the image. Bit depth is determined by an analog-to-digital converter (ADC), which is an

integral component of every digital imaging system. Because the binary system is used, bit depth is expressed as 2 to the power of n, or the number of bits (2^n). A larger bit depth allows a greater number of shades of gray to be displayed on a computer monitor. For example, a 12-bit depth (2^{12}) can display 4096 shades of gray, a 14-bit depth can display 16,384 shades of gray, and a 16-bit depth can display 65,536 shades of gray. A system that can digitize

BOX 5.2 Binary Digits

Computers operate and communicate through the binary number system, which uses combinations of zeros and ones to process and store information. A digital transistor can be operated in two states: off (0) or on (1). Each 0 and 1 is called a **bit** and refers to the computer's basic unit of information. When 8 bits are combined, they form a **byte**, and 2 bytes form a word.

Binary digits are used to display the brightness level (grayscale) of a digital image. The greater the number of bits, the greater the number of shades of gray that can be displayed, and the quality of the image is improved.

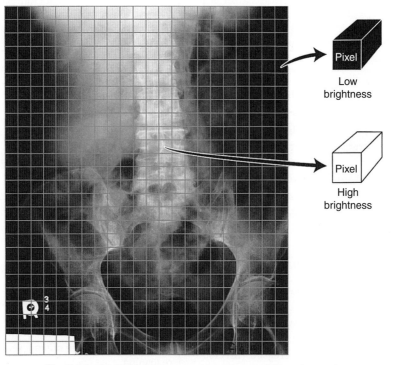

Fig. 5.3 Each pixel value represents a volume of tissue imaged.

and display a greater number of shades of gray has better *contrast resolution*. An image with increased contrast resolution increases the visibility of anatomic details and the ability to distinguish among small anatomic areas of interest (Fig. 5.4).

⚡ IMPORTANT RELATIONSHIP

Pixel Bit Depth and Contrast Resolution

The greater the pixel bit depth (i.e., 16-bit), the more precise the digitization of the analog signal and the greater the number of shades of gray available for image display. Increasing the number of shades of gray available to display in a digital image improves its contrast resolution.

A digital image is composed of discrete information in the form of pixels that display various shades of gray. As previously mentioned, the greater the number of pixels in an image matrix, the smaller is their size. An image consisting of a greater number of pixels per unit area, or pixel density, provides improved spatial resolution. In addition to its size, the pixel spacing, or the distance measured from the center of a pixel to an adjacent pixel, determines the pixel pitch (Fig. 5.5). Smaller-sized pixels have decreased pixel pitch and improved spatial resolution.

⚡ IMPORTANT RELATIONSHIP

Pixel Density and Pitch and Spatial Resolution

Increasing pixel density and decreasing pixel pitch increases spatial resolution. Decreasing pixel density and increasing pixel pitch decreases spatial resolution.

Spatial Frequency and Spatial Resolution

Spatial resolution in digital imaging is primarily limited to the size of the pixel displayed; however, when measuring an imaging system's ability to resolve small objects, it is important to understand the concept of spatial frequency and its relationship with spatial resolution. Spatial frequency can be defined by the unit of line pairs per millimeter (lp/mm). A resolution test pattern is a device used to record and measure line pairs (Fig. 5.6). Anatomic details are composed of large and small objects, and radiographic images display these details as variations from white to black brightness levels. Small objects have higher spatial frequency, and large objects have lower spatial frequency. It is more difficult to accurately image small anatomic objects

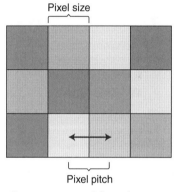

Fig. 5.5 The distance measured from the center of a pixel to an adjacent pixel determines the pixel pitch or spacing. (From Johnston JN, Fauber TL. *Essentials of Radiographic Physics and Imaging.* 3rd ed. St. Louis: Elsevier; 2020.)

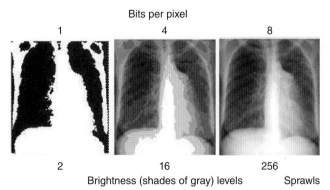

Fig. 5.4 Pixel bit depth determines the shades of gray displayed on the monitor. The greater the bit depth a digital system can display, the greater is the contrast resolution displayed in the image. (From Sprawls P. *The Physical Principles of Medical Imaging Online,* 2nd ed. http://www.sprawls.org/ppmi2.)

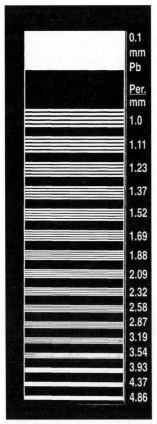

Fig. 5.6 A resolution test pattern will record and measure line pairs per millimeter. (Courtesy Fluke Biomedical.)

(high spatial frequency) than to image large ones (low spatial frequency). An imaging system that can resolve a greater number of lp/mm (higher spatial frequency) has increased spatial resolution (Fig. 5.7). In digital imaging systems, the ability to resolve or demonstrate a specific spatial frequency is directly impacted by the size of the pixel. The images of the wrist (Fig. 5.8) demonstrate the impact that pixel size has on the spatial resolution visualized in an image.

⚡ IMPORTANT RELATIONSHIP
Spatial Frequency and Spatial Resolution

The unit of measure for spatial frequency is lp/mm. Increasing the number of lp/mm resolved by the imaging system (higher spatial frequency) results in improved spatial resolution.

Dynamic Range

The dynamic range of an imaging system refers to the ability of an IR to accurately capture the range of photon intensities that exit the patient. Digital IRs have a wide dynamic range (Fig. 5.9). In practical terms, this wide dynamic range means that a small degree of underexposure or overexposure would still result in diagnostic image quality. This characteristic of digital receptors is advantageous in situations where automatic exposure

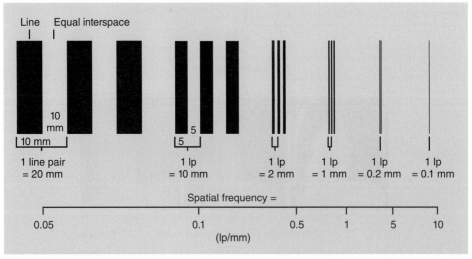

Fig. 5.7 A line pair is a high-contrast line separated by an interspace of equal width. The spatial frequency is shown for each of the line pairs. (From Bushong SC. *Radiologic Science for Technologists*. 10th ed. St. Louis: Mosby; 2013.)

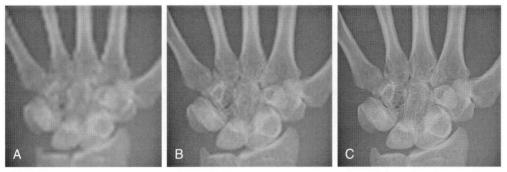

Fig. 5.8 Images showing how pixel size affects spatial resolution. **A,** Image with 20 pixels/cm; therefore the pixel size is larger, and the spatial resolution is poor. **B,** Image with 40 pixels/cm. **C,** Image with 100 pixels/cm; therefore the pixel size is smaller than in images **A** and **B,** and the spatial resolution is improved. (Courtesy Andrew Woodward.)

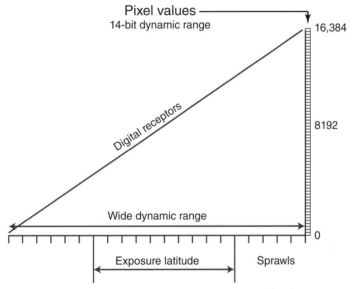

Fig. 5.9 The dynamic range of an imaging system refers to the ability of an image receptor to accurately capture the range of photon intensities exiting the patient. Exposure latitude is the range of exposure intensities that produce a diagnostic image without under- or overexposure. (Modified from Sprawls P. *Physical Principles of Medical Imaging Online*. http://www.sprawls.org/resources.)

control (AEC) may not be available, such as in mobile radiography. However, radiographers must make considerable effort to select exposure techniques that produce diagnostic images without insufficient or excessive exposure to the IR. Although digital receptors have a wide dynamic range, exposure latitude refers to the range of exposures that should be used to produce a diagnostic image (see Fig. 5.9) and is likely established by the preferences or needs of the imaging department.

During digitization of the image, a numerical value is assigned to the pixel that represents an x-ray intensity based on the attenuation characteristics of that volume of tissue. Equipment with a larger pixel bit depth means the image displayed has a wide grayscale, and this illustrates the wide dynamic range of the digital receptor. As noted in Fig. 5.9, the digital IR can accurately capture more than 16,000 x-ray intensities exiting the patient. To display that range of brightness levels (grayscale), the pixel bit depth is 14. If the digital IR can capture over 65,000 x-ray intensities exiting the patient, the bit depth would be 16, and contrast resolution is improved compared with the 14-bit digital system.

Processing the digital data yields a radiographic image that can be viewed on a display monitor and altered in various ways. Even if optimal exposure techniques are not used, the image rescaling that occurs during the processing stage can produce images with the appropriate brightness levels. Digital image processing and display are discussed in detail in Chapter 6.

The ability of the IR to capture a wide range of exit photon intensities does not mean a quality image is always created. Although lower-than-necessary x-ray exposures can be detected and processed, image quality suffers because there is insufficient exposure to the IR, and quantum noise results. The computer can process the data resulting from an IR exposed to higher-than-necessary radiation and produce a quality image but at the expense of patient overexposure. It is the responsibility of the radiographer to select the amount of exposure necessary to produce a diagnostic digital image (exposure latitude).

 IMPORTANT RELATIONSHIP

Digital Receptors, Dynamic Range, and Exposure Latitude

Digital IRs have a wide dynamic range, that is, they can accurately capture a wide range of x-ray intensities exiting the patient. The computer then processes the raw pixel data to compensate for an exposure error and create a diagnostic radiographic image. However, lower- or higher-than-necessary exposure techniques do not guarantee a quality digital image. Exposure latitude is the range of exposures that should be used to produce a diagnostic image.

❗ RADIATION PROTECTION ALERT

Digital Receptors and Dynamic Range

Because digital IRs have a wide dynamic range, a quality image can be produced when using more radiation exposure than necessary. Radiographers must take extra precautions to not unnecessarily overexpose patients and select exposure techniques within the exposure latitude established by the department.

Dose Monitoring

Air kerma (kinetic energy released in matter) specifies the intensity of x-rays at a given point in air at a known distance from the focal spot or source of x-rays. DR systems use dose area product (DAP) as an indicator of exposure. DAP is a measure of exposure in air, followed by computation to estimate the absorbed dose to the patient. It is measured by a DAP meter embedded in the collimator. The DAP value depends on the exposure factors and field size and reflects both the dose to the patient and the total volume of tissue being irradiated. Kerma area product (KAP) is the same as DAP and is the product of the total air kerma and the area of the x-ray beam at the entrance of the patient. Units of DAP or KAP are expressed in micro, milli, or centigray per area squared but can vary by manufacturer. DAP and KAP provide indicators of patient radiation risk and may be documented in the patient's record.

Modulation Transfer Function

As previously stated, a radiographic image displays a range of brightness levels (grayscale) based on the variation in radiation intensities exiting the tissue. Anatomic detail is best visualized when the brightness level of the object is different than its surrounding tissue (high contrast). Larger-sized objects (low spatial frequency) are more easily visualized. As the size of the object decreases, it attains higher spatial frequency and becomes more difficult to visualize in a radiographic image. Modulation transfer function (MTF) is a measure of the imaging system's ability to display the contrast and spatial resolution of anatomic objects varying in size, and the value will be between 0 (no difference in brightness levels) and 1.0 (maximum difference in brightness levels).

The goal of any recording system, including radiography, is to create a copy of the original with as much accurate detail as possible. Modulation transfer function (MTF) is a method for numerically expressing a recording system's ability to exactly copy an original. This concept came from the recording industry many years ago as the intent was to produce a vinyl record of a performer's voice with as much truthful fidelity as possible. In doing so, the recording created a sound as good as if the listener were standing next to the performer and hearing the music live, with no disturbances. When this was achieved, the recording was equal to the live voice and a number of 1 was assigned to this MTF assessment. This same measure has been adopted by other industries such as telephones and paper copiers.

MIND IMAGE

Creating a Copy

When you make a paper copy of a document using a copier, you want a copy that is as close as possible to the original. As a copying system, everything must work exactly as designed by the copier engineers. The closer the copy is to the original document, the higher its quality. The same can be said for producing a medical image of a patient. It is an imaging system.

MTF is a numerical expression of a recording system to recreate an image with optimum contrast and spatial resolution. An MTF of 1 (100%) would signify the image of an object that exactly represents its features in terms of contrast and spatial resolution. An MTF of 1 is easier to achieve with large objects having a low spatial frequency. It is more difficult to visualize smaller objects having high spatial frequency, and therefore most digital imaging systems' MTFs measure lower than 1.0. MTF of a system is assessed and quantified using test instruments that measure spatial and contrast resolution.

IMPORTANT RELATIONSHIP

Modulation Transfer Function and Anatomic Detail

MTF is a measure of the imaging system's ability to accurately display small anatomic objects having a high spatial frequency. An imaging system that has a high MTF can display anatomic detail with improved visibility.

Detective Quantum Efficiency

Detective quantum efficiency (DQE) is a measurement of the efficiency of an IR in converting the x-ray exposure into a usable electronic signal that can be converted to a quality radiographic image. If an IR system can convert x-ray exposure into a quality image with 100% efficiency (meaning no information loss), the DQE would measure 100% or 1.0. However, no imaging system has 100% conversion efficiency. Nevertheless, the higher the DQE of a system, the lower the radiation exposure required to produce a quality image, thereby decreasing patient exposure. The system's DQE value is impacted by the type of material used in the IR to capture the exit radiation (e.g., DQE is higher for DR compared with CR IRs) and the energy of the x-ray beam (e.g., DQE is higher for

amorphous selenium [a-Se] receptors at higher kilovoltage peak levels compared with amorphous silicon that uses cesium iodide [CsI] as a scintillator). The DQE is also impacted by spatial frequency and MTF. Some conversion efficiency is lost when imaging at higher spatial frequencies; therefore DQE is directly proportional to the MTF of the detector.

IMPORTANT RELATIONSHIP

Detective Quantum Efficiency and X-ray Exposure

An IR with a higher DQE requires less x-ray exposure to produce a quality radiographic image when compared to an IR with a lower DQE value.

Signal-to-Noise Ratio

Signal-to-noise ratio (SNR) is a method of describing the strength of the radiation exposure compared with the amount of noise apparent in a digital image. Noise is a concern with any electronic data set, in this case, digital image noise. Because the photon intensities are converted to an electronic signal that is digitized by the ADC, the term *signal* refers to the strength or amount of radiation exposure captured by the IR to create the image. The varying x-ray intensities exiting the patient are converted to varying signal strengths. Increasing the SNR improves the quality of the digital image; this means that the strength of the signal is high in comparison with the amount of noise, and therefore image quality is improved. Decreasing the SNR means that there is increased noise compared with the strength of the signal, and therefore the quality of the radiographic image is degraded. *Quantum noise* results when there are too few x-ray photons captured by the IR to create the raw image data. In addition to quantum noise, sources of noise include the electronics that capture, process, and display the digital image. Manufacturers have designed circuit components to minimize this type of electronic noise.

The ability to visualize anatomic tissues is affected by the SNR. Noise interferes with the signal strength just as background static would interfere with the clarity of music heard. When the digital image displays increased noise, regardless of the source, anatomic details have decreased visibility.

IMPORTANT RELATIONSHIP

Signal-to-Noise Ratio and Image Quality

Increasing the SNR increases the visibility of anatomic details, whereas decreasing the SNR decreases the visibility due to the presence of objectionable noise.

 IMPORTANT RELATIONSHIP

Contrast-to-Noise Ratio and Image Quality

Increasing the CNR increases the visibility of anatomic details, whereas decreasing the CNR decreases the visibility.

Contrast-to-Noise Ratio

Contrast-to-noise ratio (CNR) is a method of describing the contrast resolution compared with the amount of noise apparent in a digital image. Just as increased noise affects the SNR and visibility of the anatomic details, it also impacts the contrast displayed within the digital image. Brightness or signal differences in the digital image are a result of varying exit radiation intensities from the attenuation of the x-ray beam in anatomic tissue (differential absorption). As previously stated, digital imaging systems have high-contrast resolution. A system with higher-contrast resolution means that anatomic tissues that attenuate the x-ray beam similarly (low subject contrast) can be better visualized. However, if the image has increased noise, the low subject contrast tissues will not be as well visualized. Digital images with a higher CNR increase the visibility of anatomic tissues (Fig. 5.10).

Different types of digital IRs use various methods of transforming the continuous exit radiation intensities into the array of discrete pixel values for image display. Some image receptor systems, such as CR, use a sampling technique whereas digital detectors have fixed detector elements (DELs) in an array that are used to capture the remnant radiation intensities.

Regardless of the type used, a major determinant of spatial resolution of digital images is sampling frequency, pixel size, DEL size, and pixel spacing.

DIGITAL IMAGE RECEPTORS AND IMAGE ACQUISITION

Two types of digital IRs are typically used in radiography: CR and DR. These IRs differ in their construction and how they acquire raw image data. After the raw image data are acquired and digitized, image processing

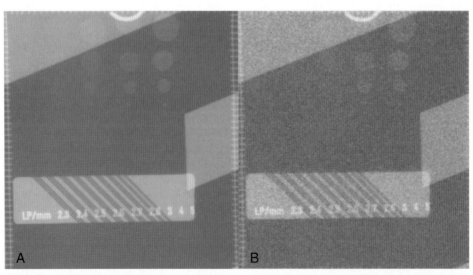

Fig. 5.10 Contrast-to-noise ratio (CNR). **A,** Image of a contrast detail phantom showing an increased CNR. Phantom objects are more visible. **B,** Image of contrast detail phantom showing a decreased CNR. Phantom objects are less visible. (Courtesy Andrew Woodward.)

and display are essentially the same, regardless of the type of IR.

Computed Radiography

CR IRs come in many sizes and can be portable and used in a table or upright x-ray unit or fixed in a dedicated chest unit. The CR IR includes a cassette that houses the imaging plate (IP) (Fig. 5.11). There is no x-ray generator connection with the CR cassette which permits them to be used with all x-ray equipment manufacturers. The radiation exiting the patient interacts with the IP, where the photon intensities are absorbed by the phosphor layer of the IP. Although some of the absorbed energy is released as visible light (luminescence), a sufficient amount of energy is stored in the phosphor to produce an invisible raw image. Luminescence is the emission of light when stimulated by radiation.

The IP consists of supporting and protective layers with the phosphor, reflective, and conductive layers sandwiched in between (Fig. 5.12). The phosphor layer is composed of barium fluorohalide crystals doped with europium, referred to as the photostimulable phosphor (PSP). This type of phosphor emits visible light

when stimulated by a high-intensity laser beam, a phenomenon termed photostimulable luminescence. CR is often referred to as storage phosphor technology since the photon energy is stored in atomic band gaps in the barium fluorohalide atomic structure.

The phosphor (active layer) may be either a turbid or structured phosphor layer. A turbid phosphor has a random distribution of phosphor crystals within the active layer and can be used with both CR and DR IRs (Fig. 5.13). A structured phosphor layer has columnar phosphor crystals within the active layer resembling needles standing on end and packed together (Fig. 5.14). The reflective layer reflects light released during the reading phase toward the photodetector. The conductive layer reduces and conducts away static electricity. The support layer is a sturdy material

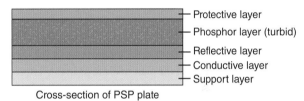

Cross-section of PSP plate

Fig. 5.12 Cross-section of a computed radiography (CR) photostimulable phosphor *(PSP)* plate. (From Johnston JN, Fauber TL. *Essentials of Radiographic Physics and Imaging.* 3rd ed. St. Louis: Elsevier; 2020.)

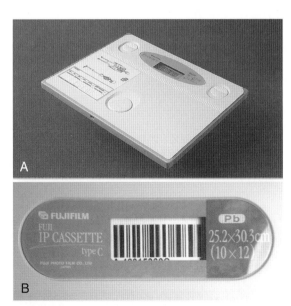

Fig. 5.11 Computed radiography (CR) image receptor. **A,** The imaging plate is housed within the cassette. **B,** CR cassette showing the barcode label to match with patient information. (From Frank, E, Long, B, Ehrlich, RA. *Radiography Essentials for Limited Practice.* 6th ed. St. Louis: Elsevier Inc.; 2021.)

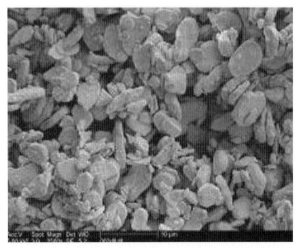

Fig. 5.13 A turbid-type phosphor layer. (From Leblans P, Vandenbroucke D, Willems P. Storage phosphors for medical imaging. *Materials.* 2011;4(6):1034-1086. https://doi.org/10.3390/ma4061034.)

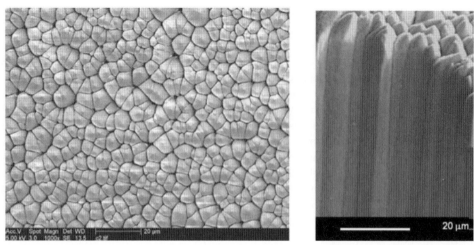

Fig. 5.14 A structured phosphor layer with columnar phosphor crystals. (From Leblans P, Vandenbroucke D, Willems P. Storage phosphors for medical imaging. *Materials.* 2011;4(6):1034-1086. https://doi.org/10.3390/ma4061034.)

to give some rigidity to the plate. Finally, the soft backing layer protects the back of the plate and assists in preventing backscatter (x-rays scattered back from the plate) from *fogging* the phosphor layer during exposure.

CR imaging requires a two-step process for image acquisition: image capture in the IP and image readout. The raw image data are formed in the PSP when the exit x-ray intensities are absorbed by the phosphor and the europium atoms become ionized by the photoelectric effect. The absorbed energy excites the electrons, elevating them to a higher-energy state, where they become stored or trapped in the conduction band (Fig. 5.15). The conduction band is an energy level just beyond the valence band (outermost energy band of an atom). The number and distribution of these trapped electrons (which form the raw image data) are proportional to the exit exposure intensity as a result of the tissue's differential x-ray absorption. Some of these excited electrons immediately return to their normal state, and the excess energy is released as visible light. A percentage of electrons remain in this higher-energy state until released during laser beam scanning of the readout stage. The acquired raw image data (released energy) are extracted from the IP phosphor layer, converted to digital data, and computer processed for image display. Exposed IPs should be processed within a relatively short amount of time (within 1 hour) because the raw image data dissipate over time (CR fading). CR fading occurs because some of the signal (released energy) captured in the

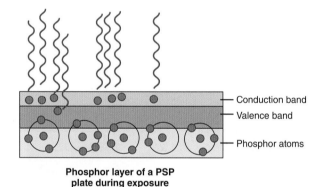

Phosphor layer of a PSP plate during exposure

Fig. 5.15 During exposure of the photostimulable phosphor *(PSP)* layer, the higher-energy electrons will become trapped in the conduction band. A percentage of the higher-energy electrons will return to their normal state and release the excess energy as visible light. (From Johnston JN, Fauber TL. *Essentials of Radiographic Physics and Imaging.* 3rd ed. St. Louis: Mosby; 2020.)

IP is lost. Nearly 25% of the stored energy in the CR PSP is lost after 8 hours so image processing in the CR reader should take place in a reasonable time frame after exposure.

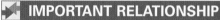 **IMPORTANT RELATIONSHIP**

Computed Radiography Image Receptors

The CR raw image data are acquired in the PSP layer of the IP. Most energy from the exit radiation intensities is stored in the PSP for extraction in the reader unit.

The exposed IP is placed in or sent to a reader unit that converts the analog data into the electronic data set for computer processing (Fig. 5.16). Reader units are available in single- or multiplate configurations. The major components of a typical reader unit are a drive mechanism to move the IP through the scanning process; an optical system, which includes the laser, beam-shaping optics, collecting optics, and optical filters; a photodetector, such as a photomultiplier tube (PMT); and an ADC. Manufacturers differ in the CR reader mechanics. Some devices move the IP, and some move the optical components. There are three important stages in digitizing the CR raw data: scanning, sampling, and quantization.

The purpose of scanning is to convert the raw image data (released energy) into an electrical signal (voltage) that can be subsequently digitized and displayed as a visible digital image. Once in the reader unit, the IP is removed from the cassette and scanned with a helium-neon laser beam or a solid-state laser diode to release the stored energy as visible light (Fig. 5.17). Absorption of the laser beam energy releases the trapped electrons,

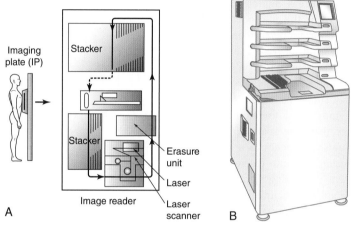

Fig. 5.16 Computed radiography (CR) reader unit. **A,** The exposed CR imaging plate *(IP)* is placed in a reader unit to release the stored raw image data and convert the analog image to an electronic data set. The reader unit also erases the exposed IP in preparation for the next exposure. **B,** Illustration of typical multi-plate reader unit.

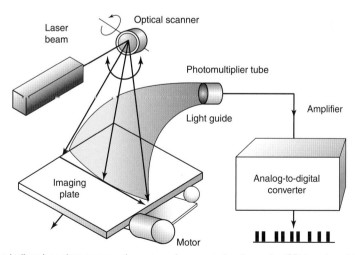

Fig. 5.17 A neon-helium laser beam scans the exposed computed radiography (CR) imaging plate (IP) to release the stored energy as visible light. The photomultiplier tube collects, amplifies, and converts the light to an electrical signal. The analog-to-digital converter converts the analog data to digital data. (Courtesy Fujifilm Medical Systems, Stamford, CT.)

and they return to a lower-energy state. During this process, the excess energy is emitted as visible light (photostimulable luminescence). The scanning of the plate results in a continuous pattern of light intensities being sent to the PMT or photodetector, whose output is directed to the ADC for sampling and quantization.

A photodetector collects, amplifies, and converts the visible light to an electrical signal proportional to the range of energies stored in the IP. The collected electronic signal values are of low voltage and therefore need to be amplified by the photodetector to travel to the ADC. The signal output from the photodetector is digitized by an ADC to produce a digital image. To digitize the analog signal from the photodetector, it must first be sampled. An important performance characteristic of an ADC is the sampling frequency, which determines how often the analog signal is reproduced in its discrete digitized form (Fig. 5.18).

As mentioned previously, small anatomic details have higher spatial frequency and would therefore need a higher sampling frequency than low spatial frequency anatomic details. The Nyquist frequency is a standard formula for converting analog data into discreet digital units to accurately represent the analog signal or electronic data in digital radiography. To accurately reproduce an image from the continuous analog signal, the sampling rate must be at least two times the highest spatial frequency in the exit x-ray intensities (signal). If the sampling frequency is too low, an improper waveform (aliasing) may result, which is considered an image artifact and reduces the visibility of small anatomic details (Fig. 5.19).

Increasing the sampling frequency of the analog signal increases the pixel density of the electronic data and improves the spatial resolution of the digital image. The closer the samples are to each other (increased sampling frequency), the smaller the sampling pitch, or distance

between the sampling points (Fig. 5.20). Increasing the sampling frequency decreases the sampling pitch and results in smaller-sized pixels. The distance between the midpoint of one pixel to the midpoint of an adjacent pixel describes the pixel pitch. Spatial resolution is improved with an increased number of smaller pixels, resulting in a more faithful digital representation of the acquired analog image.

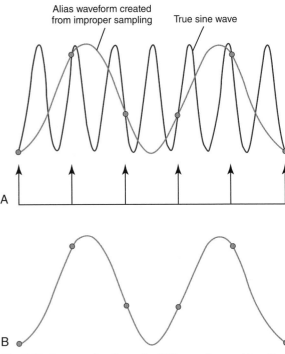

Fig. 5.19 Computed radiography (CR) sampling and its effect on the digital data. **A,** The sampling points of the analog waveform. **B,** The improper digital waveform *(alias)* that results from low sampling frequency.

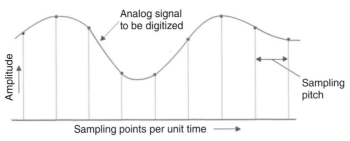

Fig. 5.18 The sampling frequency determines the distance between the midpoint of one sampling point and the midpoint of an adjacent sampling point.

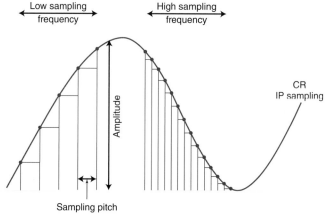

Fig. 5.20 Computed radiography *(CR)* sampling frequency and sampling pitch. *IP,* Imaging plate. (Courtesy Richard Sanders).

 IMPORTANT RELATIONSHIP

Sampling Frequency and Spatial Resolution

Increasing the sampling frequency results in more sampling points and decreased sampling pitch, which improves the spatial resolution of the digital image. Decreasing the sampling frequency results in fewer sampling points and increased sampling pitch and decreased spatial resolution.

 IMPORTANT RELATIONSHIP

Image Receptor Size and Matrix Size

For a fixed matrix size CR system, using a smaller IR for a given exposure FOV results in improved spatial resolution of the digital image. Increasing the size of the IR for a given exposure FOV results in decreased spatial resolution.

Manufacturers of CR equipment vary in the method of sampling IPs of different sizes. Some manufacturers fix the sampling frequency to maintain a fixed spatial resolution, whereas others vary the sampling frequency to maintain a fixed matrix size. If the spatial resolution is fixed, the image matrix size is simply proportional to the IP size. A larger IP has a larger matrix to maintain spatial resolution (Fig. 5.21). If the matrix size is fixed, changing the size of the IP would affect the spatial resolution of the digital image. For example, under a fixed matrix size system, changing from a 35 × 43-cm (14 × 17-inch) IR size to a 25 × 30-cm (10 × 12-inch) IR would result in improved spatial resolution for the same exposure FOV (Fig. 5.22). Spatial resolution is improved because to maintain the same matrix size and number of pixels, the pixels must be smaller in size. It is recommended to use the smallest IR size reasonable for the anatomic area of interest.

Another important ADC performance characteristic is the degree of quantization or pixel bit depth, which controls the number of gray shades or contrast resolution

of the image. During the process of quantization, each pixel, representing a brightness value, is assigned a numerical value. Quantization reflects the precision with which each sampled point is recorded. As previously discussed, the pixel size and pitch determine the spatial resolution, and the pixel bit depth determines the system's ability to display a range of shades of gray to represent anatomic tissues. Pixel bit depth is fixed by the choice of ADC, and CR systems manufactured with a greater pixel bit depth (i.e., 16-bit [in which 2^{16} bits can display 65,536 shades of gray]) improve the contrast resolution of the digital image.

Before the IP is returned to service, the plate is exposed to an intense white light to release any residual energy that could affect future exposures. PSPs can be reused and are estimated to have a life of 10,000 readings before requiring replacement. Advancements in PSP material, laser beam technology, and dual-sided IP scanning will continue to improve the process of CR image acquisition. CR has provided an excellent transitional technology as medical imaging strives toward digital radiography (DR).

FIXED SAMPLING FREQUENCY

Large matrix

Small matrix

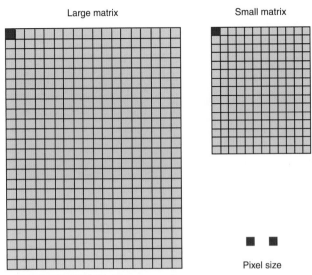

Pixel size

Fig. 5.21 Fixed sampling frequency. A fixed sampling frequency will maintain a fixed spatial resolution. A larger imaging plate (IP) size will have a larger matrix to maintain the same pixel size. Note: Pixel size is not to scale and is used for illustration only.

FIXED MATRIX SIZE

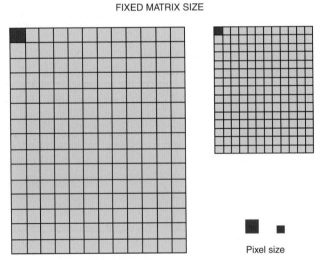

Pixel size

Fig. 5.22 Fixed matrix size. A fixed matrix size will vary the sampling frequency for a different imaging plate (IP) size. A larger IP size results in a larger pixel size and decreased spatial resolution. Note: Pixel size is not to scale and is used for illustration only.

Digital Radiography

DR IRs have a self-scanning readout mechanism that uses an array of x-ray detectors that receive the exit radiation and convert the varying x-ray intensities into proportional electronic signals for digitization (Fig. 5.23). In contrast to CR, which requires a two-step image acquisition process and results in a longer delay between image capture and image readout, DR imaging combines the two processes. As a result, DR images are available almost instantly after exposure. However, DR receptors are more fragile and much more expensive than CR IRs. Several types of electronic detectors are available for DR.

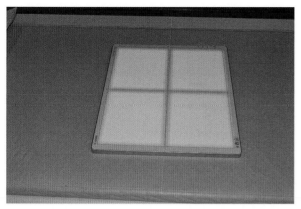

Fig. 5.23 Digital radiography (DR) detector (panel) with x-ray light field illuminating the exposure area. (Courtesy Randy Griswold).

Flat-Panel Detectors

Flat-panel detectors (FPDs) are solid-state IRs that use a large-area active matrix array of electronic components ranging in size from 43 × 35 to 43 × 43 cm (17 × 14 to 17 × 17 inches). FPDs are constructed with layers to receive x-ray photons and convert them to electrical charges for storage and readout (Fig. 5.24). Signal storage, signal readout, and digitizing electronics are integrated into the flat-panel device. The top layer is composed of an x-ray converter, the second layer houses the thin-film transistor

(TFT) array, and the third layer is a glass substrate. The TFT array is divided into square detector elements (DELs), each having a capacitor to store electrical charges and a switching transistor for readout. Electrical charges are separately read out from each DEL. The electronic signal is then sent to the ADC for digitization.

Each DEL is essentially a charge-collection device with a fixed dimension, expressed in microns, and is the functional unit of the detector as far as signal collection. DEL sizes can range among manufacturers and as the DEL size gets smaller, spatial resolution increases. DEL sizes currently range from 200 microns to as small as 60 microns (100 microns = 0.1 mm). Spatial resolution is expressed in line pairs per mm (lp/mm) and can vary based on the DEL size. For example, a DEL size of 125 microns yields 4.0 lp/mm in expected spatial resolution, whereas a DEL size of 75 microns yields 6.7 lp/mm in expected spatial resolution

Advancements in DEL technology have incorporated the ADC within the DEL. Digitizing the electronic signal within the DEL creates a more accurate signal. Having the analog electronic signal digitized before it leaves the DEL reduces its susceptibility to external disturbances. That is, the digital signal is not impacted by extraneous energy such as magnetic or radiofrequency (R/F) disturbances in the surroundings. These energy disturbances can distort the original signal values.

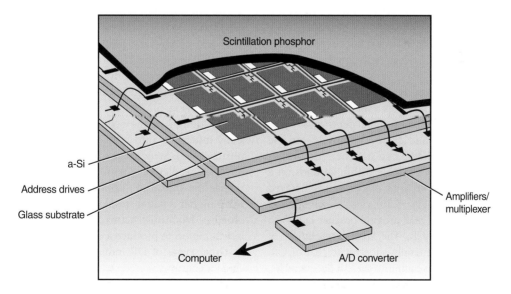

Fig. 5.24 Flat-panel detector (FPD) array. *A/D,* Analog-to-digital; *a-Si,* amorphous silicon. (From Johnston JN, Fauber TL. *Essentials of Radiographic Physics and Imaging.* 3rd ed. St. Louis: Mosby; 2020.)

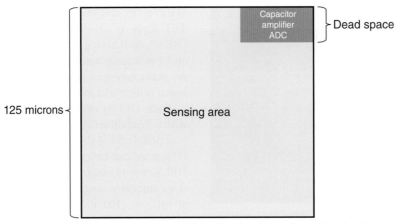

Fig. 5.25 Simple diagram of a detector element (DEL) with 125-micron dimension showing x-ray sensitive (sensing) area. *ADC,* Analog-to-digital converter. (Courtesy Randy Griswold).

The DEL has an x-ray-sensitive (sensing) area representing each pixel in the image matrix (Fig. 5.25). The pixel is therefore smaller than the DEL and can only capture a percentage of the x-rays reaching the detector. This percentage of x-ray capture (~80%–95%) is known as the fill factor. Although FPDs with smaller DELs have smaller pixel sizes represented on the visible image and therefore improved spatial resolution, the fill factor is decreased and becomes a limitation. Efforts to further decrease the size of the DEL for improved spatial resolution would require more radiation exposure to reach the IR to create the digital image. However, advancements in FPD technology, such as increasing the fill factor to more than 95% and improved detector materials, generally require less radiation exposure for optimum image quality.

The detector system can be integrated into a radiographic table or upright unit or as a stand-alone cassette, referred to as a panel. Flat-panel digital detectors are also available as mobile IRs and can be removed from the table and used on the tabletop or a stretcher. After exposure, the digital image is available within seconds on a viewing monitor, and no separate reader unit is involved for image processing (Fig. 5.26). Flat-panel systems are highly dose efficient and provide quicker access to images compared with CR. The spatial resolution of flat-panel receptors is generally superior to that of CR. Because a pixel detector is built into the DR flat-panel IR, the size and pitch of the pixel are determined by the fixed DEL dimension. Therefore spatial resolution for flat-panel

detector IRs is limited to the DEL size and pitch. A system that uses a smaller DEL size has improved spatial resolution. FPDs are manufactured in two different ways to create electrical charges proportional to the x-ray exposure: indirect and direct conversion methods.

Indirect Conversion Detectors

Indirect conversion detectors use a scintillator such as CsI or gadolinium oxysulfide (Gd_2O_2S) to convert the remnant radiation into visible light. This phosphor-type material used in a scintillator produces light following the absorption of the x-rays. The visible light, in proportion to the x-ray exposure, is then converted to electrical charges by photodetectors (layer of amorphous silicon in the TFT array). The electrical charges are temporarily stored by capacitors in the TFT array before being digitized by the ADC and processed in the computer (Fig. 5.27).

The design of the scintillator used to convert the x-ray intensities into visible light can be structured or unstructured. Structured scintillator phosphors (in the form of needles or columns), usually crystalline CsI, reduce the spread of visible light, thus yielding images with higher spatial resolution than that of images obtained from unstructured scintillators and requiring less radiation to produce a quality image.

Other types of DR indirect conversion detectors include a charge-coupled device (CCD) and the complementary metal oxide semiconductor (CMOS). The CCD is very light sensitive and can respond to very low light

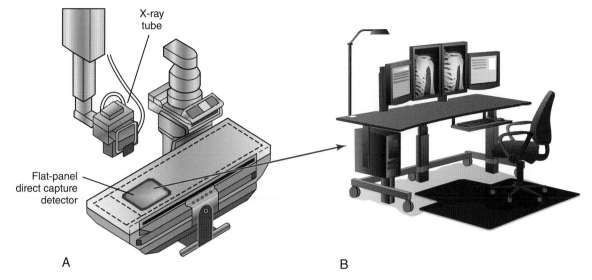

Fig. 5.26 **A,** Flat-panel detector fixed in x-ray table. **B,** Digital images sent to a computer workstation.

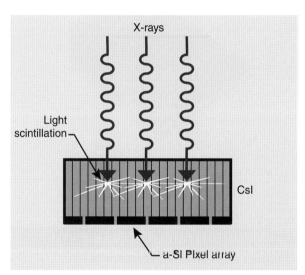

Fig. 5.27 Flat-panel detector (FPD)–indirect conversion. *a-Si,* Amorphous silicon; *CsI,* cesium iodide. (Modified from Bushong SC. *Radiologic Science for Technologists.* 10th ed. St. Louis: Mosby; 2013.)

intensities. It also has a wide dynamic range and can respond to a wide range of light intensities. The scintillator for this form of indirect capture is a CsI phosphor plate. A scintillator is a material that absorbs x-ray energy and emits visible light in response. CsI is a hygroscopic material (it readily absorbs moisture) that must be hermetically

sealed to avoid water absorption and prevent rapid degradation but is otherwise a high-efficiency scintillation material. The CsI phosphor plate may be coupled to the CCD using either a fiberoptic bundle or an optical lens system (Fig. 5.28). With this form of indirect capture, x-rays are absorbed by the scintillator and converted to light. This light energy is then transmitted to the CCD, where it is converted to an electronic signal and sent to the computer workstation for processing and display. Because there are currently technical limits to how large a single CCD device can be, an x-ray receptor may consist of an array of closely spaced CCDs. One challenge of this design is the seams at which the CCDs are joined (called *tiling* or *tiled*). Tiling is a process in which several CCD detectors adjoin to create one larger detector. This process results in seams with unequal response. This is addressed with computer preprocessing correction software that interpolates (averages) the pixel values along the seams (flat-field correction), in effect making the seams disappear.

Serving a similar purpose as the CCD is the CMOS. CMOS devices are signal-collection devices that use scintillators in a crystalline silicon matrix. Each DEL has its own amplifier, photodiode, and storage capacitor and is surrounded by transistors (Fig. 5.29). They do not have quite the light sensitivity or resolution of CCDs, but they use a fraction of the power to run, are very inexpensive to manufacture, and are improving. The newest versions

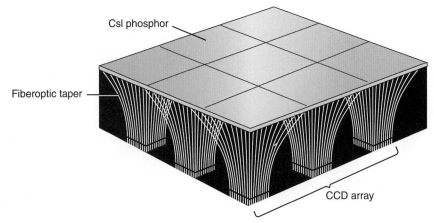

Fig. 5.28 The basic components of a charge-coupled device *(CCD)* array. The cesium iodide *(CsI)* phosphor plate is coupled to the CCD using fiberoptic bundles. (From Johnston JN, Fauber TL. *Essentials of Radiographic Physics and Imaging.* 3rd ed. St. Louis: Elsevier; 2020.)

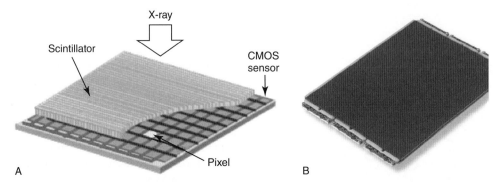

Fig. 5.29 A, Complementary metal oxide semiconductor *(CMOS)* detector array layers. **B,** CMOS device. (Part **A** courtesy RIKEN and JASRI. Part **B** courtesy Teledyne DALSA.)

have very fast image acquisition times because of their random pixel access capabilities. This feature also makes for AEC functions that are not as easy to achieve with CCDs. Creation of CMOS detectors of large enough size for general radiography has been its limitation, but this is changing. Recent advances in CMOS technology, particularly the creation of crystal light tubes that prevent light spread and methods for increasing their size, make them applicable for radiographic imaging.

Indirect conversion detectors are so named because they involve a two-stage process of converting x-ray intensities first to visible light and then to electrical charges during image acquisition. The electrical signals are then directed to amplifiers and the ADC to produce a raw digital image.

◤ IMPORTANT RELATIONSHIP

Indirect Conversion Detectors in Digital Radiography

Indirect conversion detectors involve a two-stage process of converting remnant x-ray intensities first to visible light and then to electrical charges. A scintillator-type material is used to absorb the x-ray energy, emit light in response, and then the light is converted to electrical signals. The electrical signals are then directed to amplifiers and the ADC to produce a raw digital image. Flat-panel TFT detectors are common in DR, but CCD and CMOS indirect conversion detectors are also used in DR.

Direct Conversion Detectors

Direct conversion detectors use an amorphous selenium (a-Se) detector to directly convert the remnant radiation to electrical charges (Fig. 5.30). To compensate for the moderately low atomic number of selenium (Z = 34), the thickness of the amorphous selenium is relatively high (1 mm). An electrical field is applied across the selenium layer to limit the lateral diffusion of electrons as they migrate toward the TFT array. By this means, excellent spatial resolution is maintained. Similar to indirect conversion detectors, the electronic charge is stored in a TFT array before it is amplified, digitized, and processed in the computer.

 IMPORTANT RELATIONSHIP

Direct Conversion Detectors in Digital Radiography

Direct conversion uses a-Se detectors to directly convert the incoming radiation exiting the patient to electrical charges. Similar to indirect conversion detectors, the electronic charge is stored in a TFT array before it is amplified, digitized, and processed in the computer.

DR Panel and Radiographic Generator Interface

It is important to remember that the TFT layer and DELs are electron charge-collection components. They

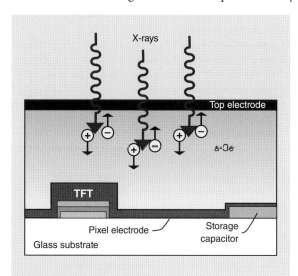

Fig. 5.30 Flat-panel detector (FPD)–direct conversion. *a-Se,* Amorphous selenium; *TFT,* thin-film transistor. (Modified from Bushong SC. *Radiologic Science for Technologists.* 10th ed. St. Louis: Mosby; 2013.)

require an electrical charge to be placed upon their photoconductive surfaces prior to x-ray exposure. This is accomplished through either a hard-wired connection (tether) or battery charge. Popular DR panels that are used for mobile examinations typically have a rechargeable battery integrated into the panel design. This battery provides a small charge to the TFTs once it is activated by the radiographer, just before exposure. Most DR system manufacturers also require direct communication with the x-ray generator known as a DR interface. This connection is typically a wireless, radio frequency (R/F) signal communication and provides an information pathway between the generator and DR panel electronics. Once the communication is "linked," a *ready* light is displayed indicating that the panel is properly charged and awaiting x-ray exposure. During exposure, charge is collected based upon radiation exposure to the DELs. Upon exposure termination, the charge values are amplified and converted by an ADC process. The electronic data are then read out on a line-by-line basis with each DEL and TFT having its own unique spatial address. The data are sent to a computer for processing, image reconstruction, and display. Following this, the TFTs are "zeroed out" with no charge and readied for the next exposure sequence. With current computer technology, this whole process takes only a few seconds before an image is displayed for viewing. It is very important to remember that the x-ray generator and DR panel must communicate with each other before, during, and after x-ray exposure. If this prerequisite condition is not established, x-ray exposure will likely be prevented. Regardless of the type of digital imaging system, the varying electrical signals are sent to the ADC for conversion into digital data. The digitized pixel intensities are patterned in the computer to form the image matrix. The image matrix is a digital composite of the varying x-ray intensities exiting the patient. Each pixel has a brightness level representing the attenuation characteristic of the volume of tissue imaged. After the varying x-ray intensities are converted to electronic data, the digital image can be processed, manipulated, transported, or stored.

QUALITY CONTROL

Ensuring the digital equipment is performing as expected is an important goal of a quality control (QC) program. Equipment acceptance testing and routine equipment maintenance are accomplished by qualified medical physicists or vendor service personnel. However, many daily, weekly, and monthly QC activities should be performed by the radiographer. In addition to the routine QC checks on the x-ray equipment discussed in other chapters, visual inspection of IRs for potential image artifacts caused by IP scratches, blood, contrast media, dirt, and damage because of daily use is necessary regardless of the type of digital imaging system. Routine cleaning (according to the manufacturer) and inspection of the digital IR by the radiographer can identify potential problems that may impact radiographic quality. DR panels are expensive and can cost tens of thousands of dollars. They typically have tolerances in terms of weight loads, bending, fluid invasion, and dropping. It is important to understand and appreciate the level of technological sophistication DR panels represent and they must be handled with professional care. Fig. 5.31 illustrates the internal components of a modern DR panel with its back protective covering removed. A damaged DR panel often is returned to the manufacturer for inspection (panel autopsy) and possible repair. If it is determined that the DR panel was damaged due to operator abuse and negligence, warranties and service contract coverage may be voided.

Engineers and manufacturers are continually improving DR panel technology. These improvements include faster and more sensitive photoconductive materials, lighter weight, greater fluid protection, and reliability.

Box 5.3 lists common QC activities for digital IRs that can be performed by the radiographer. Most of these QC checks evaluate the performance of the digital imaging system and the display monitor. QC checks specific to the performance of the display monitor will be discussed in Chapter 6.

BOX 5.3 Quality Control Check: Digital Imaging Systems

Manufacturers of digital imaging equipment have developed quality control (QC) procedures specific to their equipment; however, there are basic universal procedures for computed radiography (CR) and digital radiography (DR) image receptors (IRs) that the radiographer can perform.

Several QC phantom devices are available to assess the performance of the photostimulable phosphor (PSP) and flat-panel detector (FPD) imaging systems.

- IRs need to be visually inspected for any dirt, blood, contrast media, or scratches that could result in image artifacts. In addition, they should be regularly cleaned according to the manufacturer's specifications.
- The sensitivity of each PSP and FPD should be routinely checked to ensure the consistency of the exposure indicator value calibration.
- Shading or uniformity evaluates brightness consistency throughout the image.
- Linearity of the system can be evaluated by proportionally increasing and decreasing the radiation exposure to the IR and validating that the exposure indicator responds accordingly.
- Contrast resolution can be measured by imaging a contrast detail phantom to assess the visibility of low-contrast objects.
- Spatial resolution can be monitored by imaging a line-pair resolution test tool.
- For CR systems, the laser beam performance can be evaluated by imaging an opaque straight-edged object and visually checking for any jitter along the edges of the object.
- The measurement tool available at the workstation should be checked for accuracy.
- The thoroughness of the imaging plate (IP) erasure function can be evaluated by performing a secondary erasure on the IP and checking for any residual exposure (ghosting).
- The FPD can be evaluated to confirm that no charges remain from the previous exposure.

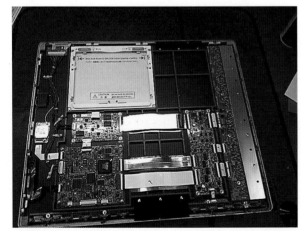

Fig. 5.31 A modern digital radiography (DR) panel backside with protective cover removed to demonstrate the precision circuitry and sophisticated design. (Courtesy Randy Griswold).

CHAPTER SUMMARY

- A digital image with a larger matrix and smaller-sized pixels has improved quality.
- The pixel size is directly related to the FOV displayed and inversely related to matrix size.
- A pixel's bit depth determines the available shades of gray to display the digital image or its contrast resolution.
- Spatial resolution is improved by increasing the pixel density and decreasing the pixel pitch.
- lp/mm is the unit of measurement for spatial frequency. Increasing the number of resolved lp/mm (higher spatial frequency) increases spatial resolution.
- Digital IRs have a wide dynamic range, which means that they can accurately capture the wide range of photon energies that exit a patient. However, lower- or higher-than-necessary exposure techniques do not guarantee a quality digital image with reasonable radiation exposure to the patient.
- Digital imaging systems with a wider dynamic range have higher pixel bit depths to display the range of grayscale. A 14-bit pixel depth system can display 16,384 shades of gray, whereas a 16-bit pixel depth system can display 65,536 shades of gray, therefore improving the quality of the displayed image.
- Radiographers should select exposure techniques within the exposure latitude of the digital imaging system and departmental standards.
- The MTF is a measure of an imaging system's ability to display contrast and spatial resolution of anatomic objects varying in size, and the value ranges between 0 (no difference in brightness levels) and 1.0 (maximum difference in brightness levels).
- DQE is a measurement of the efficiency of an IR in converting the x-ray exposure it receives to a quality radiographic image. The higher the DQE of a system, the lower the radiation exposure required to produce a quality image, and therefore, patient exposure is decreased.
- SNR is a method of describing the strength of the radiation exposure compared with the amount of noise apparent in a digital image. When the digital image displays increased noise, regardless of the source, anatomic details will have decreased visibility.
- CNR is a method of describing the contrast resolution compared with the amount of noise apparent in a digital image. Digital images having a higher CNR will increase the visibility of anatomic tissues.
- CR and DR IRs differ in their construction and how they acquire the raw image data. After the invisible image is acquired and the raw data are digitized, image processing and display are essentially the same for CR and DR.
- In CR, the IP has a photostimulable phosphor layer that absorbs the remnant radiation and excites electrons, which become elevated to a higher-energy state and get trapped.
- The exposed IP is placed in a reader unit where the trapped electrons are released during the laser beam scanning, and the excess energy is emitted as visible light. A photodetector collects, amplifies, and converts the visible light to an electrical signal proportional to the range of energies stored in the IP.
- The signal output from the photodetector is digitized by an ADC to produce a digital image.
- The sampling frequency in CR determines how often the analog signal is reproduced in its discrete digitized form. Increasing the sampling frequency increases the pixel density of the digital data and improves the spatial resolution of the digital image.
- After data extraction, CR IPs must be erased by exposure to an intense white light to release any residual energy before reuse.
- In contrast to CR, DR IRs combine image capture and readout.
- Signal storage, signal readout, and digitizing electronics are integrated into a solid-state FPD.
- FPDs use both indirect and direct conversion methods to create proportional electrical charges that are sent to the ADC for conversion to digital data.
- Indirect conversion detectors use a scintillator to convert the exit radiation to visible light, and then the visible light is converted to electrical charges for storage in the TFTs.
- The size of the DEL is inversely related to the number of lp/mm resolved in the digital image and affects spatial resolution. Smaller-sized DELs will resolve more lp/mms and increase spatial resolution.
- Other indirect conversion detectors include CCDs and CMOS.
- Direct conversion detectors directly convert the remnant radiation into electrical charges for storage in the TFTs. There is no scintillating phosphor layer.

- After the varying x-ray energies are converted to the electronic data set, the digital image can be computer processed, manipulated, transported, or stored.
- DR IRs require a communication interface between the x-ray generator and computer in order for exposure initiation and data readout and reconstruction.
- Routine quality control checks on the digital imaging system should be performed by the radiographer.

REVIEW QUESTIONS

1. Which of the following would improve spatial resolution?
   A. Small matrix and large pixel size
   B. Decreased pixel density and increased pixel pitch
   C. Large matrix and large pixel size
   D. Large matrix and increased pixel density
2. The type of image receptor (IR) that uses a photo-stimulable phosphor to acquire the raw image data is _____.
   A. an intensifying screen
   B. a flat-panel detector
   C. computed radiography
   D. digital radiography
3. Which of the following is used to extract the raw image data from a CR imaging plate (IP)?
   A. Laser beam
   B. Photomultiplier tube
   C. Analog-to-digital converter
   D. Thin-film transistor
4. Which of the following will improve the spatial resolution of the digital image?
   A. Decreased sampling frequency and increased sampling pitch
   B. Decreased sampling frequency and decreased sampling pitch
   C. Increased sampling frequency and increased sampling pitch
   D. Increased sampling frequency and decreased sampling pitch
5. Which of the following would improve the spatial resolution of the digital image for a given exposure field of view (FOV)?
   A. A fixed matrix size and larger IP
   B. A decreased sampling frequency and larger IP
   C. A small matrix size and larger pixel size
   D. A fixed matrix size and small IP
6. What is the process of assigning a numerical value to represent a brightness value?
   A. Dynamic range
   B. Signal-to-noise ratio
   C. Quantization
   D. Spectral sensitivity
7. Which of the following pixel bit depths would display a greater range of shades of gray to represent anatomic tissues?
   A. 8 bit
   B. 10 bit
   C. 14 bit
   D. 16 bit
8. Small anatomic detail has _____.
   A. decreased pixel density
   B. increased spatial resolution
   C. high spatial frequency
   D. low signal-to-noise ratio
9. Digital imaging systems have a wide dynamic range.
   A. True
   B. False
10. _____ refers to the range of exposures that should be used to produce a diagnostic image.
    A. Modulation transfer function
    B. Bit depth
    C. Exposure latitude
    D. Dynamic range
11. A lower signal-to-noise ratio (SNR) improves the quality of a digital image.
    A. True
    B. False
12. Decreasing the displayed FOV for a given matrix size will decrease the size of the pixels and increase spatial resolution.
    A. True
    B. False
13. Which of the following is a measurement of the efficiency of an IR in converting the x-ray exposure it receives to a quality radiographic image?
    A. DAP
    B. MTF
    C. DQE
    D. SNR

14. A higher sampling frequency during CR raw image data digitization will _____.
    A. increase spatial resolution
    B. decrease pixel density
    C. increase pixel pitch
    D. increase CNR

15. A 16-bit digital system would have a narrow dynamic range compared to a 12-bit system.
    A. True
    B. False

16. Which of the following provide an indication of patient radiation risk during a radiographic procedure?
    A. DQE
    B. DAP
    C. KAP
    D. B and C only

17. Digital detectors that require a two-stage process to acquire and digitize the raw image data include _____.
    A. flat-panel detectors indirect conversion
    B. CCD
    C. CMOS
    D. all the above

18. Image artifacts can be caused by _____.
    A. dirty CR IPs
    B. low sampling frequency
    C. increased pixel density
    D. A and B

19. Which of the following DEL dimensions in microns would demonstrate a greater number lp/mm of spatial resolution?
    A. 60
    B. 75
    C. 125
    D. 175

20. Prior to the x-ray exposure, what needs to occur to a DR detector?
    A. The battery needs to be charged
    B. The IP plate must be erased
    C. It must be scanned to identify any surface artifacts
    D. An electrical charge is placed on its photoconductive surface

21. DR panels that are used for mobile examinations generally use a _____.
    A. wireless communication link with the x-ray system
    B. hard-wired, electrical connection to a room outlet
    C. rechargeable battery for the TFT
    D. A and C

6

Digital Image Processing, Display, and Health Information Management

CHAPTER OUTLINE

Digital Image Processing
  Histogram Creation and Analysis
  Automatic Rescaling
  Lookup Table Application
  Exposure Indicator
Digital Imaging Artifacts
Image Display
  Postprocessing

Display Characteristics
Artificial Intelligence
Health Information Management
  Health Informatics
  Medical Image Management and Processing
    System
  Transmission, Storage, and Archives
Privacy and Security

OBJECTIVES

After completing this chapter, the reader will be able to perform the following:

1. Define all the key terms in this chapter.
2. State all the important relationships in this chapter.
3. State the purpose of digital image processing.
4. Identify preprocessing corrections performed on the raw image data.
5. Describe the construction of a histogram.
6. Explain histogram analysis, automatic rescaling, and lookup tables and their role during image processing to create a quality digital image.
7. Differentiate among the vendor-specific and the universal standard types of exposure indicators (EIs).
8. Acknowledge the critical role EIs have when assessing digital image quality.
9. Recognize default and postprocessing operations and their impact on image display.
10. Comprehend how over- and reprocessing image data could reduce the diagnostic and archival quality of the data.

11. Identify the important features of monitors that may affect the quality of the displayed image.
12. Explain the difference between luminance and luminance ratio.
13. Recognize the collaboration among technology systems such as electronic health records (EHRs), health information systems, radiology information systems (RISs), and medical image management and processing system (MIMPS).
14. Define health informatics and its role in providing radiology services.
15. Define MIMPS and state the major components.
16. Explain the role of Digital Imaging and Communications in Medicine (DICOM) in MIMPS.
17. Recognize the challenges of teleradiology, data transmission, storage, archives, and security.
18. Recognize the role of Health Insurance Portability and Accountability Act (HIPAA) in protecting health information.

KEY TERMS

alternative algorithms
artificial intelligence (AI)
aspect ratio
automatic rescaling

contrast enhancement
contrast resolution
data management
deviation index (DI)

digital image processing
Digital Imaging and
  Communications in
  Medicine (DICOM)

Acquisition of the invisible image can be accomplished with different types of image receptors (IRs), most commonly computed radiography (CR) and digital radiography (DR), as discussed in Chapter 5. After the raw image data (released energy) are extracted from the digital receptor and converted to digital (electronic) data (digitization), the image must be computer processed before its display and diagnostic interpretation. This chapter describes how digital data are processed to reproduce a quality image for display on a computer monitor. When displayed on a computer monitor, there is tremendous flexibility in altering the appearance of the digital image. In digital form, images can be transmitted, stored, and archived. Managing imaging data is an enormous responsibility, and important issues regarding health information management (HIM) are briefly discussed in this chapter.

DIGITAL IMAGE PROCESSING

The term digital image processing refers to various computer algorithms (mathematical computations) applied to electronic data for the purpose of optimizing the image for display. Although many digital image processing operations are proprietary (manufacturer specific) and outside the scope of this textbook, several commonly used processing methods are described. Generally, digital image processing can be described in stages, preprocessing to prepare the data for processing and display, and default (preset) or postprocessing, which includes computer operations available before and after the image is displayed.

When the released energy from the IR is digitized, several preprocessing operations occur to the raw data to account for flaws or imperfections in the electronic data set and to prepare the image data for processing and display. Bad or dead pixel and flat-fielding corrections are just two examples of computer operations applied to the raw image data. Because of the electronic components of a DR IR, imperfections can lead to artifacts and malfunctioning pixels (bad or dead pixels). Software corrections can be applied to account for these imperfections, which only occur with DR-type IRs. Flat-fielding correction is a process of correcting the nonuniformity of pixel values throughout the entire image. The anode heel effect discussed in Chapter 3 is an example of how pixel values can become nonuniform across the digital IR.

Following preprocessing, processing of digital data involves several operations to prepare the raw image for display: histogram creation and analysis, automatic rescaling, and lookup table (LUT) application. These processes are applied to all digital data including CR and DR. Although CR and DR acquire the raw image differently, both systems create an electronic data set of signal values that need to be computer processed. To create a quality digital image for display, the signal values need to be assembled and analyzed.

Histogram Creation and Analysis

The first step in processing digital data is histogram creation and analysis. The computer creates a histogram (or graphic representation of a data set) of the image that includes all the pixel values that represent the invisible image (released energy) after the software corrections were applied and sometimes referred to as the *exposure* histogram. The x-axis represents the range of pixel values assigned, and the y-axis represents the number (frequency) of pixels for each value (Fig. 6.1). The location of the graph along the x-axis represents image brightness levels, and the shape of the graph represents image contrast (grayscale).

With computed radiography, the entire CR imaging plate (IP) is scanned to extract the invisible image from the photostimulable phosphor, and the computer identifies the exposure field brightness levels and the edges of the collimated image so all the exposure data outside the collimated image can be excluded (exposure field

recognition and segmentation). Ideally, all four edges of a collimated field should be recognized. If at least three edges are not identified, all data, including raw exposure or scatter outside the x-ray field, may be included in the histogram, resulting in a histogram processing error. See Fig. 6.2 for an example of a processing error.

In newer CR imaging systems, the collimated borders may not have the same impact on data processing as in older CR systems. Processing errors are less likely to occur with DR IRs than with CR IRs because the image data are extracted only from the exposed detector elements (DELs); however, the collimated edges of the image still need to be recognized.

 IMPORTANT RELATIONSHIP

Corrections and Histogram Creation

Several operations occur on the raw image data to prepare for further processing to display a quality image. Software corrections can be applied to account for imperfections (bad or dead pixels) that only occur with DR-type IRs, and flat fielding is a process of correcting the nonuniformity of pixel values throughout the entire image. A histogram is created that represents the range of digital pixel values versus the relative prevalence of the pixel values in the invisible image. Scanning the entire CR IR to identify the exposure field brightness levels and the edges of the collimated image (exposure field recognition and segmentation) is necessary to identify only the image data representing the anatomic area.

Histogram Analysis

Histogram analysis is an important processing technique to identify the edges of an image and assess the exposure data (pixel values) before image processing and display. The location and shape of the exposure histogram are impacted by the anatomic area imaged, the exposure technique, positioning, and collimation. The computer analyzes the histogram using processing algorithms and compares it with a preestablished (reference) histogram specific to the anatomic part being imaged. This process is called histogram analysis. The computer software has stored histogram models, each having a shape characteristic of the selected anatomic region and projection. These stored histogram models have values of interest (VOIs), which determine the range of the histogram data set that should be included in the displayed image (Fig. 6.3).

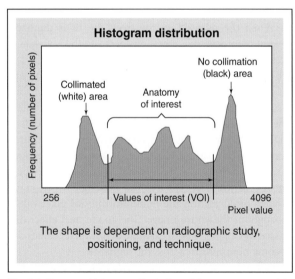

Fig. 6.1 Exposure histogram. Illustration of the raw exposure data histogram before processing. The exposure data outside the collimated image need to be excluded from the histogram to prevent a processing error. (Modified from Seibert JA. [1999]. Physics of Computed Radiography, AAPM 1999 Annual Meeting, Nashville [PowerPoint slides]. Retrieved from https://www.aapm.org/meetings/99AM/pdf/2795-64903.pdf, accessed June 17, 2019.)

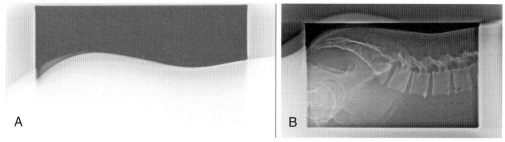

Fig. 6.2 Histogram analysis error. **A,** Poor-quality computed radiography (CR) image resulting from a histogram error caused by incorrect collimation. **B,** Image showing correctly collimated borders resulting in a quality CR image. (Courtesy Andrew Woodward.)

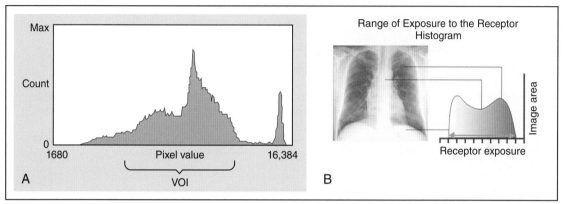

Fig. 6.3 A, The histogram represents the number of digital pixel values versus the relative prevalence of those values in the latent image. The x-axis represents the amount of exposure and the y-axis the incidence of pixels for each exposure level. **B,** Range of exposure to the receptor histogram. Each image has its own histogram. *VOI,* Value of interest. (**A,** Modified from Cesar LJ: Computed radiography: its impact on radiographers, Radiol Technol. 68(3):225-232, 1997. **B,** modified from Sprawls P. Physical Principles of Medical Imaging Online. 2nd ed. http://www.sprawls.org/ppmi2.)

⚡ IMPORTANT RELATIONSHIP

Histogram Analysis

> During histogram analysis, the exposure histogram is compared with a stored (reference) histogram for that anatomic part; VOIs are identified in preparation for image processing and display.

Automatic Rescaling

Computer processing is used to maintain consistent image brightness despite over- or underexposure of the IR (Fig. 6.4). This procedure is known as automatic rescaling. The computer rescales the image based on the comparison of the histograms. Fig. 6.5 is an example of how the brightness and contrast of the exposure histogram can be rescaled to match the reference histogram to display a quality radiographic image. Although automatic rescaling is a convenient feature, radiographers should be aware that rescaling errors can occur because of positioning and collimation errors and with image artifacts, such as a hip prosthesis, and can result in poor-quality digital images. Rescaling will also compensate for patient overexposure which is looked upon poorly by the profession and discouraged. Rescaling will not compensate for image noise due to underexposure. This will be discussed more in Chapter 7.

Lookup Table Application

Lookup table (LUT) application provides a method of processing the image data, based on the reference

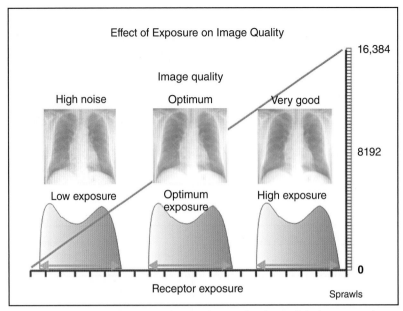

Fig. 6.4 Effect of exposure on image quality. Automatic rescaling is used during processing to maintain a consistent image brightness despite over- or underexposure of the image receptor (IR). (Modified from Sprawls P. Physical Principles of Medical Imaging Online. 2nd ed. http://www.sprawls.org/ppmi2.)

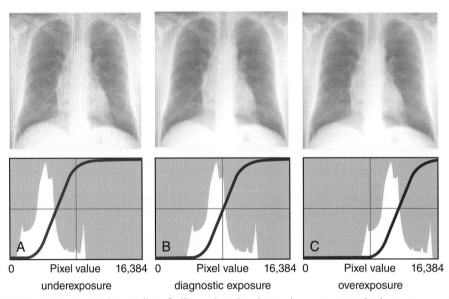

Fig. 6.5 Histogram automatic rescaling. **A,** Illustration showing underexposure to the image receptor (IR). Notice the location of the histogram and lookup table (LUT) graph along the x-axis and the shape of the LUT graph. **B,** Illustration showing how the histogram and LUT graph have been rescaled to display an improved quality image. **C,** Illustration showing overexposure to the IR. Notice the location of the histogram and LUT curve along the x-axis and the shape of the LUT curve before its rescaling in **B**. The LUT graph is created in **A** and **C** for illustration only.

histogram, to transform the image data into a quality image for display. Because digital IRs have a linear exposure response and a wide dynamic range, raw data images exhibit low contrast and must be altered to improve the visibility of anatomic structures. LUTs provide the means to alter the brightness and grayscale of the digital image using computer algorithms. Additionally, LUTs vary between manufacturers so an image of a body part from one vendor may have a different appearance when compared to another. Similarly, a body part's appearance can be altered if different LUTs are applied to its histogram. It is important that the correct LUT is used for the body part being examined.

 IMPORTANT RELATIONSHIP

Applied LUTs

It is important that the correct LUT be applied to the body part imaged. If an incorrect LUT is applied to the histogram of the body part imaged, its appearance could be jeopardized for display.

LUTs also provide a means to adjust the contrast or grayscale necessary to adequately view the anatomic region. Fig. 6.6 visually compares pixel values of the original image with those of a processed image. If the image is not altered, the graph would be a straight line. If the original image is altered, the original pixel values would be different in the processed image, and the graph would no longer be a straight line but resemble an S-shaped curve (Fig. 6.7). For example, each pixel value could be altered to display the digital image with a change in contrast (grayscale). New pixel values would be calculated that result in the image being displayed with higher contrast (Fig. 6.8). Fig. 6.9 shows the original image, the graph after changes in the pixel values, and the processed higher-contrast image. LUTs provide a method of processing digital images to change the displayed brightness and contrast required for each anatomic area (Fig. 6.10).

 IMPORTANT RELATIONSHIP

Lookup Tables

LUTs provide the means to alter the original pixel values to improve the brightness and contrast of the displayed image.

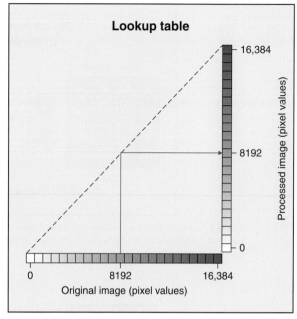

Fig. 6.6 Straight line graph demonstrating no change in the pixel values from the original to the processed image. (Modified from Sprawls P. Physical Principles of Medical Imaging Online. 2nd ed. http://www.sprawls.org/ppmi2.)

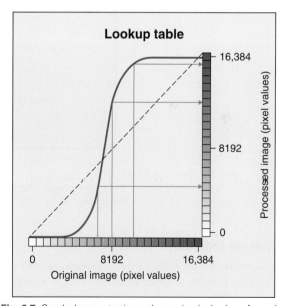

Fig. 6.7 Graph demonstrating a change in pixel values from the original image to the processed image. The shape of the graph resembles an S-shaped curve. (Modified from Sprawls P. Physical Principles of Medical Imaging Online. 2nd ed. http://www.sprawls.org/ppmi2.)

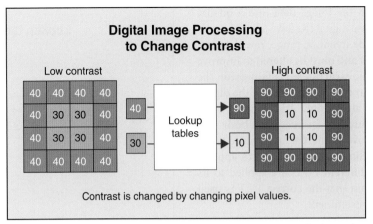

Fig. 6.8 Lookup table (LUT) altering the pixel values of a low-contrast image to display an image with higher contrast. (Modified from Sprawls P. Physical Principles of Medical Imaging Online. 2nd ed. http://www.sprawls.org/ppmi2.)

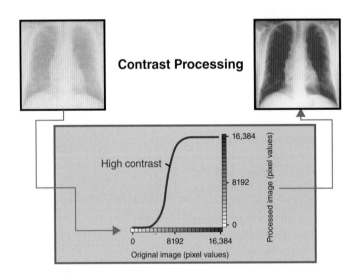

Fig. 6.9 The original low-contrast chest image is altered to have higher contrast. The graph shows a change in the pixel values from the original image. (Modified from Sprawls P. Physical Principles of Medical Imaging Online. 2nd ed. http://www.sprawls.org/ppmi2.)

Exposure Indicator

An important feature of digital image processing, both CR and DR, is its ability to create an image with the appropriate amount of brightness. As a result of the histogram analysis, pixel values of interest (VOIs) are identified and the average value of the VOIs is used to determine the exposure to the IR. A numerical value, known as the exposure indicator (EI), is assigned to this midpoint VOI and can be used to assess the image quality as it relates to IR exposure. It is important to understand that the EI value is not a measure of radiation exposure to the patient, but rather exposure to the IR. The calculation of an EI value is complex, proprietary, and the result of collaborative efforts among industry experts and beyond the scope of this text. The expression of an EI value may be direct with x-ray exposure or indirect, depending upon the

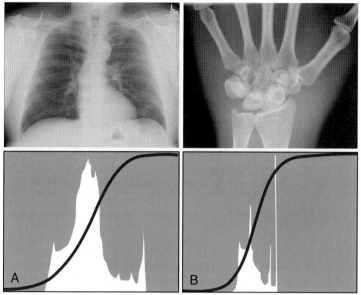

Fig. 6.10 A, Chest image with its histogram and lookup table (LUT) graph, which differs from **B,** image of the wrist with its histogram and LUT graph. (Courtesy Andrew Woodward.)

manufacturer. For example, Carestream, Philips, Siemens, and Canon exposure indicator values increase as exposure to the IR increases. With Fuji, a term known as the sensitivity number (S) is used and this number decreases as exposure increases. Optimal ranges of the exposure indicator values are vendor specific and vary among the types of procedures, such as abdomen and chest imaging versus extremity imaging. It is very important for the radiographer to clearly understand which system is being used in a department and the relationship between the number value and IR exposure. A decision to repeat an image should be based on the quality of the displayed image and departmental standards in addition to the EI value.

IMPORTANT RELATIONSHIP

Image Repeat

A decision to repeat an image should be based on the quality of the displayed image and departmental standards in addition to the EI value.

Because EI values are not standardized between manufacturers, a universally accepted term known as a deviation index (DI) was established and adopted in 2008 by the International Electrotechnical Commission (IEC) and the American Association of Physicists in Medicine (AAPM). The AAPM Report No. 116, published soon after, provided guidelines for DI ranges and subsequent actions for image exposures within the DI ranges. More recently, the AAPM published Report No. 232 and revised some of the recommendations stated in the 116 Report.

The deviation index (DI) is a value that reflects the difference between the desired or target exposure to the IR (EI_t) and the actual exposure to the IR (EI). A DI of 0 would indicate there is no difference between the desired (EI_t) and the actual EI and is the recommended target exposure. DIs range from −3 to +3 and labeled as standard deviations (SDs) above and below the target DI of 0. DIs greater than +1.0 SD are considered overexposed. A DI of +3.0 SD has excessive exposure by a factor of 2 or 100% more than the EI_t. DIs less than −1.0 SD are considered underexposed and a DI of −3.0 SD has insufficient exposure by ½ or 50% of the EI_t.

It is well understood that underexposure of the IR may produce an image with quantum noise. The challenge for radiographers is to determine whether the amount of noise visible on the displayed image is unacceptable. This decision should be based on several factors, such as the type of imaging procedure, age of the patient, and departmental standards. If the DI is less than −2 SD below the target DI of 0, and the decision is made to repeat the image, then increasing the exposure to the IR by a factor of 2 (generally double the original milliamperage-seconds [mAs]) would be considered a sufficient change to reduce the visible quantum noise.

Repeating a digital image for an overexposure is not as straightforward as for underexposure. Because digital detectors have a wide dynamic range, image quality can be maintained for overexposures, within limits. If the DI is more than +2 SD above the target DI of 0, the decision to repeat the image should not be made solely on the DI value. If the displayed image demonstrates saturation or the desired anatomy is not visible, repeating the image may be necessary. If a decision is made to repeat the image, decreasing the exposure to the IR by a factor 2 (generally half the mAs) would be considered a sufficient change. It is important to note that repeating an image due to overexposure further increases the radiation dose to the patient and therefore should be clinically warranted.

 RADIATION PROTECTION ALERT

Image Repeat for Overexposure

It is important to note that repeating an image due to overexposure further increases the radiation dose to the patient and therefore should be clinically warranted.

It is important for radiographers to have accurate information about the exposure to the IR when considering a repeat image. The calibration of the equipment, automatic exposure control (AEC), and EI_t values for each anatomical area will determine whether the DI provided to the radiographer is an accurate assessment of exposure to the IR. It cannot be overemphasized that the quality of the image and departmental standards must be considered in addition to the DI before choosing to repeat a radiographic image.

 IMPORTANT RELATIONSHIP

Exposure Indicator

The exposure indicator (EI) provides a numeric value indicating the level of radiation exposure to the digital IR. These values may be vendor specific and have a direct or inverse relationship to the IR exposure. A universal standard exposure indicator (DI) has been developed and provides the radiographer with important information about the IR exposure.

 IMPORTANT RELATIONSHIP

Deviation Index

DIs range from −3 to +3 and labeled as standard deviations (SDs) above and below the target DI of 0. DIs greater than +1.0 SD are considered overexposed. A DI of +3.0 SD has excessive exposure by a factor of 2 or 100% more than the EI_t. DIs less than −1.0 SD are considered underexposed and a DI of −3.0 SD has insufficient exposure by ½ or 50% of the EI_t.

It is important to note that all EIs, even the recommended standard DI, have limitations. Variables such as collimation, kilovoltage peak (kVp), and centering may influence the EI, and therefore the level of noise and image quality should be evaluated along with the EI or DI value. Departments establish target EI values (EI_t) as a standard for acceptable image quality, regarding IR exposure. Target EI numbers vary based on body part and examination needs and are developed in conjunction with radiologists, medical physicists, and quality control (QC) staff. These EI_t values are to assess the overall department image quality and adherence to optimization of radiological protection by department officials. The radiographer needs to be knowledgeable about the EI value on the equipment being used in digital imaging and how exposure techniques can be altered to correct exposure errors. In addition, the department standards should be followed for how over- and underexposures are to be handled before repeating the image.

The radiographer should monitor the exposure indicator values as a guide for proper exposure techniques. If the exposure indicator value is within the acceptable range, adjustments can be made for contrast and brightness with postprocessing display functions, and this will not degrade the image. However, if the exposure is outside of the acceptable range, attempting to adjust the image data with postprocessing display functions would not correct for improper IR exposure and may result in noisy or suboptimal images that should not be submitted for interpretation.

 IMPORTANT RELATIONSHIP

Improper IR Exposures

Attempting to adjust the image data with postprocessing display functions would not correct for improper IR exposure and may result in noisy or suboptimal images that should not be submitted for interpretation.

The radiographer has a role in the selection of the appropriate anatomic part and projection before computer processing. This step prepares the computer for the type of data being supplied for histogram analysis. If the radiographer selects a part other than the imaged one, a histogram analysis error may occur. In addition, any errors that occur, such as during data extraction from the IR or rescaling during computer processing, could affect the exposure indicator and provide a false value. It is important for radiographers not only to consider the exposure indicator value carefully but also to recognize its limitations.

⚠️ RADIATION PROTECTION ALERT

Exposure Indicators

> The radiographer should strive to select techniques that result in exposure indicator values falling within the indicated optimum range for the corresponding digital imaging system. However, the radiographer also needs to recognize the limitations of exposure indicators for providing accurate information. The radiographer should assess the exposure indicator along with image quality before considering a repeat image.

Some of the newer digital imaging systems provide a mechanism for the radiographer to reprocess the image data using a different Lookup table to improve its presentation at the display monitor, known as alternative algorithms. Selecting an alternative anatomical region or projection will apply a different algorithm to the original image data, and the reprocessed image will be displayed with a change in brightness and/or contrast at the radiographer's workstation. This could prevent the need for a repeat image causing additional exposure to the patient. However, the reprocessed image is not assured to have improved quality and if sent to the medical image management and processing system (MIMPS, discussed later) for display on the radiologist's workstation, it would limit their ability to further postprocess and manipulate the image because some of the original image data are lost. Additionally, information about the reprocessing of the original image data would be identified on the displayed image and could cause problems with storage and retrieval of the imaging procedure. Use of alternative algorithms is not a standard practice for radiographers and should only be performed within the established policies of the department.

Depending on the software available, a digital image can be additionally manipulated in a variety of ways. The following are common default (preset) or postprocessing techniques:

1. Dual-energy subtraction (Fig. 6.11) is a technique that can remove superimposed structures so that the anatomic area of interest becomes more visible. Because the image is in a digital format, the computer can subtract selected brightness values to create an image without superimposed structures.

2. Contrast enhancement (Fig. 6.12) is a postprocessing technique that alters the pixel values to increase image contrast.

3. Edge enhancement (also known as high-band pass filtering) (Fig. 6.13) is a postprocessing technique that improves the visibility of small, high-contrast structures. However, image noise may be slightly increased.

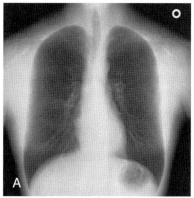 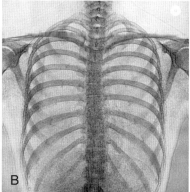

Fig. 6.11 Subtraction postprocessing techniques. **A,** Skeletal areas are removed. **B,** Lungs and soft tissue are removed.

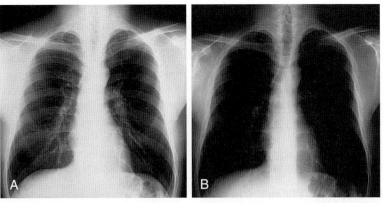

Fig. 6.12 Postprocessing adjustment in radiographic contrast. **A,** Longer-scale contrast typical of chest radiography. **B,** Contrast has been adjusted to present a higher scale.

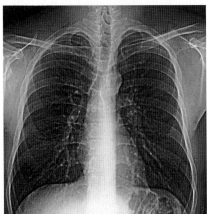

Fig. 6.13 A radiographic image demonstrates an *edge-enhancement* postprocessing technique.

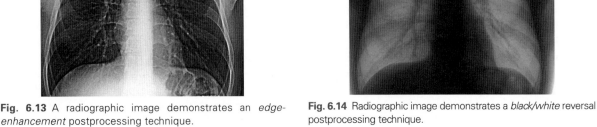

Fig. 6.14 Radiographic image demonstrates a *black/white* reversal postprocessing technique.

4. Inversion (also known as black/white reversal) (Fig. 6.14) is a postprocessing technique that reverses the grayscale from the original image.
5. Smoothing (also known as low-band pass filtering) (Fig. 6.15) is a postprocessing technique that suppresses image noise (quantum noise). However, visible spatial resolution is degraded.
6. Equalization (Fig. 6.16) is a postprocessing function whereby underexposed areas (light areas) are made darker and overexposed areas (dark areas) are made lighter. The effect is an image that appears to have lower contrast so that dense and lucent structures can be better seen within the same image.

Other postprocessing functions include region of interest (ROI), which provides the calculation of selected pixel values within the area of interest to provide quantitative information about the tissue. Additional software can provide stitching of multiple images into one image for viewing anatomic areas such as for a scoliosis series or leg-length examination.

A word of caution is warranted regarding postprocessing: overuse of these functions can drastically and negatively alter the original data set, which is the digital image. Overwriting the original image with a postprocessed replica may reduce the diagnostic and archival quality of the data. One should also keep in mind that in many facilities, the radiographers' workstations use monitors of significantly lower quality and viewing conditions that are very different compared with the radiologists' workstations. How an image looks on the radiographer's workstation in a brightly lit work area may be very different from the way it looks on the radiologist's

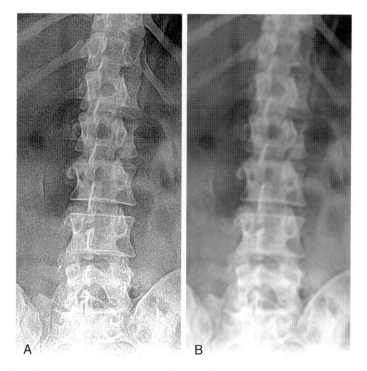

Fig. 6.15 Smoothing (also known as low-band pass filtering). **A,** Image without applying smoothing processing. **B,** Image after smoothing processing. (Courtesy Andrew Woodward.)

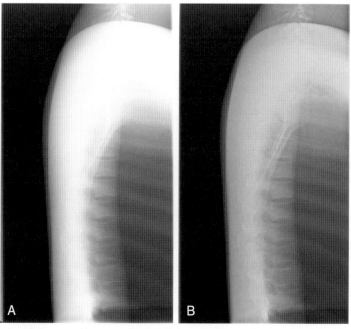

Fig. 6.16 Equalization. **A,** Image without equalization. **B,** Image with equalization. (Courtesy Andrew Woodward.)

high-resolution monitor in a darkened reading room. Therefore care should be taken in the postprocessing of an image before forwarding it for interpretation.

Advancement in digital image processing continues to improve image quality and diagnostic interpretation. Grid subtraction and grid replacement software algorithms are just two examples of these software advancements. Grids are discussed in Chapter 8 and improve image quality by removing scatter (fog) that serves no useful purpose and only degrades image quality. However, the use of grids provides challenges in terms of grid artifacts, grid positioning errors, and increased radiation exposure to the patient. Computer software is being developed that can remove unwanted artifacts caused by the grid pattern (grid subtraction), such as the moiré effect, or remove the scatter radiation (fog) visualized in a digital image produced without a grid (scatter correction software). There are many radiographic procedures that could prevent the use of a grid especially during mobile or operating room procedures caused by grid alignment challenges. Advancements in computer software algorithms can remove the scatter radiation and display the digital image with improved grayscale (contrast).

DIGITAL IMAGING ARTIFACTS

Digital imaging artifacts occur for various reasons and generally have a bright or dark appearance. The complexity of the electronics involved in creating the digital image often makes it difficult to isolate the cause of the problem because the level of brightness of digital artifacts does not necessarily provide an indication of the source. Digital artifacts may be classified as equipment or procedural (discussed in Chapter 4). Equipment artifacts typically involve detectors (CR plate, thin-film transistor array), occurring during image data extraction before the analog-to-digital converter (ADC) or during the ADC process and subsequent signal processing performed by the computer up to the point of image display. Examples of CR detector–related artifacts include IP stains, particulates, scratches, cracks, and fogging. Artifacts occurring during data extraction on CR systems are related to issues with the laser optics, transport mechanisms, light guide, and laser sampling and stationary grid frequencies. CR detector artifacts can also occur from an erasure error or if the technologist improperly centers the CR to table grid. See Fig. 6.17 for examples of CR artifacts.

DR detector artifacts may be related to the calibration of an individual DEL, row, or column of the detector matrix. Artifacts occurring during data extraction are related to electronic readout mechanisms associated with the rows and columns of the DELs comprising the detector matrix. See Fig. 6.18 for examples of DR artifacts. If the source of the artifact is not related to the detector or extraction of image data up to the ADC, the remaining sources are likely to be the electronic

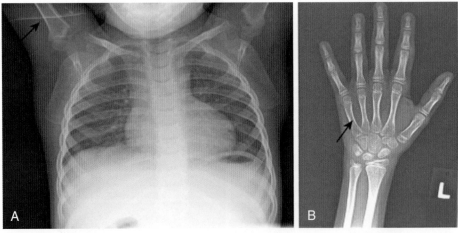

Fig. 6.17 Computed radiography (CR) image artifacts. **A,** *Bright lines* in the shoulder region as a result of scratches on the imaging plate. **B,** *Bright specs* between the fourth and fifth metacarpals as a result of dirt on the image plate. (Courtesy Andrew Woodward.)

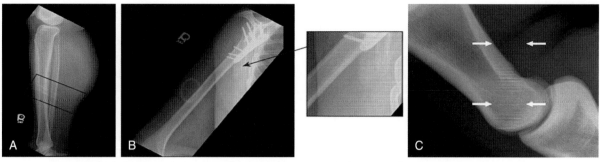

Fig. 6.18 Digital radiography image artifacts. **A,** Erasure error. **B,** Improper alignment of central ray and image receptor (IR) in a Bucky table. **C,** An example of radiofrequency (RF) interference (between the *white arrows*) caused by a breakdown in RF shielding in a flat-panel digital radiography system. (**C,** From Vet Radiology Ultrasound, Volume: 49, Issue: s1, Pages: S48-S56, First published: 10 January 2008, DOI: (10.1111/j. 1740-8261.2007.00334.x).)

components starting within the ADC and subsequent circuits that are involved with transmitting the digital signal to the computer for processing or processed image data sent to the display monitor. A discussion of artifacts related to the electronic readout mechanisms or occurring within the ADC and subsequent components of the imaging system is beyond the scope of this book.

IMAGE DISPLAY

After computer processing, the digital image is ready to be displayed for viewing. The quality of the digital image is also affected by important features of the display monitor, such as its luminance and resolution, and viewing conditions such as ambient lighting and monitor placement. Specialized postprocessing software is used at the display workstation to aid the radiologist in image interpretation. In addition to soft-copy viewing, the digital image can be saved to transportable storage media or printed on specialized film by a laser printer.

Postprocessing

Postprocessing functions are computer software operations available to the radiographer and radiologist that allow manual manipulation of the displayed image. These functions allow the operator to manually adjust many presentation features of the image to enhance the diagnostic value.

Electronic Masking

After the image is processed, regions viewed on the image can be altered further by electronic masking, also known

as *shuttering*. For example, when the area of interest is properly collimated, the image may display increased brightness surrounding the radiation-exposed field. This region of brightness provides no useful information and can be removed from the displayed image, which is automatic in newer digital equipment. In addition, electronic masking can remove regions surrounding the exposure field that provide no useful information and potentially impact the histogram analysis. However, it is not within the standards of practice for radiographers to make decisions about removing information within the radiation-exposed field. Proper collimation before radiation exposure is important and should not be replaced with electronic masking. A properly collimated x-ray field preexposure and automatic electronic masking of the bright intensities outside the radiation-exposed field should show a thin white line around the edges of the image, which indicates the image was collimated smaller than the size of the IR. Electronic masking has no effect on the overall image quality (removing scatter) or on patient exposure.

> ### IMPORTANT RELATIONSHIP
> #### *Electronic Masking*
>
> Proper collimation before radiation exposure is important and should not be replaced with electronic masking. It is not within the standards of practice for radiographers to make decisions about removing information within the radiation-exposed field.

Displayed Brightness

Because the image is composed of numerical data, the brightness level displayed on the computer monitor can be easily altered to visualize the range of the recorded anatomic structures. This adjustment is accomplished using a basic windowing function. The window level (or center) sets the midpoint of the range of brightness levels visible in the image. Changing the window level on the display monitor allows the image brightness to be increased or decreased throughout the entire range (Fig. 6.19). When the range of brightness displayed is less than the maximum, the processed image presents only a subset of the total information contained within the computer (Fig. 6.20).

 IMPORTANT RELATIONSHIP

Window Level and Image Brightness

A relationship exists between window level and image brightness on the display monitor. Changing the window level on the display monitor allows the image brightness to be increased or decreased throughout the entire range.

Displayed Contrast

The number of different shades of gray that can be stored and displayed by a computer system is termed grayscale. Contrast resolution is another term associated with digital imaging and is used to describe the ability of the imaging system to distinguish between objects that exhibit similar brightness levels because they attenuate the x-ray beam similarly. An important distinguishing characteristic of a digital image is its improved contrast resolution. As previously mentioned, the brightness level of a pixel is determined by the bit depth or number of bits (i.e., 12, 14, or 16), which affects the number of shades of gray available for image display. Increasing the number of shades of gray increases the contrast resolution within the image. An image with increased contrast resolution, when optimally windowed, increases the visibility of very subtle anatomic features.

After the digital image is processed, radiographic contrast can be adjusted to vary the visualization of the area of interest; this is necessary because the contrast resolution of the human eye is limited. Window width is a basic control that adjusts the radiographic contrast. Because the digital image can display shades of gray ranging from black to white, the display monitor can vary the range or number of shades of gray visible on the image to show the desired anatomy. Adjusting the range of visible shades of gray varies the image contrast (Fig. 6.21). When the entire number of shades of gray is displayed (wide window width), the image has lower contrast; when a smaller number of shades of gray is displayed (narrow window width), the image has higher contrast (Fig. 6.22).

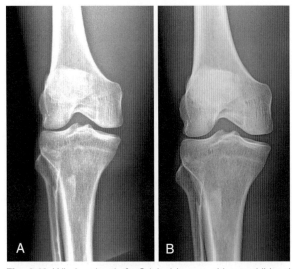

Fig. 6.19 Window level. **A,** Original image without additional postprocessing. **B,** Image with a change in the window level to make the image displayed with less brightness (darker).

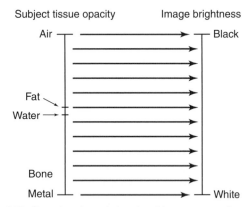

Fig. 6.20 Changing the window level increases or decreases the image brightness throughout the range of tissue opacities recorded in the image. (Modified from Kuni C: Introduction to Computers and Digital Processing in Medical Imaging, Chicago, 1988, Year Book Medical Publishers.)

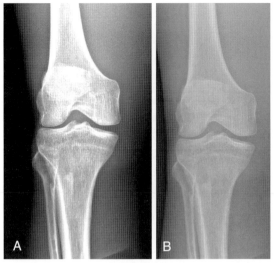

Fig. 6.21 Window width. **A,** Original image without additional postprocessing. **B,** Image with an increase in window width displaying decreased (lower) contrast.

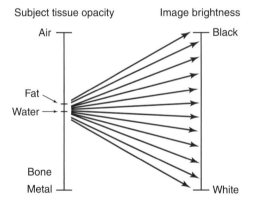

Fig. 6.22 Changing the window width increases or decreases the range of visible brightness levels. A narrow window width decreases the range of brightness levels and increases contrast. A wider window width increases the range of brightness levels and reduces contrast. (Modified from Kuni C: Introduction to Computers and Digital Processing in Medical Imaging, Chicago, 1988, Year Book Medical Publishers.)

In digital imaging, an inverse relationship exists between window width and image contrast. A wide window width displays an image with lower contrast than the same area of interest displayed with a narrow window width.

The center or midpoint of the window level and the width of the window determine the brightness and contrast of the displayed image (Fig. 6.23). Fig. 6.24 demonstrates how the image is altered when the window level is changed for a given window width.

 IMPORTANT RELATIONSHIP

Window Width and Image Contrast

A narrow (decreased) window width displays higher radiographic contrast, whereas a wider (increased) window width displays lower radiographic contrast.

The ability to optimize image display in real time using the window level and width controls is a major advantage of soft-copy viewing of digital images. It is important to note that, generally, windowing does not alter the original stored pixel values of an image but rather alters only how they are displayed. However, more complex image manipulations available on primary display monitors use preset LUTs for windowing (level and width) and other operations. It is advised to save the original image and one for display so complex operations on the display image will not affect the original image.

Display Characteristics

As previously discussed, the quality of the digital image is affected by its acquisition parameters and subsequent computer processing. In addition, the quality of the digital image is affected by the performance of the display monitor. The quality of display monitors may not be equal among all those used for viewing digital images. Monitors used by radiologists for diagnostic interpretation, referred to as *primary*, must be of higher quality than the monitors used only for routine image review (*secondary*). However, the radiographer's monitor should be of sufficiently high quality to accurately discern all the image quality characteristics before sending the image to the radiologist for diagnostic interpretation. Display monitors used for radiographic diagnostic interpretation are typically monochrome high-resolution monitors and can be set to portrait or landscape formats and configured with one, two, or four monitors (Fig. 6.25). The construction of common display monitors used in routine imaging is discussed in Chapter 10.

Several important features of display monitors (used in digital radiography) affect their performance. Digital images are captured and processed to display a specific matrix size. As previously discussed, an image created with a large matrix having many smaller-sized pixels improves the spatial resolution of the digital image (pixel image). If the monitor used for viewing the digital image cannot display a matrix of that size (because it has too few display pixels), the image quality is decreased.

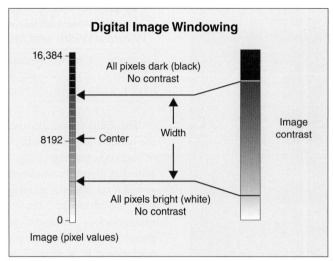

Fig. 6.23 The level or center of the window and the window width change the visual display of the digital image. (Modified from Sprawls P. *Physical Principles of Medical Imaging Online*. 2nd ed. http://www.sprawls. org/ppmi2.)

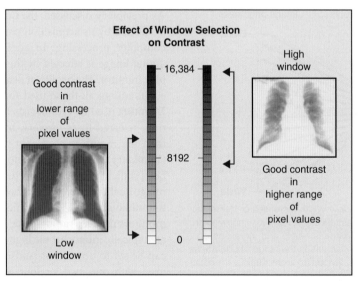

Fig. 6.24 Changing the window level for a chest x-ray varies the visibility of the anatomic detail or contrast for both low- and high-brightness levels. (Modified from Sprawls P. *Physical Principles of Medical Imaging Online*. 2nd ed. http://www.sprawls.org/ppmi2.)

A high-resolution 5-megapixel (2048 × 2560 pixels) display monitor used for diagnostic interpretation will provide improved visualization of the imaging system's high spatial resolution. Although, displays with 3-megapixel (1500 × 2000 pixels) are sufficient for routine diagnostic interpretation. However, the display size (dimensions) along with the pixel pitch is another method to assess the capabilities of the display monitor. A display monitor having diagonal dimensions of 53 cm (21 inches) is adequate for viewing images sized 35 × 43 cm (14 × 17 inches) with a recommended pixel pitch of 0.200 mm at a standard

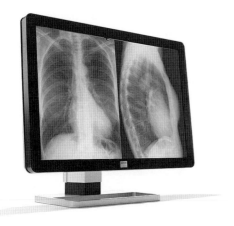

Fig. 6.25 A set of portrait display monitors used for soft-copy viewing. (©Barco.)

viewing distance of about 60 cm (24 inches). According to the ACR-AAPM-SIIM Technical Standards for Electronic Practice of Medical Imaging (2022), suitable visualization of the entire digital image will occur when the diagonal display distance is 80% of the viewing distance. At a 66-cm (26-inch) viewing distance, 80% would yield a 53-cm (21-inch) diagonal-sized display monitor. However, depending on the type of device used to display the digital image (workstation, tablet, laptop), the display dimensions and viewing distances could change.

 IMPORTANT RELATIONSHIP

Display Monitor

A high-resolution 5-megapixel (2048 × 2560 pixels) display monitor will provide improved visualization of the imaging system's high spatial resolution. In addition, a display monitor having diagonal dimensions of 53 cm (21 inches) is adequate for viewing images sized 35 × 43 cm (14 × 17 inches) with a recommended pixel pitch of 0.200 mm at a standard viewing distance of about 60 cm (24 inches).

Another important display feature is the aspect ratio (width-to-height dimension). Display monitors with 3:4 or 4:5 aspect ratios are appropriate for viewing radiographic digital images. Newer display monitors may have a wider format such as 16:9 or 16:10, which would provide for the presentation of multiple images on a single display, similar to dual monitors.

Because anatomic tissue is visualized using various brightness levels, the amount of light emitted from the monitor (luminance) affects the quality of the displayed image. Luminance is a measurement of the light intensity (brightness) emitted from the surface of the monitor and is expressed in units of candela per square meter (cd/m^2). There are different measurements of luminance: ambient, minimum, maximum, and ratio. Ambient luminance is the light that reflects off the display surface from the room (ambient) lighting after the monitor has been turned off and is added into the other measurements. Primary display monitors should exhibit a minimum luminance of 1.0 cd/m^2 and a maximum luminance of 350 cd/m^2. A ratio of the maximum to minimum luminance, luminance ratio (LR), is recommended to be greater than 250, and a display monitor with an LR of 350 has improved image contrast.

 IMPORTANT RELATIONSHIP

Display Monitor Luminance

Luminance is a measurement of the light intensity (brightness) emitted from the surface of the monitor and is expressed in cd/m^2. Primary display monitors should exhibit a minimum luminance of 1.0 cd/m^2 and a maximum luminance of 350 cd/m^2. A ratio of the maximum to minimum luminance, LR, is recommended to be greater than 250, and a display monitor with an LR of 350 has improved image contrast.

The contrast resolution of a digital image is determined by the pixel bit depth. A digital imaging system capable of displaying 16,384 shades of gray (14 bits) requires a monitor capable of displaying a large grayscale range. Monitors that have a higher LR can display a greater grayscale range. It is recommended that display monitors used for image interpretation have a minimum graphic bit depth of 8, yielding 256 shades of gray. The display of digital images must be consistent among the monitors used within and outside the health care system. The Grayscale Standard Display Function (GSDF) is the Digital Imaging and Communications in Medicine (DICOM) recommended standard for consistent display characteristics such as grayscale appearance and image quality and should not vary by more than 10%.

Additional concerns of display monitors include geometrical distortions, such as concavity and convexity; veiling glare, which adversely affects image contrast; and display noise, which is typically a result of statistical fluctuations or luminance differences in the image. Routine quality control (QC) of the display monitor is just as important as monitoring the digital imaging acquisition and processing devices. Box 6.1 describes QC methods for evaluating display monitors.

A display workstation is simply a desktop computer that allows for the retrieval and viewing of medical images from one of the modalities or storage components of the MIMPS previously known as PACS (Fig. 6.28). The quality and function of one of these stations depend on the user. The software loaded to each display station also depends on the user. For general viewing by noninterpreting physicians and other health care workers, a very basic package allowing minimal adjustment may be

---

BOX 6.1 Quality Control Check: Display Monitor

Quality control (QC) test devices for evaluating the performance of the display monitor include the American Association of Physicists in Medicine (AAPM) TG18-QC test pattern (Fig. 6.26) and the Society of Motion Picture and Television Engineers (SMPTE) test pattern (Fig. 6.27). Several aspects of a display monitor can be evaluated with these test patterns, including geometric distortion, luminance, resolution, contrast resolution, noise, and veiling glare.

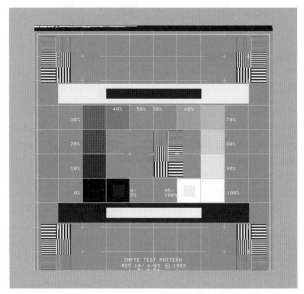

Fig. 6.27 The Society of Motion Picture and Television Engineers (SMPTE) test pattern. (Bushong SC. *Radiologic Science for Technologists.* 9th ed. St. Louis, MO: Mosby, Inc., an affiliate of Elsevier Inc.; 2008.)

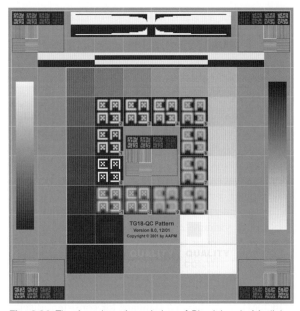

Fig. 6.26 The American Association of Physicists in Medicine (AAPM) TG18-QC test pattern. (Johnston J, Fauber T. *Essentials of Radiographic Physics and Imaging.* St. Louis: Mosby, Inc., an affiliate of Elsevier Inc.; 2012.)

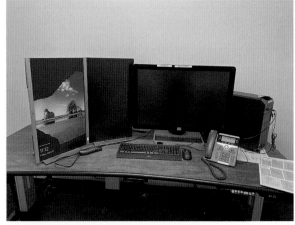

Fig. 6.28 Primary workstation. A digital display monitor workstation. (© Bellin Memorial Hospital, Inc.)

all that is available. QC display stations and interpreting stations have greater functions and capabilities, such as more advanced image manipulation, windowing (level and width), annotation, patient demographic information, cropping, panning, and magnification (zoom). Even among radiographers, each may have access to different functions protected by login and password to limit which aspects of a medical image may be changed, and by whom, to prevent accidentally damaging or negatively altering the record.

 IMPORTANT RELATIONSHIP

Display Workstation

A display workstation is simply a desktop computer that allows for the retrieval and viewing of medical images from one of the modalities or storage components of the MIMPS. QC display stations and interpreting stations have greater function and capability, such as more advanced image manipulation, windowing (level and width), annotation, patient demographic information, cropping, panning, and magnification (zoom). In addition to other standards of communication, DICOM specifies information included as a header on digital images (DICOM header), and the GSDF is the DICOM recommended standard for consistent display characteristics, such as grayscale appearance and image quality.

ARTIFICIAL INTELLIGENCE

Because the nature of a medical image is now digital, any number of computer processing applications can be used to enhance the interpretability of these images. Considerable research is now being conducted to use Artificial Intelligence (AI) algorithms for image analysis. Much of this research has been done outside of the medical world and is now being applied to medical images. AI originated within the US Department of Defense through its worldwide network of satellite communications to monitor global intelligence activities. Using pattern-recognition computer programs, AI is used extensively now in other nonmilitary applications, including medical imaging.

Because medical images are essentially digital data sets with defined boundaries, specific patterns can be recognized on these images that can represent identified pathological conditions. AI is now being used as an aid for radiologists in image interpretation for disease states

such as chest tumors and pneumonia, bone fractures, and breast lesions. AI will not replace the radiologist but assist in the routine interpretive tasks they face on an everyday basis. AI will eventually be used by radiographers as an aide to assess image quality in terms of collimation, positioning, and signal-to-noise levels.

HEALTH INFORMATION MANAGEMENT

The modern health care industry is very information-intensive and comprises a variety of care and treatment settings. Safe and efficient patient care through coordination and communication of the patient's health information acquired in the delivery of health care services is vital in all areas of health care. Interprofessional collaboration using technology systems such as electronic health records (EHRs), health information systems, and medical image management and processing system (MIMPS), previously known as picture archival and communication system (PACS), require interoperability and management within and outside of the health care facility. Health information management (HIM) within health care facilities involves the management of the medical record and the data contained within. Health informatics and data management, components of the HIM system, are utilized in the acquisition, storage, retrieval, transmission, and display of digital images from multiple imaging modalities and throughout health care systems.

Health Informatics

Health informatics, also known as radiology informatics within radiology departments, involves data management for radiology services both within and outside the health care system. Data management is a complex system-wide effort to ensure that people, equipment, and processes are in place to expand health care information transmission and improve patient outcomes. Radiology informatics facilitates the accurate collection, documentation, maintenance, and protection of health information. Maintaining complete and accurate health information is essential for clinical diagnosis and reimbursement. Application of electronic health information with digital images (acquisition, storage, retrieval, and transmission) and their interpretation are also referred to as clinical informatics.

Personal information is gathered from patients as they seek treatment in a health care facility that will assist in their care. Information gathered from the patient (demographic data, relevant history, service type, etc.) is

IMPORTANT RELATIONSHIP

Health Information Management

Health information management (HIM) involves the management of the medical record and the data contained within. Health informatics and data management, components of the HIM system, are utilized in the acquisition, storage, retrieval, transmission, and display of digital images from multiple imaging modalities and throughout health care systems.

considered protected health information (PHI). PHI is any health-related information collected, stored, and shared that can be linked to an individual. This information is collected and stored in the hospital information system (HIS). The HIS allows for patient information to be shared within the health care facility during service. Individual medical record numbers are assigned by the HIS and allow for the tracking/management of the patient's electronic medical record (EMR).

The electronic medical record (EMR) is a digital record with the ability to store, share, and manage PHI within a single health care organization. The patient's EMR is specific to the health care organization and can be shared with other organizations in its entirety or individual components. Similar to the EMR, the electronic health record (EHR) also manages patient medical information but is a comprehensive record that comprises medical records from all health care encounters throughout the patient's lifetime, regardless of the institution or organization. To ensure interoperability across organizations, the American Recovery and Reinvestment Act (ARRA) and the Health Information Technology for Economic and Clinical Health Act (HITECH) of 2009 set requirements for EMR/EHR systems and provided financial incentives to health care organizations to adopt EMR/EHR systems. These acts also required health care organizations to switch over to certified EMR/EHR system by January 2015.

Multiple components of the HIS integrate with the EMR as part of an encompassing system that manages several departmental operations. If the patient is scheduled for a radiology procedure, some of this patient information becomes a part of the radiology workflow and is stored in the radiology information system (RIS). The RIS is similar to the HIS but specific to the radiology department and manages the radiology examination orders, scheduling, tracking, billing, and reports. All this electronic information (demographics, relevant history, digital images, and interpretations) is included

in the HIS/RIS and available to authorized personnel at the facility. The RIS communicates with the medical image management and processing system (MIMPS) to share the required patient information to be documented on the images acquired.

 IMPORTANT RELATIONSHIP

Patient Health Information

Patient health information is collected and stored in the HIS and shared with the RIS. The EMR is a digital record with the ability to store, share, and manage PHI within a single health care organization. The EHR is the system for patient PHI that can be shared outside the facility and among many health care systems.

The organization's revenue cycle includes activities from benefit verification to reimbursement for services provided, involving patient registration, claim submission, and communication with patients, insurance providers, and government payers such as Medicare and Medicaid. The facilitation of accurate billing and reimbursement procedures based on health diagnosis and treatment is achieved using a comprehensive coding system. The International Classification of Diseases, 10th Edition, Clinical Modification (ICD-10-CM) is the coding system used for diagnosis coding, whereas the Current Procedural Terminology, 4th Edition (CPT-4) is used for ambulatory and ancillary services (radiology, laboratory, etc.). These medical codes are integrated into the HIS as part of the collective patient medical record.

Medical Image Management and Processing System

The medical image management and processing system (MIMPS), previously known as picture archival and communication system (PACS), is a networked computer system designed for digital imaging that can receive, store, archive, distribute, and display digital images. The major components of MIMPS include the control server, digital communication networks, the imaging modality systems, display workstations, and archival capabilities for storage and retrieval. An integrated local network system links the control server with the RIS/HIS so that images, patient data, and interpretations can be viewed simultaneously by people at different workstations (Fig. 6.29). The interoperability of the MIMPS with the various modality vendors is achieved using a high-level universal communication standard. Integrating the Healthcare Enterprise (IHE)

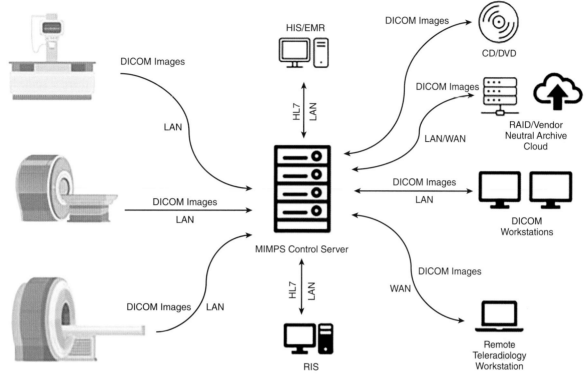

Fig. 6.29 Communication among the computer system for medical information (RIS), the computer systems for imaging (input modalities), radiology workstations, and archive storage. Referring physicians can receive radiology reports, patient data, and radiographic images through the Internet (web server). *DICOM,* Digital Imaging and Communications in Medicine; *EMR,* electronic medical record; *HIS,* hospital information system; *HL7,* Health Level Seven standard; *LAN,* local area network; *MIMPS,* medical image management and processing system; *RAID,* redundant array of independent disks; *RIS,* radiology information system; *WAN,* wide area network. (Courtesy Chad Dall).

"is an initiative by health care professionals and industry to improve the way computer systems in health care share information. IHE promotes the coordinated use of established standards such as DICOM and HL7 (discussed later) to address specific clinical needs in support of optimal patient care."

IMPORTANT RELATIONSHIP

Medical Image Management and Processing System

A MIMPS is a computer system designed for digital imaging that can receive, store, archive, distribute, and display digital images. The major components of MIMPS include the imaging modalities, digital communication networks, display workstations, and archival capabilities for storage and retrieval.

The Health Level Seven standard (HL7) is a communication standard for the sharing of medical information across various platforms. Digital Imaging and Communications in Medicine (DICOM) is an international communication standard for information sharing between MIMPS and imaging modalities to transmit, store, retrieve, print, process, and display medical imaging information. All digital image data management equipment should conform to the DICOM standard so that the features and performance of the devices are consistent throughout health care systems. In addition to other standards of communication, DICOM specifies information included as a header on digital images (DICOM header), such as accession number, patient name and identification number, date and time of examination, radiographic procedure, and the total number of images in the study. It is also recommended that exposure-related information be included in the DICOM header such as kVp, milliamperage-seconds, exposure indicator, and any post- or reprocessing of the digital data. Connectivity and communication among these systems are necessary for radiology to realize the full potential of health informatics. A well-integrated system would improve patient care through cost-effective, reliable, secure, and timely delivery of patient and digital imaging information.

As the complexity of medical images and patient data has grown, new approaches to MIMPS have developed. One challenge has been the expansion and maintenance of MIMPS systems, access to and storage of data over decades, and changes in vendors. One latest solution is the trend toward vendor neutral archives (VNAs). VNAs allow for images and data from different systems and in different formats to be stored using a singular system on a common infrastructure. VNAs may be used as replacements for existing MIMPS to avoid very expensive transition costs. They may also be used to consolidate several systems that exist within a single facility or across a system of facilities. Another growing trend is the creation of health information exchanges (HIEs) for the purpose of sharing patient information across systems and creating networks of service providers.

 IMPORTANT RELATIONSHIP

Digital Communication Networks

DICOM is an international communication standard for information sharing between MIMPS and imaging modalities to transmit, store, retrieve, print, process, and display medical imaging information. HL7 is a communication standard for medical information. Connectivity and communication among these systems are necessary for radiology to realize the full potential of imaging informatics. IHE promotes the coordinated use of established standards such as DICOM and HL7 to address specific clinical needs in support of optimal patient care.

Transmission, Storage, and Archives

Transmission of medical images and patient information occurs across digital electronic lines, fiberoptic cables, and wireless networks. The physical and/or wireless networks are considered part of the organization's local area network (LAN). The LAN allows data to be transferred with the organization, to outside clinics, and to a radiologist's home. A wide area network (WAN) is utilized if data/images are required at remote locations. To improve the transmission/storage of the imaging

data, compression may be used. Image compression can be reversible or irreversible. Reversible (lossless) compression means that there is no loss of image data as the image is restored at the end user. Lossless compression ratios are typically around 2:1, but under 8:1. Irreversible (lossy) compression means that there is some loss of image data as the image is restored at the end user. Lossy compression ratios are typically above 10:1. However, lossy compression is only used in circumstances in which the loss of image data does not impact the job of the end user. If lossy compression is used, the image displayed must be labeled as such, and irreversible compression cannot be used for diagnostic interpretation of images.

Teleradiology is the transmission of diagnostic images for interpretation outside the facility (offsite) from where the imaging data are acquired. It can be used for preliminary diagnosis for referring and emergency department physicians, after-hours interpretations and consultations, and subspecialty expertise (e.g., cardiovascular or neuroradiology), and it can solve manpower issues such as vacations and rural facilities having limited access to radiologists. There is a growing number of large companies using radiologists for teleradiology both within and outside the United States. Although teleradiology can address many of the challenges facing imaging departments as described previously, some issues need to be considered. Because of the nature of teleradiology, communication among imaging professionals could be problematic with radiologists interpreting imaging studies outside the radiology department (teleradiologists). Communication needs between teleradiologists and imaging professionals include providing timely and relevant patient information, the ability to answer questions regarding the procedure, and maintaining standard QC practices. The practice of teleradiology should maintain the same high standards, safety, and quality as onsite radiology services.

Poor communication can have negative results and impact the patient's care and outcomes. Having onsite radiologists is preferred; however, there is a need for teleradiology, and it can serve a valuable supplemental purpose in radiology.

One of the biggest challenges of a MIMPS is storage. With increasingly complex modalities supplying large image files (data sets) into the system, the demand for storage is ever increasing. Policies and procedures are also needed to effectively and appropriately archive

IMPORTANT RELATIONSHIP

Teleradiology

Teleradiology is the practice of diagnostic image interpretation outside the facility (offsite) from where the imaging data are acquired. Communication needs between teleradiologists and the imaging professionals include providing timely and relevant patient information, the ability to answer questions regarding the procedure, and maintaining standard QC practices. The practice of teleradiology should maintain the same high standards, safety, and quality as onsite radiology services.

IMPORTANT RELATIONSHIP

Transmission, Storage, and Archive

Transmission devices need to have the capacity to handle the volume of images delivered within a reasonable time frame and can check for errors. To improve the transmission of the data to the various end users of the imaging data, compression (reversible or irreversible) may be used. Policies and procedures are also needed to effectively and appropriately archive (current and previous exams) and store digital image data for years.

(current and previous exams) and store digital image data according to local, state, and federal guidelines. This is further complicated by patient privacy requirements to store images and data for years. There is also the requirement to address disaster recovery processes. This involves the requirement to duplicate all files in a remote location so that recovery is possible in the event of a disaster and the primary files are lost.

To support this ever-increasing demand for data storage, MIMPS has taken on new directions. Traditionally, MIMPS was created and maintained within the organization's facilities. This required the purchase and maintenance of very large computer servers and storage systems. The current trend is to address storage space and expense using cloud-based technology. This process consists of offsite storage and servers supported by a secure network and third-party vendor. This also shifts the disaster recovery requirement to the vendor along with the maintenance and storage equipment purchase. The user basically pays for the service and storage space as needed. There are also hybrid versions of this configuration whereby the facility maintains current image and patient data in house and longer-term storage externally or in the cloud. The advantages and disadvantages of these systems are facility dependent and change according to the imaging volume, facility size, and need for access. The speed of access, for example, depends on connectivity speed and file size.

QC activities are equally important for digital image data management. According to the ACR-AAPM-SIIM *Technical Standard for Electronic Practice of Medical Imaging* (revised in 2022), "Any facility using a digital image data management system must have documented policies and procedures for monitoring and evaluating the effective management, safety, and proper performance of acquisition, digitization, processing, compression, transmission, display, archiving, and retrieval functions of the system. The quality assurance (QA) program should be designed to maximize the quality and accessibility of diagnostic information." QC activities for digital image data management, including compression, transmission, archiving, and retrieval functions of the system, are beyond the scope of this textbook and would most likely be performed by an imaging informatics professional.

PRIVACY AND SECURITY

Security of PHI is an ever-growing concern in health care and radiology. Policies and procedures must be in place and adhered to by all health care workers who have access to PHI. The Health Insurance Portability and Accountability Act (HIPAA) and the HITECH Act are two key legislative acts that have sought to protect PHI from being misused and to provide privacy and security to PHI. HIPAA, enacted in 1996, included privacy and security provisions to ensure that PHI is used appropriately, timely, and securely by all who have access. HIPAA was enacted before the vast adoption of EMRs, so updated provisions were added to ensure electronic transfers of PHI were also held to the same privacy and security standards. The HITECH Act enhanced these protections as health care organizations were required to transition to EMR/EHR systems. Some of the recommended procedures that will ensure privacy and security include anonymization (patient-identifiable information is removed from the PHI) if performing clinical research, authentication to verify the identity of the user of PHI, authorization (which limits access to PHI for approved users only, maintaining records of interactions with PHI [auditing]), and confidentiality to prevent unauthorized users from access to PHI. Cybersecurity protocols are increasingly being updated by health care IT departments to protect against hacking and other malicious attempts at accessing PHI.

Radiographers have routine access to PHI in the performance of their duties and must take responsibility for adhering to the department's policies and procedures. Patients must be confident that radiographers have the skills to perform their imaging procedures and believe that their PHI will be secure.

 IMPORTANT RELATIONSHIP
Security of Patient Health Information

Radiographers have routine access to PHI in the performance of their duties and must take responsibility for adhering to the department's policies and procedures. Patients must be confident that radiographers have the skills to perform their imaging procedures and believe that their PHI will be secure.

CHAPTER SUMMARY

- Digital image processing refers to various computer algorithms applied to digital data for the purpose of optimizing the image for display.
- Preprocessing operations such as bad or dead pixel and flat-fielding corrections occur to the raw data to prepare the image data for processing and display.
- A histogram is a graphic representation of the image data set. This graph includes all the pixel values that represent the latent image after the software corrections were applied. The location of the graph along the x-axis represents image brightness levels, and the shape represents image contrast or grayscale.
- Histogram analysis is an important processing technique used to identify the edges of the image and assess the exposure data (pixel values) prior to image processing and display.
- The computer analyzes the histogram using processing algorithms and compares it with a preestablished (reference) histogram specific to the anatomic part being imaged.
- Automatic rescaling is a process employed to maintain a consistent image brightness despite over- or underexposure.
- During histogram analysis, the exposure indicator provides a numerical value that indicates the level of radiation exposure to the digital IR.
- The deviation index (DI) is a value that reflects the difference between the desired or target exposure to the IR (EI_t) and the actual exposure to the IR (EI). A DI of 0 would indicate there is no difference between the desired (EI_t) and the actual EI and is the recommended target exposure.
- After histogram analysis, LUTs provide the means to alter the original pixel values to improve the brightness and contrast of the image.

- Default and postprocessing functions, such as electronic masking, window level and width, subtraction, contrast enhancement, edge enhancement, smoothing, and equalization, allow manipulation of the displayed image.
- Display monitors provide soft-copy viewing of digital radiographs. Primary monitors are high-quality monitors used for diagnostic interpretation.
- Important features regarding display monitors used for interpretation include viewing conditions, matrix size, pixel pitch, luminance, luminance ratio (LR), and contrast resolution.
- QC activities are important to ensure that digital radiographic equipment and systems are functioning properly.
- Health informatics and data management, components of health information management (HIM) system, are utilized in the acquisition, storage, retrieval, transmission, and display of digital images from multiple imaging modalities and throughout health care systems.
- Patient health information is collected and stored in the HIS and shared with the RIS.
- The EMR is a digital record with the ability to store, share, and manage PHI within a single health care organization. The EHR is the system for patient PHI that can be shared outside the facility and among many health care systems.
- MIMPS, previously known as PACS, is a networked computer system designed for digital imaging modalities and can receive, store, archive, distribute, and display digital images.
- DICOM is a communication standard for information sharing among MIMPS, imaging modalities, and display, and HL7 is a communication standard for medical information.

- Image compression may be used to transmit image data but should be reversible so no data are compromised or lost prior to diagnostic interpretation.
- Teleradiology is the practice of diagnostic image interpretation outside the facility from where the imaging data are acquired.
- Digital data storage has challenges and requires policies and procedures to effectively and appropriately archive and store digital image data.
- HIPAA and HITECH Act establish standards for PHI privacy protection.
- Security protocols regarding PHI must be in place and adhered to by all health care workers.

REVIEW QUESTIONS

1. Which of the following is defined as a graphic representation of the pixel values?
   A. Automatic rescaling
   B. Values of interest
   C. Histogram
   D. Exposure indicator
2. What process is employed to maintain consistent digital image brightness for over- or underexposure?
   A. Automatic rescaling
   B. Histogram
   C. Exposure indicator
   D. Lookup tables (LUTs)
3. Which of the following is not a numerical value indicating the level of radiation exposure to a digital image receptor (IR)?
   A. Sensitivity number
   B. Exposure indicator
   C. Window level
   D. Deviation index
4. Which of the following may impact the location and shape of the histogram?
   A. Exposure technique
   B. Positioning
   C. Collimation
   D. A and C only
   E. A, B, and C
5. What digital process alters image brightness and grayscale to improve the visibility of anatomic structures?
   A. Automatic rescaling
   B. Histogram analysis
   C. Exposure indicator
   D. LUTs
6. Maintaining a low level of ambient lighting can improve soft-copy viewing of digital images.
   A. True
   B. False
7. Display monitors used for soft-copy viewing of digital images should have _____.
   A. increased ambient lighting
   B. decreased matrix size
   C. high pixel pitch
   D. high luminance
8. Which of the following is not a function during postprocessing of a displayed digital image?
   A. Histogram analysis
   B. Electronic masking
   C. Windowing
   D. Edge enhancement
9. Wider window width _____.
   A. increases brightness
   B. decreases brightness
   C. increases contrast
   D. decreases contrast
10. What postprocessing technique suppresses image noise?
    A. Edge enhancement
    B. Equalization
    C. Inversion
    D. Smoothing
11. What is the communication standard for information sharing between MIMPS and imaging modalities?
    A. DQE
    B. DICOM
    C. SMPTE
    D. HL7
12. The deviation index (DI) is a value that reflects the difference between the desired or target exposure to the IR and the actual exposure to the IR.
    A. True
    B. False
13. A DI of −1.75 reflects underexposure to the IR.
    A. True
    B. False

14. Which of the following may occur if the DI value is greater than +3.0 SD?
    A. Excessive noise visible
    B. Saturation
    C. Patient overexposure
    D. B and C only
    E. A, B, and C
15. What standard was enacted to protect privacy and confidentiality of patient's health information?
    A. Digital Imaging and Communication in Medicine
    B. Health Insurance Portability and Accountability Act
    C. Protected health information
    D. Integrating the Healthcare Enterprise
16. To transmit and store large amounts of imaging data efficiently, what may occur?
    A. Compression
    B. Disaster recovery
    C. Teleradiology
    D. Vendor neutral archives
17. Which system is designed to receive, store, archive, and transmit digital images?
    A. Electronic Medical Record
    B. Health Level Seven
    C. Medical Image Management and Processing System
    D. Health Information System
18. What international standard is required to transmit, store, retrieve, and display medical images across health care systems?
    A. Digital Imaging and Communication in Medicine
    B. Health Level Seven
    C. Current Procedural Terminology
    D. Health Information Management
19. Which information system supports radiology-specific patient information regarding orders, reports, and schedules?
    A. HIS
    B. HIM
    C. PHI
    D. RIS
20. Which information system is a digital record of private health information regarding a patient's health within a health care organization?
    A. Electronic Medical Record
    B. Medical Image Management and Processing System
    C. Teleradiology
    D. Data Management

Exposure Technique Factors

CHAPTER OUTLINE

OBJECTIVES

After completing this chapter, the reader will be able to perform the following:

1. Define all the key terms in this chapter.
2. State all the important relationships in this chapter.
3. Explain the relationship between milliamperage (mA) and exposure time with radiation production and image receptor (IR) exposure.
4. Calculate changes in milliamperage and exposure time to change or maintain exposure to the IR.
5. Describe the effect of changes in mA and exposure time on digital images.
6. Recognize how to correct factors for an exposure error.
7. Explain how kilovoltage peak (kVp) affects radiation production and IR exposure.
8. Calculate changes in kVp to change or maintain exposure to the IR.
9. Describe the effects of changes in kVp on digital images.
10. Recognize the factors that affect spatial resolution and distortion.
11. Calculate changes in mAs for changes in source-to-image-receptor distance.
12. Calculate the magnification factor and the percent of magnification.
13. Describe the use of grids and beam restriction and their effect on IR exposure and image quality.
14. Calculate changes in mAs when adding or removing a grid.
15. Recognize patient factors that may affect IR exposure.
16. Identify exposure factors that can affect patient radiation exposure.
17. State exposure technique modifications for the following considerations: body habitus and patient thickness.
18. Recognize the importance of exposure techniques in imaging for pathology.

KEY TERMS

15% rule
body habitus
direct square law
exposure maintenance formula

inverse-square law
magnification factor (MF)
object-to-image-receptor distance
    (OID)

source-to-image-receptor distance
    (SID)
source-to-object distance (SOD)

In Chapter 3, variables that affect both the quantity and the quality of the x-ray beam are presented. Milliamperage (mA) and exposure time affect the quantity of radiation produced, and kilovoltage affects both the quantity and the quality. Chapter 4 emphasizes that a good-quality radiographic image accurately represents the anatomic area of interest. The characteristics evaluated for displayed image quality are brightness, contrast, spatial resolution, distortion, and noise. This chapter focuses on exposure techniques and the use of accessory devices and their effects on the radiation reaching the patient, image receptor (IR), and the image processed and displayed. Radiographers have the responsibility of selecting the combination of exposure factors to produce a diagnostic-quality image. Knowledge of how these factors affect the exposure to the IR individually and in combination assists radiographers in producing a radiographic image with the amount of information desired for a diagnosis. In addition, the patient should be exposed to the least amount of radiation reasonable to produce a diagnostic-quality image. This chapter discusses all the primary and secondary factors and their effects on the radiation reaching the patient, IR, and displayed image quality.

PRIMARY FACTORS

The primary exposure technique factors selected by the radiographer on the control panel are mA, exposure time (s), and kilovoltage peak (kVp). Depending on the type of control panel, mA and exposure time may be selected separately or combined as one factor, milliamperage-seconds (mAs). Regardless, it is important to understand how changing each factor separately or in combination affects the radiation reaching the patient, IR, and the radiographic image.

Milliamperage and Exposure Time

The quantity of radiation exiting the x-ray tube and reaching the patient affects the amount of remnant radiation reaching the IR. The product of mA and exposure time is directly proportional to the quantity of x-rays produced (Fig. 7.1). When an anatomic part is adequately penetrated, the exposure to the IR will increase in proportion to increases in the quantity of x-rays (Fig. 7.2). Conversely, when the quantity of x-rays is decreased, the exposure to the IR decreases. Therefore exposure to the IR can be increased or decreased by adjusting the amount of radiation (mAs).

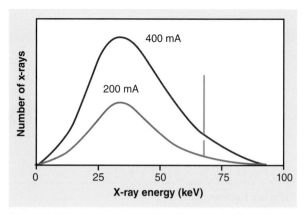

Fig. 7.1 Milliamperage *(mA)* and radiation quantity. Changing the mA results in a proportional change in the quantity (amplitude) of x-rays produced. (From Johnston JN, Fauber TL. *Essentials of Radiographic Physics and Imaging.* 3rd ed. St. Louis: Mosby; 2020.)

✚ IMPORTANT RELATIONSHIP
mAs and Quantity of Radiation

> As mAs increases, the quantity of radiation reaching the IR increases. As mAs decreases, the amount of radiation reaching the IR decreases.

Because the mAs is the product of mA and exposure time, increasing either mA or time will increase the amount of radiation exposure to the IR.

▶ MATHEMATICAL APPLICATION
Adjusting mA or Exposure Time

> 200 mA × 0.100 s = 20 mAs
>
> To increase the mAs to 40, one could use the following formulas:
>
> 400 mA × 0.100 s (100 ms) = 40 mAs
>
> 200 mA × 0.200 s (200 ms) = 40 mAs

As demonstrated in the Mathematical Application, mAs can be doubled by doubling either the mA or the exposure time. A change in either milliamperage (mA) or exposure time (s) proportionally changes the mAs. To maintain the same mAs, the radiographer must increase the mA and proportionally decrease the exposure time or decrease the mA and proportionally increase the exposure time.

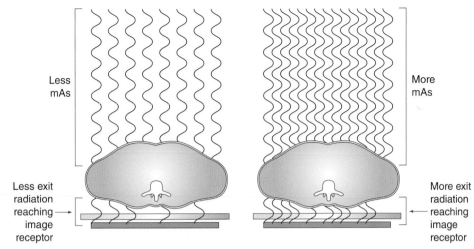

Fig. 7.2 Milliamperage-seconds *(mAs)* and radiation exposure. As the quantity of x-rays is increased mAs, the exposure to the image receptor (IR) proportionally increases.

 IMPORTANT RELATIONSHIP

mA and Exposure Time

mA and exposure time have an inverse proportional relationship when maintaining the same mAs.

 MATHEMATICAL APPLICATION

Adjusting mA and Exposure Time to Maintain mAs

200 mA × 100 ms (0.100 s) = 20 mAs

To maintain mAs, use the following formulas:

400 mA × 50 ms (0.050 s) = 20 mAs

100 mA × 200 ms (0.200 s) = 20 mAs

It is important for the radiographer to determine the appropriate mAs level needed to produce a diagnostic image. This is not an easy task because there are so many variables that can affect the required mAs. For example, single-phase generators produce less radiation with the same mAs compared with high-frequency generators. A patient's age, the general condition of the patient, and the thickness of the anatomic part also affect the mAs required for a procedure. In addition, IRs respond differently for a given mAs level. For example, mAs does not control the amount of brightness displayed within a digital image. Digital IRs can detect a wider range of radiation intensities (wider dynamic range) exiting the patient and therefore are not dependent on the mAs. However, exposure errors can adversely affect the quality of a digital image. If the mAs is too low (low exposure to the digital IR), image brightness is adjusted during computer processing (histogram automatic rescaling) to achieve the desired level. Even after adjusting the level of brightness, there may be increased quantum noise visible within an image (Fig. 7.3). If the selected mAs is too high (high exposure to the digital IR), the brightness can also be adjusted; however, the patient will receive more radiation than necessary. Therefore it is critical that the radiographer select mAs values that will reduce quantum noise and maintain reasonable patient radiation exposures. Because digital IRs have a wide dynamic range, mAs values need to be carefully selected to stay within the image receptor's exposure latitude.

 IMPORTANT RELATIONSHIP

mAs and Digital Image Brightness

The level of mAs does not control image brightness when using digital IRs. During computer processing, image brightness is maintained when the mAs is too low or too high. A lower-than-needed mAs produces an image with increased quantum noise, and a higher-than-needed mAs exposes a patient to unnecessary radiation.

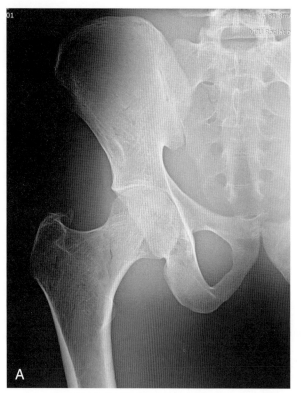 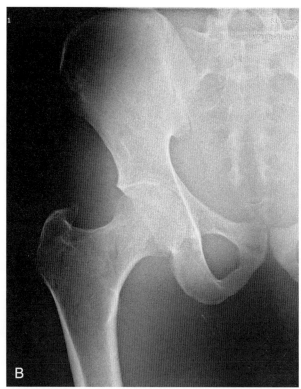

Fig. 7.3 A, Radiographic image obtained with high milliamperage-seconds (mAs) showing decreased quantum noise. **B,** Radiographic image obtained with low mAs showing increased quantum noise. (From Johnston JN, Fauber TL. *Essentials of Radiographic Physics and Imaging,* 3rd ed. St. Louis: Elsevier; 2020.)

The brightness of a digital image can be altered during image processing; hence, information about the exposure to the IR is important. Manufacturers of each type of digital system specify the expected range of x-ray exposure sufficient to produce a quality image. An exposure indicator (EI) is displayed on the processed image to indicate the level of x-ray exposure received (remnant exposure) on the digital IR. It is important for the radiographer to consider the indicated value because exposure errors, as previously stated, affect the quality of the digital image and the radiation dose to the patient. Exposure errors are not obvious by simply looking at the digital image because the digital data are normalized to provide images with diagnostic brightness levels (Fig. 7.4). Most manufacturers of digital IRs suggest a range for the exposure indicator on the basis of the radiographic procedure. If the exposure indicator value falls outside this range, exposure to the digital IR, image quality, and patient exposure could be affected.

⚡ IMPORTANT RELATIONSHIP
Exposure Indicator Value

An exposure indicator (EI) is displayed on the processed digital image to indicate the level of x-ray exposure received (remnant exposure) on the IR. If the exposure indicator value falls outside the manufacturer's suggested range, exposure to the digital IR, image quality, and patient exposure could be affected.

Generally, for repeat images necessitated by exposure errors, the mAs is adjusted by a factor of 2; therefore a minimum change involves doubling or halving the mAs. If a radiographic image must be repeated because of another error, such as positioning, the radiographer may use the opportunity to make an adjustment in the exposure to the IR to produce an image of diagnostic quality. A radiographic image repeated because of insufficient or excessive exposure requires a change in mAs by a factor of at least 2.

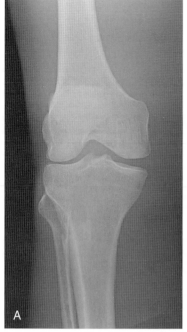 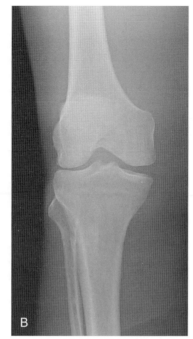 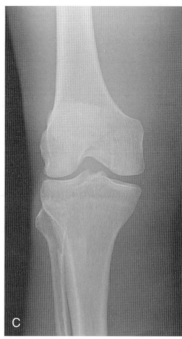

Fig. 7.4 Exposure errors can be computer adjusted to maintain image brightness. **A,** Image created with sufficient milliamperage-seconds (mAs). **B,** Image created with insufficient mAs, resulting in increased quantum noise visible. **C,** Image created with excessive mAs, resulting in decreased quantum noise visible. The exposure indicator value reflected the exposure errors to the image receptor (IR) for images **B** and **C**. (From Johnston JN, Fauber TL. *Essentials of Radiographic Physics and Imaging*. 3rd ed. St. Louis: Mosby; 2020.)

To best visualize the anatomic area of interest, the selected mAs must produce a sufficient amount of radiation that reaches the IR. An excessive or insufficient amount of mAs adversely affects image quality and patient radiation exposure. The radiographer should be diligent in monitoring exposure indicator values to ensure that quality images are obtained with the lowest reasonable radiation dose to the patient.

Kilovoltage Peak

The kVp affects the exposure to the IR because it alters the amount and penetrating ability of the x-ray beam (Fig. 7.5). The area of interest must be adequately penetrated before the mAs can be adjusted to produce a quality radiographic image. When adequate penetration is achieved, increasing the kVp further results in more radiation reaching the IR (Fig. 7.6). In addition to affecting the amount of radiation exposure to the IR, the kVp affects subject contrast displayed in the image.

 IMPORTANT RELATIONSHIP

kVp and the Radiographic Image

Increasing or decreasing the kVp changes the amount of radiation exposure to the IR and the subject contrast produced within the image.

Kilovoltage Peak and Exposure to the Image Receptor

Because kVp affects the amount of radiation reaching the IR, its effect on the digital image is similar to the effect of mAs. Assuming that the anatomic part has been adequately penetrated, too much radiation reaching the IR (within reason) will still produce a digital image with the appropriate level of brightness as a result of computer adjustment during image processing; however, the patient will be overexposed. Similarly, too little radiation reaching the IR (within reason) will produce a digital image with the appropriate level of brightness,

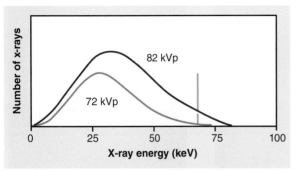

Fig. 7.5 Kilovoltage peak *(kVp)* and radiation quality and quantity. Increasing the kVp from 72 to 82 shows an increase in the quantity of x-rays (amplitude), and the x-ray emission shifts toward the right, indicating an increase in the energy or quality of the beam. (From Johnston JN, Fauber TL. *Essentials of Radiographic Physics and Imaging.* 3rd ed. St. Louis: Mosby; 2020.)

but the increased quantum noise will decrease the image quality.

A diagnostic-quality image (Fig. 7.7A) was produced using 70 kVp at 2 mAs. Fig. 7.7B was produced using 50 kVp at 2 mAs, and Fig. 7.7C was produced using 93 kVp at 2 mAs. Although the brightness was adjusted by the computer, the exposure indicator for each of the images varied greatly and reflected the exposure to the IR. When a kVp that is too low is selected, the brightness is adjusted, but quantum noise may be visible. Additionally, when a kVp that is too high is selected without an appropriate decrease in mAs, the image brightness is adjusted, but patient exposure may be increased because of increased x-ray quantity and scatter within the tissues. Although brightness can be

computer adjusted when using a kVp that is too high, increased scatter radiation can also reach the IR and may adversely affect image quality.

Excessive or insufficient radiation exposure to the digital IR, as a result of the mAs or kVp, should be reflected in the exposure indicator value.

◢ IMPORTANT RELATIONSHIP
Exposure Errors in Digital Imaging

kVp and mAs exposure errors should be reflected in the exposure indicator value; however, image brightness can be maintained during computer processing.

❗ RADIATION PROTECTION ALERT
Excessive Radiation Exposure and Digital Imaging

Although the computer can adjust image brightness for technique exposure errors, routinely using more radiation than required for the procedure in digital radiography unnecessarily increases patient exposure. Even though the digital system can adjust overexposure, it is an unethical practice to knowingly overexpose a patient.

Kilovoltage is not a factor that is typically manipulated to vary the amount of IR exposure because the kVp also affects subject contrast. However, it is sometimes necessary to manipulate the kVp to maintain the required exposure to the IR. For example, using mobile x-ray equipment may limit the choice of mAs settings, and the

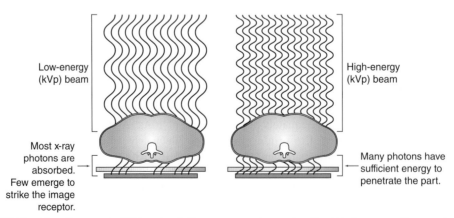

Fig. 7.6 The kilovoltage peak *(kVp)* and radiation exposure. Increasing the kVp increases the penetrating power of the radiation and increases the exposure to the image receptor (IR).

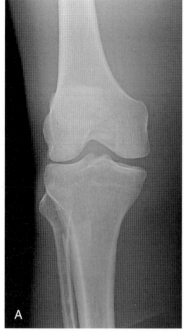
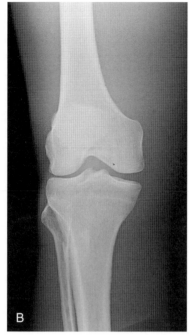
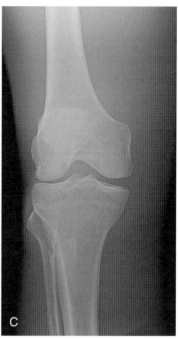

Fig. 7.7 A, Image produced using 70 kVp at 2 mAs. **B,** Image produced using 50 kVp at 2 mAs, resulting in higher subject contrast and computer adjusted to maintain brightness but increased quantum noise visible. **C,** Image produced using 93 kVp at 2 mAs, resulting in lower subject contrast and computer adjusted to maintain brightness, but patient exposure is increased. (From Johnston JN, Fauber TL. *Essentials of Radiographic Physics and Imaging.* 3rd ed. St. Louis: Mosby; 2020.)

radiographer must adjust the kVp to maintain sufficient exposure to the IR.

Maintaining or adjusting exposure to the IR can be accomplished with kVp using the 15% rule. The 15% rule states that increasing or decreasing the kVp by 15% has the same effect as doubling or halving the mAs; for example, increasing the kVp from 82 to 94 (15%) produces a similar exposure to the IR as increasing the mAs from 10 to 20.

⚡ IMPORTANT RELATIONSHIP

kVp and the 15% Rule

A 15% increase in kVp has the same effect on exposure to the IR as doubling the mAs. A 15% decrease in kVp has the same effect on exposure to the IR as halving the mAs.

Increasing the kVp by 15% increases the exposure to the IR unless the mAs is decreased. In addition, decreasing the kVp by 15% decreases the exposure to the IR unless the mAs is increased.

▶ MATHEMATICAL APPLICATION

Using the 15% Rule

To increase exposure to the IR, multiply the kVp by 1.15 (original kVp + 15%):

$$75\,kVp \times 1.15 = 86\,kVp$$

To decrease exposure to the IR, multiply the kVp by 0.85 (original kVp − 15%):

$$75\,kVp \times 0.85 = 64\,kVp$$

To maintain exposure to the IR, when increasing the kVp by 15% (kVp × 1.15), divide the original mAs by 2:

$$75\,kVp \times 1.15 = 86\,kVp \text{ and } mAs / 2$$

When decreasing the kVp by 15% (kVp × 0.85), multiply the mAs by 2:

$$75\,kVp \times 0.85 = 64 \text{ and } mAs \times 2$$

! RADIATION PROTECTION ALERT

kVp/mAs

Whenever possible, a higher kilovoltage and lower mAs should be used to reduce patient exposure. Increasing kilovoltage requires a lower mAs to maintain the desired exposure to the IR and decreases the radiation dose to the patient. For example, changing kVp from 75 to 86 when imaging a pelvis is a 15% increase and would require half the mAs needed for the original 75 kVp. Higher kVp increases the beam penetration; therefore less radiation is needed to achieve a desired exposure to the IR.

Kilovoltage Peak and Subject Contrast

Altering the penetrating power of the x-ray beam affects its absorption and transmission through the anatomic tissue being radiographed. Higher kVp increases the penetrating power of the x-ray beam and results in less absorption and more transmission in the anatomic tissues, which results in less variation in the x-ray intensities exiting the patient (lower subject contrast). As a result, images with lower subject contrast (more shades of gray) are produced (Fig. 7.8). When a low kVp is used, the x-ray beam penetration is decreased, resulting in more absorption and less transmission, which results in greater variation in the x-ray intensities exiting the patient. This produces an image with higher subject contrast (Fig. 7.9).

IMPORTANT RELATIONSHIP

kVp and Subject Contrast

A high kVp results in less absorption and more transmission in anatomic tissues, which results in less variation in the x-ray intensities exiting (remnant) the patient, producing lower subject contrast. A low kVp results in more absorption and less x-ray transmission in the anatomic tissues but with more variation in the x-ray intensities exiting the patient, resulting in higher subject contrast.

Changing the kVp affects the beam's absorption and transmission as it interacts with anatomic tissue; however, using a higher kVp reduces the total number of interactions and increases the amount of x-rays transmitted. In these interactions, Compton scattering increases, photoelectric absorption decreases, and more scatter exits the patient. It is important to understand that in addition to

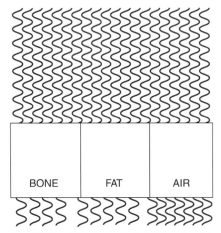

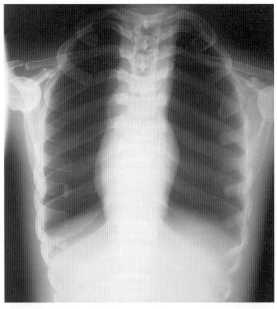

Fig. 7.8 The kilovoltage peak (kVp) and exit-beam intensities. Higher kVp increases the penetrating power of the x-ray beam and results in less absorption and more transmission in the anatomic tissues, resulting in less variation in the x-ray intensities exiting the patient. As a result, images with lower subject contrast are produced.

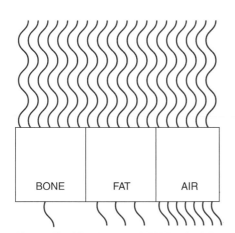
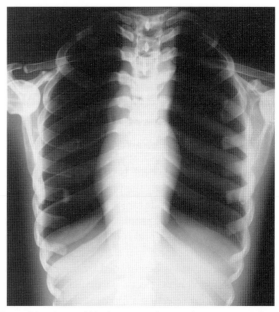

Fig. 7.9 The kilovoltage peak (kVp) and exit-beam intensities. Lower kVp decreases the x-ray beam penetration, resulting in more absorption and less transmission, which results in greater variation in the x-ray intensities exiting the patient. As a result, images with higher subject contrast are produced.

kVp affecting subject contrast, increasing kVp increases the amount of scatter (fog) reaching the IR and consequently decreases radiographic contrast.

 IMPORTANT RELATIONSHIP

Kilovoltage, Scatter Radiation, and Displayed Image Contrast

At higher kVp, more x-rays are transmitted with fewer overall interactions; however, a greater proportion of the interactions are from Compton scattering (fog) than photoelectric absorption, which decreases the displayed image contrast. Decreasing the kVp will increase photoelectric absorption and increase the number of interactions, but the proportion of Compton scattering (fog) will decrease compared with photoelectric absorption, increasing radiographic contrast.

The level of radiographic contrast desired and the kVp selected depend on the type and composition of the anatomic tissue, the structures that must be visualized, and (to some extent) the diagnostician's preference. For most anatomic regions, an accepted range of kVp provides an appropriate level of subject contrast. As long as the selected kVp is sufficient to penetrate the anatomic part, image contrast can be further adjusted by the computer to display the desired contrast for the anatomic region.

Radiographic images are generally not repeated because of contrast errors. If a repeat radiograph is necessary and kVp is to be adjusted either to increase or decrease the level of subject contrast, the 15% rule provides an acceptable method of adjustment. In addition, whenever a change of 15% is made in the kVp to maintain the exposure to the IR, the radiographer must adjust the mAs by a factor of 2. The selection of kVp alters its absorption and transmission through the anatomic part, regardless of the type of IR used; therefore the selection of kVp is important to producing a quality image. Exposure techniques using higher kVp with lower mAs settings are recommended in digital imaging because display contrast is primarily controlled during computer processing. Computer processing and windowing the displayed image will overcome some of the negative impacts of higher kVp, such as lower subject contrast and increase in scatter radiation.

SECONDARY FACTORS

Many secondary or influencing factors affect the x-ray beam, amount of radiation reaching the IR, and image quality. It is important for the radiographer to understand their effects individually and in combination.

Focal Spot Size

On the control panel, the radiographer can select whether to use a small or large focal spot size. On some equipment, the focal spot size will be automatically applied based on the mA selected. The physical dimensions of the focal spot on the anode target in x-ray tubes used in standard radiographic applications usually range from 0.5 to 1.2 mm. Small focal spot sizes are usually 0.5 or 0.6 mm, and large focal spot sizes are usually 1 or 1.2 mm. Focal spot size is determined by the filament size. When radiographers select a particular focal spot size, they are actually selecting a filament size that is energized during x-ray production. Lower mA settings are associated with the small filament, whereas higher mA settings energize the large filament. Focal spot size is an important consideration for the radiographer because it affects spatial resolution (Fig. 7.10).

IMPORTANT RELATIONSHIP
Focal Spot Size and Spatial Resolution

As focal spot size increases, unsharpness increases and spatial resolution decreases; as focal spot size decreases, unsharpness decreases and spatial resolution increases.

Generally, the smallest available focal spot size should be used for every exposure. However, exposure is limited for a small focal spot size. When a small focal spot is used, the heat created during the x-ray exposure is concentrated into a smaller area and could cause tube damage. The radiographer must weigh the importance of improved spatial resolution for a particular examination or anatomic part against the amount of radiation exposure used. Modern radiographic x-ray generators are equipped with safety circuits that prevent an exposure from being made if the exposure exceeds the tube-loading capacity for the selected focal spot size. Repeated exposures made just under the x-ray tube limit over a long period can still jeopardize the life of the x-ray tube.

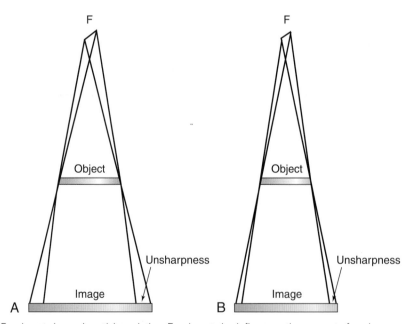

Fig. 7.10 Focal spot size and spatial resolution. Focal spot size influences the amount of unsharpness recorded in the image. As focal spot size changes, so does the amount of unsharpness. **A,** Larger focal spot. **B,** Smaller focal spot.

Source-to-Image-Receptor Distance

The distance between the radiation source and the IR, known as source-to-image-receptor distance (SID), affects the amount of radiation reaching the patient and subsequently the IR. Because of the divergence of the x-ray beam, the intensity of the radiation varies at different distances.

This relationship between distance and x-ray beam intensity is best described by the inverse-square law. This law states that the intensity of an x-ray beam is inversely proportional to the square of the distance from the source. Because beam intensity varies as a function of the square of the distance, SID affects the quantity of radiation reaching the IR. As SID increases, the x-ray intensity becomes spread over a larger area, decreasing the overall intensity of the x-ray beam reaching the IR (Fig. 7.11).

 IMPORTANT RELATIONSHIP

SID and X-ray Beam Intensity

As SID increases, the x-ray beam intensity becomes spread over a larger area. This decreases the overall intensity of the x-ray beam reaching the IR.

 MATHEMATICAL APPLICATION

Inverse-Square Law Formula

$$\frac{I_1}{I_2} = \frac{(D_2)^2}{(D_1)^2}$$

If the intensity of radiation at an SID of 100 cm (40 inches) is equal to 4 mGy (400 mR), what is the intensity of radiation when the distance is increased to 180 cm (72 inches)?

$$\frac{4\ \text{mGy}}{X} = \frac{(180\ \text{cm})^2}{(100\ \text{cm})^2};\ 4\ \text{mGy} \times 10{,}000 = 40{,}000$$

$$= 32{,}400\ X;\ \frac{40{,}000}{32{,}400} = X;\ 1.24\ \text{mGy} = X$$

Because increasing the SID decreases x-ray beam intensity, the mAs must be accordingly increased to maintain proper exposure to the IR. When the SID is decreased, the beam intensity increases; therefore the mAs must be accordingly decreased to maintain proper exposure to the IR.

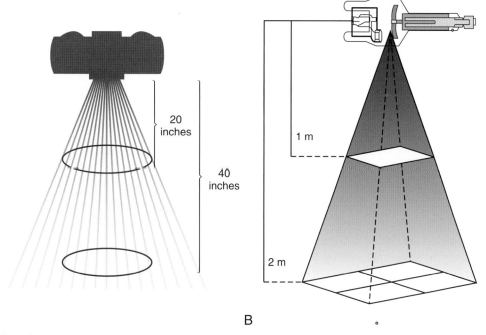

Fig. 7.11 Source-to-image-receptor distance (SID) and radiation intensity. **A** and **B,** Changing SID and its effect on the intensity of the x-ray beam reaching the image receptor (IR, **A**) and on the divergence of the beam **B.**

IMPORTANT RELATIONSHIP

SID and mAs

> Increasing the SID requires the mAs to be increased to maintain exposure to the IR, and decreasing the SID requires a decrease in the mAs to maintain exposure to the IR.

Maintaining consistent radiation exposure to the IR when the SID is altered requires the mAs to be adjusted to compensate. The direct square law or exposure maintenance formula provides a mathematical calculation for adjusting the mAs when changing the SID.

 MATHEMATICAL APPLICATION

Direct Square Law or Exposure Maintenance Formula

$$\frac{mAs_1}{mAs_2} = \frac{(SID_1)^2}{(SID_2)^2}$$

Optimal exposure to the IR is achieved at an SID of 40 inches (100 cm) using 25 mAs. The SID must be increased to 72 inches (180 cm). What adjustment of mAs is needed to maintain exposure to the IR?

$$\frac{25}{X} = \frac{(40)^2}{(72)^2};\ 1600X = 129,600;\ \frac{129,600}{1600};$$
$$X = 81\ mAs$$

Optimal exposure to the IR is achieved at an SID of 120 cm (48 inches) using 15 mAs. The SID must be decreased to 90 cm (36 inches). What adjustment of mAs is needed to maintain exposure to the IR?

$$\frac{15}{X} = \frac{(120\ cm)^2}{(90\ cm)^2};\ 14,400X = 121,500; = \frac{121,500}{14,400}$$
$$= X = 8.4\ mAs$$

Standard distances are used in radiography to provide more consistency in radiographic quality. Most diagnostic radiography is performed at an SID of 100, 120, or 180 cm (40, 48, or 72 inches). Certain circumstances, such as trauma or mobile radiography, do not permit the use of standard distances. In these circumstances, the radiographer must determine the change needed in the mAs to obtain a quality radiograph. When a 180 cm

(72 inch) SID cannot be used, adjusting the SID to 140 cm (56 inches) requires about half the mAs. When a 100 cm (40 inch) SID cannot be used, adjusting the SID to 140 cm (56 inches) requires twice the mAs. This quick method of calculating mAs changes should produce sufficient exposure to the IR.

In addition to altering the intensity of radiation, SID affects size distortion and spatial resolution. As the distance between the source and the IR increases, the diverging x-rays become more perpendicular to the object being radiographed and thus reduce the size distortion (magnification) produced on the image (Fig. 7.12).

 IMPORTANT RELATIONSHIP

SID, Size Distortion, and Spatial Resolution

> As SID increases, size distortion (magnification) decreases, and spatial resolution increases; as SID decreases, size distortion (magnification) increases, and spatial resolution decreases.

Standard distances for SID are used in radiography to accommodate equipment limitations. Except for chest and cervical spine radiography, a 100 (40 inch) or 120 cm (48 inch) SID is standard. A greater 180 cm

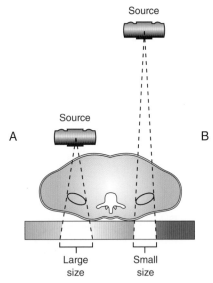

Fig. 7.12 Source-to-image-receptor distance (SID) and size distortion. **A** and **B,** A long SID creates less magnification than a short SID. The image in **A** is larger than that in **B** because the object is closer to the source.

(72 inch) SID, such as that used for chest imaging, decreases the magnification of the heart and records its size more accurately. Increasing the SID from the standard distances may be recommended for positions that result in increased object-to-image-receptor distance (OID). For example, increase the SID when imaging the cervical spine between 150 (60 inches) and 180 cm (72 inches) for positions that have an increased OID, such as the lateral and oblique positions. Increasing the SID improves spatial resolution.

Object-to-Image-Receptor Distance

When distance is created between the object being radiographed and the IR, known as object-to-image-receptor distance (OID), a decrease in beam intensity may result. As the exit radiation continues to diverge, less overall intensity of the x-ray beam reaches the IR. Decreasing the exposure to the IR may require an increase in the mAs to compensate.

When sufficient distance between the object and IR exists, an air gap is created, also reducing the amount of scatter radiation from striking the IR (Fig. 7.13). Whenever the amount of scatter radiation reaching the IR is reduced, the displayed image contrast is increased. The amount of OID required to increase image contrast depends in part on the percentage of scatter radiation exiting the patient. For anatomic areas that produce a high percentage of scatter radiation, more OID is needed to increase image contrast than for anatomic areas that produce less scatter.

In addition to affecting the intensity of radiation reaching the IR, the OID affects the amount of size distortion (magnification) and spatial resolution. Optimal spatial resolution is achieved when the OID is zero. However, this OID cannot realistically be achieved in radiographic imaging because there is always some distance created between the area of interest and the IR. As the remnant beam leaves the patient, it continues to diverge. When distance is created between the area of interest (within the body) and the IR, the diverging exit beam records the anatomic part with increased size distortion or magnification (Fig. 7.14).

 IMPORTANT RELATIONSHIP

OID, Size Distortion, and Spatial Resolution

Increasing the OID increases magnification and decreases the spatial resolution, whereas decreasing the OID decreases magnification and increases the spatial resolution.

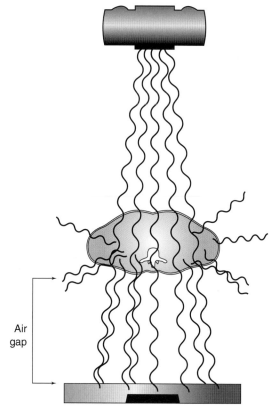

Fig. 7.13 Object-to-image-receptor distance (OID) and air gap. The distance created between the object and the image receptor (IR) reduces the amount of scattered radiation reaching the IR.

OID is a factor that affects the intensity of radiation reaching the IR, image contrast, magnification, and spatial resolution. The distance between the area of interest and the IR has the greatest effect on the amount of size distortion. The radiographer must position the area of interest as close to the IR as possible to minimize the distortion. Although the OID necessary to adversely affect image quality has not been standardized, the radiographer should minimize the OID whenever possible. In certain situations, it is difficult to minimize OID because of factors or conditions beyond the radiographer's control. In these situations, size distortion can still be reduced by increasing the SID.

Calculating Magnification

To observe the effect of distance (SID and OID) on size distortion, it is necessary to consider the magnification factor (MF). This factor indicates how much size distortion or magnification is demonstrated on a radiographic

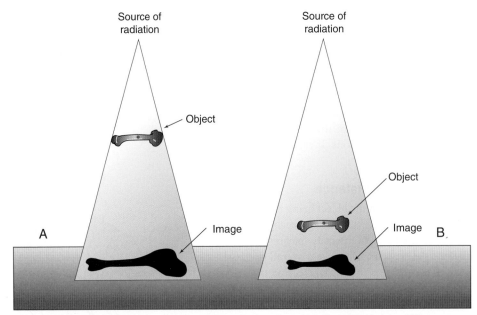

Fig. 7.14 Object-to-image-receptor distance (OID) and size distortion. **A** and **B,** A long OID creates more magnification than a short OID. The image in **A** is larger than that in **B** because the object is farther from the image receptor (IR).

image. The MF can be mathematically expressed by the following formula:

$$MF = SID \div SOD$$

Source-to-object distance (SOD) refers to the distance from the x-ray source (focal spot) to the object being imaged. SOD can be mathematically expressed as follows:

$$SOD = SID - OID$$

SOD is demonstrated in Fig. 7.15.

An MF of 1 indicates no magnification, meaning that the image size matches the true object size. True object size on an image is impossible to achieve because some magnification exists on every image. MF values greater than 1 can be expressed as percentages of magnification. For example, an MF of 1.15 indicates that the image size is 15% larger than the object size.

 MATHEMATICAL APPLICATION

Magnification Factor

An anteroposterior projection (AP) of the knee is produced with an SID of 100 cm (40 inches) and an OID of 7.5 cm (3 inches). SOD is equal to 92.5 cm (37 inches). What is the MF?

$$SOD = SID - OID, \quad MF = \frac{100}{92.5}; \quad MF = 1.081$$
$$92.5 = 100 - 7.5$$

In the case of the Mathematical Application for MF, an MF of 1.081 means that the image size is 8.1% (0.081 × 100) larger than the true object size. It should be noted that the MF computed here is a minimum. A 7.5 cm (3 inch) OID implies that the posterior surface of a patient's knee was 7.5 cm (3 inches) away from the IR for an AP projection. Anatomy that is anterior to the posterior surface of the knee, such as the patella, is farther away from the IR and is magnified even more.

Central Ray Alignment

Shape distortion of the anatomic area of interest can occur from inaccurate central ray (CR) alignment of the x-ray tube, the part being radiographed, or the IR. Any misalignment of the CR among these three factors alters the shape of the part recorded on the image.

For example, Fig. 7.16 demonstrates shape distortion when the anatomic part and the IR are misaligned. In addition, shape distortion can occur if the CR of the

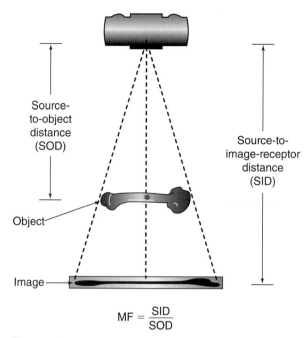

$$MF = \frac{SID}{SOD}$$

Fig. 7.15 Source-to-object distance *(SOD)*. The SOD is the distance between the source of the x-ray and the object being radiographed. *MF,* Magnification factor; *SID,* source-to-image-receptor distance.

primary beam is not directed to enter or exit the anatomy as required for the particular projection or position (off-centering). This shape distortion occurs because the path of individual photons in the primary beam becomes more divergent as the distance increases from the CR. The radiographer must properly control alignment of the x-ray tube, part, and IR and must properly direct the CR to minimize shape distortion. A right-angle (orthogonal) relationship between the IR, part, and CR is preferred to minimize shape distortion. In addition to creating shape distortion, CR angulation and misalignment of the tube, part, and IR could affect the exposure to the IR. For example, when the CR is angled, the distance between the source of the radiation and the IR is increased. Generally, when the CR is angled, the SID is accordingly decreased to maintain exposure to the IR. If misalignment occurs among the tube, part, or IR, the distance from the source of radiation and the IR or the part, and the IR, could be increased or decreased. This change could affect the amount of exposure to the IR, and the mAs may need adjustment.

IMPORTANT RELATIONSHIP
Minimizing Shape Distortion

A right-angle (orthogonal) relationship between the IR, part, and CR is preferred to minimize shape distortion. Shape distortion of the anatomic area of interest can occur from inaccurate central ray (CR) alignment of the x-ray tube, the part being radiographed, or the IR. Any misalignment of the CR among these three factors alters the shape of the part recorded on the image.

Grids

A radiographic grid is a device that is placed between the part of interest and the IR to absorb scatter radiation exiting the patient. Limiting the amount of scatter radiation that reaches the IR improves the quality of the displayed image. Much of the scatter radiation exiting the patient does not reach the IR when absorbed by a grid (Fig. 7.17). The effect of less scatter, or unwanted exposure, on the image is to increase the displayed image contrast. Grids are typically used only when the anatomic part is 10 cm (4 inches) or greater in thickness, and more than 60 kVp is needed for the exam.

IMPORTANT RELATIONSHIP
Grids, Scatter, and Contrast

Placing a grid between the anatomic part and the IR absorbs scatter radiation exiting the patient and increases the displayed image contrast.

The more efficient a grid is in absorbing scatter, the greater is its effect on radiographic contrast. Grids also absorb a certain amount of the transmitted radiation exiting the patient and therefore reduce the amount of radiation reaching the IR.

IMPORTANT RELATIONSHIP
Grids and IR Exposure

Adding, removing, or changing a grid requires an adjustment in mAs to maintain radiation exposure to the IR.

When grids are used, the mAs must be adjusted to maintain exposure to the IR. In addition, the more efficient a grid is in absorbing scatter, the greater is the increase in

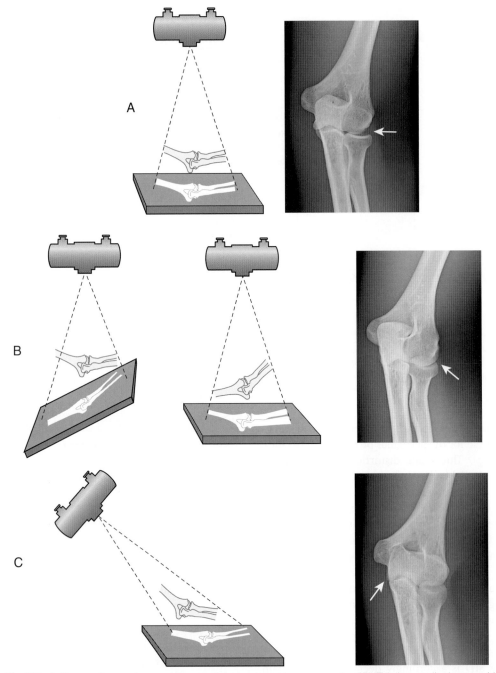

Fig. 7.16 A, Proper alignment among the x-ray tube, part, and image receptor (IR). This is a quality image with minimal distortion. Note the proper alignment of the radial head with the capitulum in the image. **B,** Improper alignment among the x-ray tube, part, and IR. The illustration on the *left* shows the IR misaligned to the part, and the one on the *right* shows the part not parallel to the IR. This image has a distorted shape because of misalignment of the part and IR. Note the improper alignment of the radial head with the capitulum in the image. **C,** Improper alignment among the x-ray tube, part, and IR. This image has shape distortion because of the central ray not being perpendicular to the part. Note the elongation of the olecranon process. (From Johnston JN, Fauber TL. *Essentials of Radiographic Physics and Imaging.* 3rd ed. St. Louis: Mosby; 2020.)

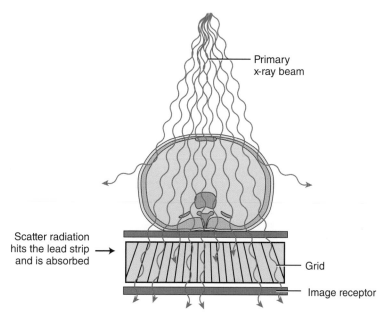

Fig. 7.17 Grids and scatter absorption. When a grid is used, much of the scatter radiation toward the image receptor (IR) is absorbed. (From Johnston JN, Fauber TL. *Essentials of Radiographic Physics and Imaging.* 3rd ed. St. Louis: Mosby; 2020.)

mAs. The grid conversion formula is a mathematical formula for adjusting the mAs for changes in the type of grid.

When a grid is added, the radiographer must multiply the mAs by the correct grid conversion factor (Table 7.1) to compensate for the decrease in exposure. When a grid is removed, the mAs must be divided by the correct conversion grid factor to compensate for the increase in exposure. When the grid ratio is changed, the following formula should be used to adjust the exposure:

$$\frac{mAs_1}{mAs_2} = \frac{\text{Grid conversion factor}_1}{\text{Grid conversion factor}_2}$$

▶ MATHEMATICAL APPLICATION

Adjusting mAs for Changes in the Grid

A quality radiographic image is obtained using 5 mAs at 70 kVp without using a grid. What new mAs is needed when adding a 12:1 grid to maintain the same exposure to the IR?

$$\frac{5 \text{ mAs}}{X} = \frac{1}{5}; \ 1X = 25; \ X = 25 \text{ mAs}$$

The new mAs produces an exposure comparable to the IR without the grid.

TABLE 7.1 Grid Conversion Chart

Grid Ratios	Grid Conversion Factor (GCF)
No grid	1
5:1	2
6:1	3
8:1	4
12:1	5
16:1	6

❗ RADIATION PROTECTION ALERT

Grid Selection

Decisions regarding the use of a grid and grid ratio should be made by balancing image quality and patient protection. To keep patient exposure as low as reasonable, grids should be used only when appropriate, and the grid ratio should be the lowest that would provide sufficient contrast improvement.

It is important to note that brightness can be computer adjusted when the mAs is not properly adjusted for adding or changing a grid (Fig. 7.18). However, without proper mAs adjustment when adding or changing a grid,

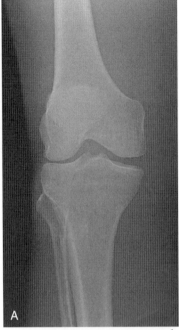
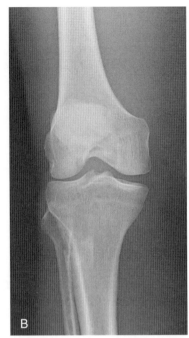
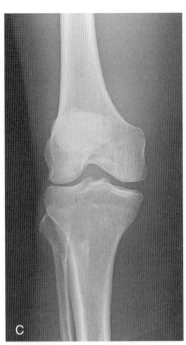

Fig. 7.18 A, A quality image created without a grid. **B,** An image created with a grid but no adjustment in milliamperage-seconds (mAs). This image has higher contrast but increased quantum noise visible. **C,** Image created with a grid and appropriate mAs adjustment. This image has higher contrast than image **A** and less quantum noise visible than image **B**. (From Johnston JN, Fauber TL. *Essentials of Radiographic Physics and Imaging.* 3rd ed. St. Louis: Elsevier; 2020.)

increased quantum noise or unnecessary patient radiation exposure could be the result.

Grid construction and efficiency are discussed in greater detail in Chapter 8.

Exposure Conversions

Situations may arise where the radiographer is tasked with changing several exposure factors simultaneously, such as during mobile imaging or in the operating room. The ability to make an adjustment in mAs correctly when changing multiple factors, that is, SID, grid, and kVp, is an important critical thinking skill.

▶ MATHEMATICAL APPLICATION

Exposure Conversions

A. Calculate the new exposure factor required to maintain a similar exposure to the IR as in the initial exposure technique.

Initial Exposure Technique		New Exposure Technique
25 mAs		_____ mAs
80 kVp	TO	68 kVp

Calculations:
  a. Decrease from 80 to 68 kVp = 15% decrease (80 × 0.85)
  b. Increase mAs × 2, 25 × 2 = 50 mAs
  c. The new mAs needed to maintain a similar exposure to the IR as the initial technique is 50

B. Calculate the new exposure factor required to maintain a similar exposure to the IR as in the initial exposure technique.

Initial Exposure Technique		New Exposure Technique
25 mAs		_____ mAs
80 kVp	TO	68 kVp
12:1 grid		No grid

Calculations:
a. Decrease from 80 to 68 kVp = 15% decrease (80 × 0.85)
b. Increase mAs × 2, 25 × 2 = 50 mAs
c. Remove 12:1 grid (GCF 5) = decrease mAs, 50 ÷ 5 = 10 mAs
d. The new mAs needed to maintain a similar exposure to the IR as the initial technique is 10

C. Calculate the new exposure factor required to maintain a similar exposure to the IR as in the initial exposure technique.

Initial Exposure Technique		New Exposure Technique
25 mAs		_____ mAs
80 kVp	TO	68 kVp
12:1 grid		No grid
40 inch (100 cm) SID		54 inch (135 cm) SID

Calculations:
a. Decrease from 80 to 68 kVp = 15% decrease (80 × 0.85)
b. Increase mAs × 2, 25 × 2 = 50 mAs
c. Remove 12:1 grid (GCF 5) = decrease mAs, 50 ÷ 5 = 10 mAs
d. Increase SID from 40 to 54 inches $= \dfrac{10 \text{ mAs}}{X} = \dfrac{40^2}{54^2}$; 10 × 2916 = 1600 X; = 29,160 ÷ 1600 = 18.2 = X
e. The new mAs needed to maintain a similar exposure to the IR as the initial technique is 18.2

Beam Restriction

Any change in the size of the x-ray field alters the amount of tissue irradiated. A larger field size (decreasing collimation) increases the amount of tissue irradiated, causing more scatter radiation to be produced, thus increasing the amount of radiation reaching the IR. The increased amount of scatter (fog) reaching the IR results in less radiographic contrast. Conversely, a smaller field size (increasing collimation) reduces the amount of tissue irradiated, the amount of scatter radiation produced, and the amount of radiation reaching the IR. The decreased amount of scatter radiation reaching the IR results in higher radiographic contrast but requires an increase in the mAs. The effect of collimation is greater when imaging large anatomic areas, performing examinations without a grid, and using a high kVp.

 IMPORTANT RELATIONSHIP
Beam Restriction and IR Exposure

Changes in beam restriction alter the amount of tissue irradiated and therefore affect the amount of exposure to the IR. The effect of collimation is greater when imaging large anatomic areas, performing examinations without a grid, and using a high kVp.

! RADIATION PROTECTION ALERT
Beam Restriction

In performing a radiographic examination, the radiographer should be aware of the anatomic area of interest and limit the x-ray field size to just beyond this area. Collimating to the appropriate field size is a basic method for protecting patients from unnecessary exposure.

Generator Output

Exposure techniques and radiation output depend on the type of generator used. Generators with more efficient output, such as three-phase or high-frequency units, require lower exposure technique settings to produce an image comparable with single-phase units (Fig. 7.19). The radiographer must be aware of the generator output when using different types of equipment, especially when

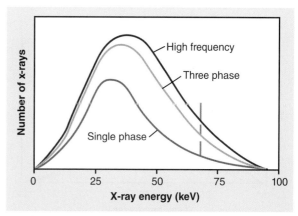
Fig. 7.19 Generators and radiation output. The quantity (amplitude) and the quality (shift to the right) of the x-ray beam are increased when using high-frequency and three-phase generators because they are more efficient in x-ray production. (From Johnston JN, Fauber TL. *Essentials of Radiographic Physics and Imaging.* 3rd ed. St. Louis: Mosby; 2020.)

performing examinations in different departments. For example, imaging a knee using a single-phase generator requires more mAs than imaging a knee using a three-phase generator. In addition, x-ray generators must be periodically calibrated to ensure that they are producing consistent radiation output.

Tube Filtration

Small variations in the amount of tube filtration should not have any effect on radiographic quality. Variability of the x-ray tube filtration should be checked as a part of routine quality control checks on the radiographic equipment. X-ray tubes with excessive or insufficient filtration may affect image quality. Increasing the amount of tube filtration increases the ratio of higher-penetrating x-rays to lower-penetrating x-rays. As a result, the average energy of the x-ray beam has been increased and can increase the amount of scatter radiation reaching the IR. The increased x-ray energy (kVp) and scatter production decrease radiographic contrast. In addition, increasing the tube filtration decreases the quantity of radiation reaching the patient (Fig. 7.20). Insufficient tube filtration increases the quantity of radiation and decreases the ratio of higher-penetrating x-rays to lower-penetrating x-rays. As a result, the average energy of the x-ray beam has been decreased, which can decrease the amount of scattered radiation reaching the IR. The decreased x-ray energy (kVp) and scatter production increase radiographic contrast. The amount

of tube filtration should not vary greatly, and therefore small changes would not have a visible effect on radiographic contrast. With digital IRs, an x-ray beam with a higher average energy is preferred and new filtration options are being employed. These include copper (Z# 29) as a filter material in combination with aluminum. The addition of copper reduces entrance skin exposure (ESE) with no visible loss in contrast resolution.

 IMPORTANT RELATIONSHIP

Tube Filtration, Radiation Quantity, and Average Energy

Increasing tube filtration decreases radiation quantity and increases the average energy of the x-ray beam. Decreasing tube filtration increases radiation quantity and decreases the average energy of the x-ray beam.

Compensating Filters

When imaging an anatomic area that varies greatly in tissue thickness, a compensating filter (discussed in Chapter 3) can be placed in the primary beam to produce a more uniform exposure to the IR. The use of compensating filters requires an increase in the mAs to maintain the overall exposure to the IR. The amount of increase in the mAs depends on the thickness and type of compensating filter. In addition, the use of a compensating filter increases the exposure to the patient and is not typically used in routine radiography.

PATIENT FACTORS

Body Habitus

Body habitus refers to the general form or build of the body, including its size. It is important for the radiographer to consider body habitus when establishing exposure techniques. There are generally four types of body habitus: sthenic, hyposthenic, hypersthenic, and asthenic (Fig. 7.21).

The sthenic body habitus is commonly called a *normal* or *average* build. The hyposthenic type refers to a similar type of body habitus as sthenic but with a tendency toward a more slender and taller build. Together, the sthenic and hyposthenic types of body habitus are, in terms of establishing radiographic techniques, classified as *normal* or *average* for the adult population.

Hypersthenic and asthenic body habitus types are more extreme. The hypersthenic body habitus refers to

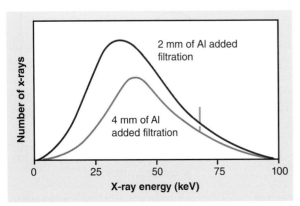

Fig. 7.20 Tube filtration and radiation output. Increasing beam filtration decreases the quantity (amplitude) and increases the quality (shift to the right) of the x-ray beam. *Al*, Aluminum. (From Johnston JN, Fauber TL. *Essentials of Radiographic Physics and Imaging.* 3rd ed. St. Louis: Mosby; 2020.)

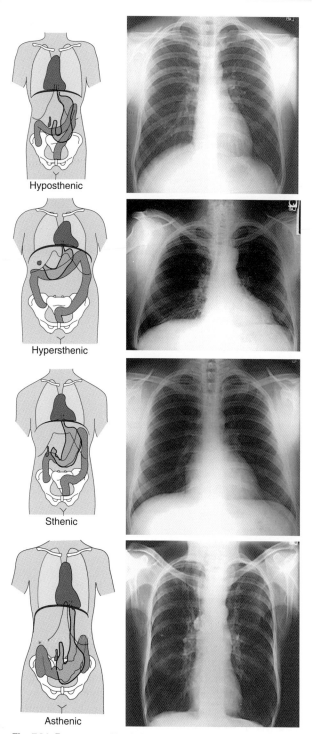

Hyposthenic

Hypersthenic

Sthenic

Asthenic

Fig. 7.21 Four types of body habitus. (From Johnston JN, Fauber TL. *Essentials of Radiographic Physics and Imaging.* 3rd ed. St. Louis: Mosby; 2020.)

a large, stocky build. These individuals have thicker part sizes compared with sthenic or hyposthenic individuals, so the exposure factors for their radiographic examinations are higher.

Asthenic refers to a very slender body habitus, and exposure factors for asthenic individuals are at the low end of technique charts because their respective part sizes are thinner than those of sthenic and hyposthenic individuals.

Part Thickness

The thickness of the anatomic part being imaged affects the amount of x-ray beam attenuation that occurs. A thick part absorbs more radiation, whereas a thin part transmits more radiation. Maintaining the exposure to the IR when imaging a thicker part requires the mAs to be accordingly increased (Fig. 7.22). In addition, when a thinner anatomic part is being radiographed, the mAs must be accordingly decreased.

Because x-rays are exponentially attenuated, a general guideline is that for every change in part thickness of 4 to 5 cm (1.6–2 inches), the radiographer should adjust the mAs by a factor of 2 (Fig. 7.23). For example, a diagnostic image is obtained using 20 mAs on an anatomic part measuring 18 cm (7 inches). The same anatomic part is radiographed in another similar patient and it measures 23 cm (9 inches). What new mAs is needed to expose the IR? Because the part thickness increased by 5 cm (2 inches), the original mAs is multiplied by 2, yielding 40 mAs. If the same part in another patient measures 28 cm (11 inches), what new mAs is needed? Because the part thickness increased by another 5 cm (2 inches), the mAs is multiplied by 2, yielding 80 mAs. This mAs is four times greater than that for the original patient's anatomic part, which measured 10 cm (4 inches) less.

As the thickness of a given type of anatomic tissue increases, the amount of scattered radiation increases, and radiographic contrast decreases. Using a higher kVp for a thicker part only adds to the increase in scatter radiation. Increased scatter radiation would continue degrading the quality of the displayed image because it creates fog, which decreases the contrast.

The amount of displayed image contrast achieved is also influenced by the composition of the anatomic part to be radiographed. As mentioned in Chapter 4, subject contrast is a category of radiographic contrast. The thickness of the tissue, effective atomic number, and cell

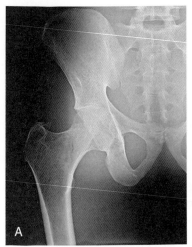
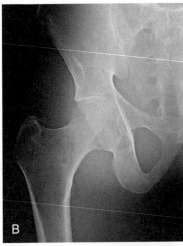
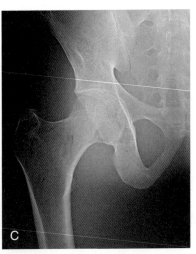

Fig. 7.22 A, A quality image. **B,** Image created with added thickness and no milliamperage-seconds (mAs) adjustment, which results in increased quantum noise visible. **C,** Image created with added patient thickness and appropriate mAs adjustment, which results in decreased quantum noise visible. (From Johnston JN, Fauber TL. *Essentials of Radiographic Physics and Imaging.* 3rd ed. St. Louis: Elsevier, Inc.; 2020.)

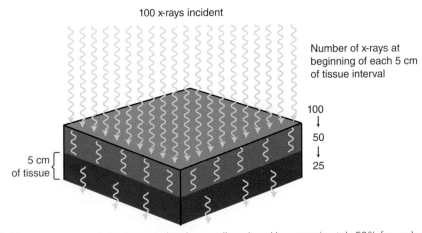

Fig. 7.23 X-rays are exponentially attenuated and generally reduced by approximately 50% for each 4 to 5 cm (1.6–2 inches) of tissue thickness. (From Johnston JN, Fauber TL. *Essentials of Radiographic Physics and Imaging.* 3rd ed. St. Louis: Mosby; 2020.)

compactness (tissue density) affect its absorption characteristics. The absorption characteristics of the anatomic tissue create the brightness levels displayed on a radiographic image. Tissues that have a higher effective atomic number absorb more radiation than tissues with a lower effective atomic number.

Anatomic structures having a wide range of tissue compositions, varying in parameters such as effective atomic number and tissue density, demonstrate high subject contrast (Fig. 7.24). Anatomic structures consisting of a similar type of tissue demonstrate low subject contrast (Fig. 7.25). The radiographer cannot control the composition of the anatomic part to be radiographed. Changing the kVp alters its absorption and transmission within anatomic tissues. Knowledge about the absorption characteristics of anatomic tissues and the effect of kVp helps the radiographer produce a desired level of subject contrast in the displayed image.

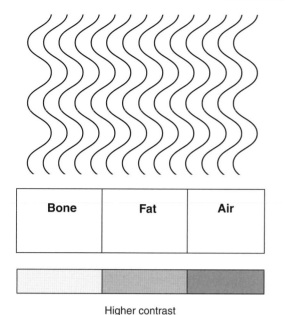

Bone	Fat	Air

Higher contrast

Fig. 7.24 Higher subject contrast resulting from great differences in radiation absorption between tissues that vary greatly in composition.

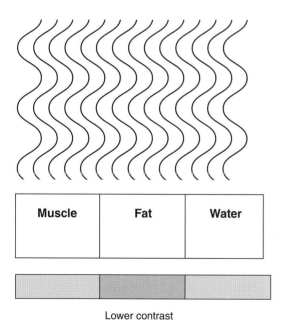

Muscle	Fat	Water

Lower contrast

Fig. 7.25 Lower subject contrast resulting from fewer differences in radiation absorption between tissues that are more similarly composed.

Imaging for Pathology

For certain radiographic examinations, the radiologist inspects the contrast resolution between fat and water-based connective tissues such as muscle and fascia. This is particularly important in studies of the elbow, knee, wrist, and ankle. The visualization of anatomical collections of fat in the form of fat stripes and pads is very important for interpretation, as they are often indirect signs of underlying pathologies indicating tissue effusion (fluid collection), soft tissue injury, and/or fractures. The excellent contrast resolution of modern digital receptors along with improved filtration improves visualization of this important fat/water contrast with decreased entrance skin exposure (ESE).

The selection of appropriate exposure factors, both kVp and mAs, is important for the visualization of low and high subject contrast substances (see Box 7.1). Fat and connective tissues have low effective atomic numbers and

---

BOX 7.1 Exposure Techniques in Digital Imaging

Exposure technique selection is important in producing a diagnostic image for interpretation. Although computer processing before and after image display can alter the visibility of anatomic detail, it cannot overcome poor exposure technique. If the amount or intensity of x-rays captured by the image receptor is too low, quantum noise results and anatomic information is compromised, even after computer processing. If the kVp is too low to penetrate the anatomic area, no amount of mAs or computer processing can make anatomic details visible. The selected kVp needs to penetrate the anatomic part and provide appropriate subject contrast to best visualize the anatomic part. Further computer processing and postprocessing of the displayed image would maximize the anatomic information visible for interpretation. Selecting excessively high kVp as a routine practice is not a best practice and should be avoided. However, routine use of a higher kVp and lower mAs, within the recommended exposure latitude, is a best practice for producing diagnostic-quality images with reasonable radiation exposure to the patient.

Exposure technique selection remains important to the unique role of radiographers in providing quality radiographic images with maximum anatomic information at radiation exposures that are optimized for the imaging procedure.

kVp, Kilovoltage peak; *mAs*, milliamperage-seconds.

tissue opacity, and consequently the contrast between them is subtle and very dependent upon photoelectric interactions occurring to create tissue contrast. Lower kVp values, generally 60 to 75 kVp for distal extremities, create a higher percentage of photoelectric interactions and an improvement in subject contrast visualization. Using a high kVp (≥90) would reduce the visibility of these tissues that attenuate the x-rays similarly, such as fat and connective tissues. As a result, differentiating between fat and connective tissue would be more difficult even with image display window adjustments. Likewise, the correct mAs level minimizes quantum noise and makes this subtle subject contrast more visible. Suboptimum mAs creates an image that is noisy and consequently will detract from the visualization of these low subject contrast tissues.

Imaging anatomic areas that are composed of many tissue substances such as the chest require the use of high kVp (>100 when using a grid) to best visualize the range of tissue opacities in the chest cavity. High kVp will produce an image with a wider range of gray shades and lower subject contrast, which is best for visualizing tissues that are both radiopaque, such as the heart, and radiolucent, such as the lungs. A lower-contrast image produces more shades of gray and fewer differences among them, which provides better visualization of anatomic tissues that vary greatly in differential absorption, such as the chest.

The quality of a radiographic image depends on a multitude of variables. Knowledge of these variables and their radiographic effect assists the radiographer in producing quality radiographs. Table 7.2 summarizes common exposure technique mathematical calculations. Table 7.3 is a chart demonstrating how the variables discussed in this chapter affect the primary beam and IR exposure, and Table 7.4 is a chart demonstrating how the variables discussed in this chapter affect image quality.

TABLE 7.2   Exposure Technique Mathematical Calculations

Exposure Technique Factor	Relationship to Maintain Exposure to Image Receptor	Formula
mAs	↑ mA and ↓ second	mA × second = mAs
kVp: 15% rule	↑ kVp and ↓ mAs	kVp × 1.15 and mAs/2 kVp × 0.85 and mAs × 2
Direct square law or exposure maintenance formula	↑ SID and ↑ mAs	$\dfrac{mAs_1}{mAs_2} = \dfrac{(SID_1)^2}{(SID_2)^2}$

Grid conversion factor (GCF):
No grid = 1
  5:1 = 2
  6:1 = 3
  8:1 = 4
  12:1 = 5
  16:1 = 6
	↑ Grid ratio and ↑ mAs	$\dfrac{mAs_1}{mAs_2} = \dfrac{GCF_1}{GCF_2}$

Magnification factor (MF)	↑ OID and ↓ SID will ↑ magnification	MF = SID ÷ SOD
Patient thickness	↑ Thickness and ↑ mAs	Every 4- to 5-cm change in thickness change mAs by a factor of 2

kVP, Kilovoltage peak; *mAs*, milliamperage-seconds; *OID*, object-to-image-receptor distance; *SID*, source-to-image-receptor distance; *SOD*, source-to-object distance.

TABLE 7.3   Exposure Factors and Their Effects on the Primary and Remnant X-ray Beams

	Primary Beam Reaching the Patient	Remnant Beam Reaching the Image Receptor
mAs		
Increasing mAs	↑ Quantity	↑ Quantity
Decreasing mAs	↓ Quantity	↓ Quantity
kVp		
Increasing kVp	↑ Quantity and quality	↑ Quantity and quality
Decreasing kVp	↓ Quantity and quality	↓ Quantity and quality
Focal Spot Size		
Smaller focal spot size	No effect	No effect
Larger focal spot size	No effect	No effect
SID		
Increasing SID	↓ Quantity	↓ Quantity
Decreasing SID	↑ Quantity	↑ Quantity
OID		
Increasing OID	No effect	↓ Quantity and scatter
Decreasing OID	No effect	↑ Quantity and scatter
CR Angle		
Increase CR Angle[a]	↓ Quantity	↓ Quantity
Grid		
Increasing grid ratio	No effect	↓ Quantity and scatter
Decreasing grid ratio	No effect	↑ Quantity and scatter
Beam Restriction		
Increasing collimation	↓ Quantity	↓ Quantity and scatter
Decreasing collimation	↑ Quantity	↑ Quantity and scatter
Generator Output		
Single-phase generator	↓ Quantity and quality	↓ Quantity and quality
High-frequency generator	↑ Quantity and quality	↑ Quantity and quality
Tube Filtration		
Adding filtration	↓ Quantity and ↑ average energy	↓ Quantity and ↑ average energy
Removing filtration	↑ Quantity and ↓ average energy	↑ Quantity and ↓ average energy
Compensating Filter		
Adding a compensating filter	↓ Quantity	↓ Quantity
Part Thickness		
Increasing part thickness	No effect	↓ Quantity
Decreasing part thickness	No effect	↑ Quantity

[a]Without a decrease in source-to-image-receptor distance (SID).

CR, Central ray; *kVP*, kilovoltage peak; *mA*, milliamperage; *mAs*, milliamperage-seconds; *OID*, object-to-image-receptor distance; *SID*, source-to-image-receptor distance.

TABLE 7.4 Exposure Technique Factors and Displayed Image Quality

INDIVIDUAL FACTOR CHANGE WITHOUT EXPOSURE TECHNIQUE COMPENSATION RESULTING IN A DIAGNOSTIC IMAGE

Exposure Factor	IR Exposure	Display Brightness[a]	Display Contrast[a,b]	Spatial Resolution	Distortion
mAs					
Increase	Increase	No effect	No effect	No effect	No effect
Decrease	Decrease	No effect	No effect	No effect	No effect
kVp[c]					
Increase	Increase	No effect	Decrease	No effect	No effect
Decrease	Decrease	No effect	Increase	No effect	No effect
Focal Spot Size					
Increase	No effect	No effect	No effect	Decrease	No effect
Decrease	No effect	No effect	No effect	Increase	No effect
SID					
Increase	Decrease	No effect	No effect	Increase	− Magnification
Decrease	Increase	No effect	No effect	Decrease	+ Magnification
OID					
Increase	Decrease	No effect	Increase[d]	Decrease	+ Magnification
Central Ray Angle					
Increase	Decrease	No effect	No effect	Decrease	+ Shape distortion
Grid Use					
Add grid	Decrease	No effect	Increase	No effect	No effect
Remove grid	Increase	No effect	Decrease	No effect	No effect
Collimation					
Increase	Decrease	No effect	Increase	No effect	No effect
Decrease	Increase	No effect	Decrease	No effect	No effect
Tube Filtration					
Excessive	Decrease	No effect	Decrease	No effect	No effect
Insufficient	Increase	No effect	Increase	No effect	No effect
Patient Thickness					
Increase	Decrease	No effect	Decrease	Decrease	+ Magnification
Decrease	Increase	No effect	Increase	Increase	− Magnification
Patient Motion	No effect	No effect	No effect	Decrease	No effect

[a]Brightness and contrast can be adjusted by the computer.
[b]Increase is higher contrast, and decrease is lower contrast.
[c]Kilovoltage peak (kVp) affects subject contrast.
[d]Increase (higher) contrast because of less scatter reaching image rector; effect dependent on anatomic region, thickness, and amount of object-to-image-receptor distance (OID).
IR, Image receptor; *mAs*, milliamperage-seconds; *SID*, source-to-image-receptor distance.

CHAPTER SUMMARY

- The product of mA and exposure time (mAs) is directly proportional to the quantity of x-rays produced and exposure to the IR.
- The mA and exposure time have an inverse relationship to maintain exposure to the IR.
- The kVp changes the penetrating power of the x-ray beam and has a direct effect on exposure to the IR.
- Changing the kVp by 15% has the same effect on exposure to the IR as changing the mAs by a factor of 2.
- A numerical value or exposure indicator is displayed on the processed digital image that indicates the level of x-ray exposure received (incident exposure) on the IR.
- The kVp has an inverse relationship with subject contrast: a high kVp creates an image with low subject contrast, and a low kVp creates an image with high subject contrast.
- Displayed image brightness and contrast are primarily controlled by computer processing in digital imaging.
- Focal spot size affects only spatial resolution. A smaller focal spot size increases spatial resolution.
- SID has an inverse-squared relationship with the intensity of radiation reaching the patient and the IR.
- Increasing OID decreases exposure to the IR.
- Decreasing SID and increasing OID increases size distortion (magnification) and decreases spatial resolution.
- Grids absorb the scatter radiation exiting the patient and increase displayed image contrast.
- Beam restriction affects the amount of tissue irradiated, scatter produced, and exposure to the IR.
- Changes in SID, grids, and patient thickness require a change in mAs to maintain the exposure to the IR.
- Generators with more efficient output, such as three-phase or high-frequency generators, require lower exposure techniques to produce the same exposure to the IR as a single-phase generator.
- Excessive or insufficient tube filtration affects the exposure to the IR and displayed image contrast.
- Exposure factors may need to be modified for body habitus and part thickness.

REVIEW QUESTIONS

1. Which of the following is accurate regarding the relationship between milliamperage (mA) and exposure time to maintain the exposure to the image receptor (IR)?
   A. Direct proportional
   B. Direct
   C. Inverse
   D. Inverse proportional

2. The exposure indicator value reflects excessive exposure to the IR. Which of the following is the best for correcting the exposure error?
   A. Decrease kVp by 50%
   B. Increase mAs by 15%
   C. Decrease mAs by 50%
   D. Decrease mAs by 15%

3. What exposure factor affects both the quality and the quantity of the x-ray beam?
   A. kVp
   B. SID
   C. mA
   D. Focal spot size

4. Which of the following is not affected by kilovoltage?
   A. Compton interactions
   B. Spatial resolution
   C. Subject contrast
   D. Radiation quantity

5. Increasing the mAs has _____ effect on brightness displayed in digital imaging.
   A. a direct
   B. a proportional
   C. an inverse
   D. no

6. Which of the following would maintain radiation exposure to the IR when the kilovoltage is decreased by 15%?
   A. Increase mAs by 15%
   B. Increase mAs by 50%
   C. Double the mAs
   D. Halve the mAs

7. A quality image is produced using 70 kVp and 25 mAs at a 100-cm (40-inch) SID. What calculated change in the exposure technique is necessary to maintain radiation exposure to the IR when the SID is increased to 140 cm (56 inches)?
   A. 60 kVp at 25 mAs
   B. 70 kVp at 12.5 mAs
   C. 70 kVp at 50 mAs
   D. 60 kVp at 50 mAs
8. Without exposure technique compensation, increasing the OID by 10 cm (4 inches) for a knee image would
   A. increase magnification and decrease exposure to the IR.
   B. increase magnification and increase contrast.
   C. decrease exposure to the IR and increase contrast.
   D. increase magnification, decrease exposure to the IR, and increase contrast.
9. A quality image is produced using 80 kVp at 10 mAs with a 6:1 ratio grid. Calculate the change in exposure technique to maintain radiation exposure to the IR when changing to a 12:1 ratio grid.
   A. 80 kVp at 17 mAs
   B. 68 kVp at 20 mAs
   C. 80 kVp at 6 mAs
   D. 92 kVp at 5 mAs
10. Which of the following factors does not affect spatial resolution?
    A. Focal spot size
    B. SID
    C. OID
    D. Grid
11. Which of the following factors does not affect the radiation exposure to the IR?
    A. Collimation
    B. Focal spot size
    C. Compensating filters
    D. Body habitus
12. What exposure factor change is recommended to maintain radiation exposure to the IR when increasing the patient thickness by 5 cm?
    A. Double the kVp
    B. Double the mAs
    C. Decrease kVp by 15%
    D. Increase mAs by 15%

EXPOSURE CALCULATIONS

13. Calculate the new exposure factor required to maintain a similar exposure to the IR as in the initial exposure technique.

Initial Exposure Technique		New Exposure Technique
10 mAs		_____ mAs
70 kVp	TO	81 kVp

CALCULATIONS

14. Calculate the new exposure factor required to maintain a similar exposure to the IR as in the initial exposure technique.

Initial Exposure Technique		New Exposure Technique
10 mAs		_____ mAs
70 kVp	TO	81 kVp
8:1 grid		12:1 grid

CALCULATIONS

15. Calculate the new exposure factor required to maintain a similar exposure to the IR as in the initial exposure technique.

Initial Exposure Technique		New Exposure Technique
10 mAs		_____ mAs
70 kVp	TO	81 kVp
8:1 grid		12:1 grid
180 cm SID		150 cm SID

CALCULATIONS

Scatter Control

CHAPTER OUTLINE

OBJECTIVES

After completing this chapter, the reader will be able to perform the following:

1. Define all the key terms in this chapter.
2. State all the important relationships in this chapter.
3. Explain how scatter radiation affects radiographic images.
4. State the purpose of beam-restricting devices.
5. Describe each type of beam-restricting device.
6. State the purpose of automatic collimators or positive beam-limiting devices.
7. Describe the purpose of a radiographic grid.
8. Describe the construction of grids, including the different types of grid patterns, dimensions, and grid focus.
9. Calculate grid ratio.
10. List the various types of stationary grids and describe the function and purpose of a moving grid.
11. Demonstrate the use of the grid conversion formula.
12. Describe the different types of grid alignment errors that can occur to cause grid cutoff.
13. Identify the factors to be considered in using a grid.
14. Recognize how beam restriction and the use of grids affect patient radiation exposure.
15. Explain the air gap technique and describe its use.

KEY TERMS

air gap technique
aperture diaphragm
automatic collimator
beam-restricting device
beam restriction
Bucky
Bucky factor

collimation
collimator
cone
convergent line
convergent (focal) point
crossed grid
crosshatched grid

cylinder
focal distance
focal range
focused grid
grid
grid cap
grid cassette

KEY TERMS—cont'd

grid conversion factor (GCF)
grid cutoff
grid focus
grid frequency
grid pattern
grid ratio

interspace material
linear grid
long dimension
moiré effect
nonfocused grid
parallel grid

positive beam-limiting device
short dimension
variable aperture
wafer grid

Controlling the amount of scatter radiation produced in a patient and ultimately reaching the image receptor (IR) is essential for creating a good-quality image. Scatter radiation is detrimental to radiographic quality because it adds unwanted exposure (fog) to the image without adding any patient information. The only radiation that is of any clinical value is the radiation that strikes the image receptor and provides anatomic information. The radiation must be at an energy level that can be converted to a usable electronic signal. Any other radiation, such as scatter, has no value and likely will add to patient exposure unnecessarily and poor image quality. Digital IRs are sensitive to lower-energy levels of radiation such as scatter, which results in increased fog (noise) in the image and reduces radiographic contrast. Although increased fog negatively impacts the quality of the image, image contrast can be computer manipulated by changing the window width. Increased scatter radiation, produced within the patient and the higher-energy scatter exiting the patient, affects the exposure to the patient and anyone within close proximity. The radiographer must act to minimize the amount of scatter radiation reaching the IR.

Beam-restricting devices and radiographic grids are tools that the radiographer can use to limit the amount of scatter radiation reaching the IR. Beam-restricting devices decrease the x-ray-beam field size and the amount of tissue irradiated, thereby reducing the amount of scatter radiation produced. Radiographic grids are used to improve radiographic image quality by absorbing scatter radiation exiting the patient, thereby reducing the amount of scatter reaching the IR. It should be noted that grids do nothing to prevent scatter *production*; they merely reduce the amount of scatter reaching the IR after scatter radiation is produced. The use of grids can be challenging in terms of positioning errors and the potential for visible grid lines and grid cutoff. In addition, the use of a grid significantly adds to the patient's radiation exposure during the procedure.

SCATTER RADIATION

Scatter radiation, as described in Chapter 4, is primarily the result of Compton interactions, in which an incoming x-ray photon loses energy and changes direction. Two major factors affect the amount and energy of scatter radiation exiting the patient: kilovoltage peak (kVp) and the volume of irradiated tissue. The volume of irradiated tissue depends on the thickness of the part and the x-ray-beam field size. Increasing the volume of irradiated tissue results in increased scatter production because there are more atoms available for Compton interactions. In addition, using a higher kVp increases x-ray transmission and reduces its overall absorption (photoelectric interactions); however, higher kVp increases the percentage of Compton interactions and the energy of scatter radiation exiting the patient. Using higher kVp or increasing the volume of irradiated tissue results in increased scatter radiation exiting the patient.

 IMPORTANT RELATIONSHIP

kVp and Scatter

The amount and energy of scatter radiation exiting the patient depends, in part, on the kVp selected. Examinations using higher kVp produce a greater proportion of higher-energy scattered x-rays than examinations using low kVp.

 IMPORTANT RELATIONSHIP

X-ray-Beam Field Size, Thickness of the Part, and Scatter

The larger the x-ray-beam field size, the greater the amount of scatter radiation produced. The thicker the part being imaged, the greater the amount of scatter radiation produced.

Volume of Tissue Irradiated and Scatter

The volume of tissue irradiated is affected by both the part thickness and the x-ray-beam field size. Therefore, the greater the volume of tissue irradiated, because of either or both factors, the greater the amount of scatter radiation produced.

BEAM RESTRICTION

It is the responsibility of the radiographer to limit the x-ray-beam field size to the anatomic area of interest. Beam restriction serves two purposes: limiting patient exposure and reducing the amount of scatter radiation produced within the patient.

The unrestricted primary beam is cone shaped and projects a round field onto the patient and IR (Fig. 8.1).

If not restricted in some way, the primary beam goes beyond the boundaries of the IR, resulting in unnecessary patient exposure. Any time the x-ray field extends beyond the anatomic area of interest, the patient receives unnecessary exposure. Federal regulations require that the size and shape of the x-ray field must not exceed the dimensions of the IR. Limiting the x-ray-beam field size is accomplished with a beam-restricting device. Located just below the x-ray tube housing, the beam-restricting device changes the shape and size of the primary beam.

The terms beam restriction and collimation are used interchangeably; they refer to a decrease in the size of the projected radiation field. The term *collimation* is used more often than the term *beam restriction* because collimators are the most popular type of beam-restricting device. Increasing collimation means decreasing the field size, and decreasing collimation means increasing the field size (Fig. 8.2).

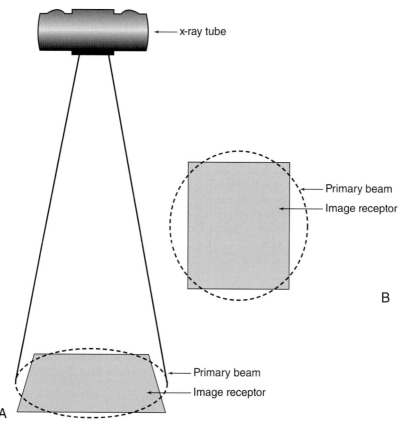

Fig. 8.1 The unrestricted primary beam is cone shaped, projecting a circular field. **A,** Side view. **B,** View from above.

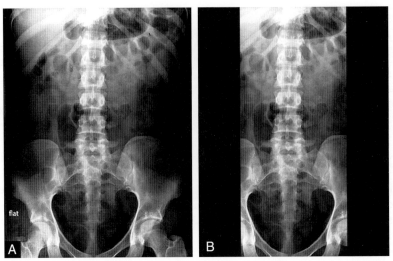

Fig. 8.2 A, Full view of the abdomen with decreased collimation when compared with B. **B,** Increased collimation of the abdominal region to image the lumbar spine. (From Bontrager K, Lapignano J. Textbook of Radiographic Positioning and Related Anatomy. 7th ed. St. Louis: Elsevier; 2010.)

 IMPORTANT RELATIONSHIP

Beam Restriction and Patient Dose

As beam restriction or collimation increases, the field size and patient dose decrease. As beam restriction or collimation decreases, the field size and patient dose increase.

! RADIATION PROTECTION ALERT

Appropriate Beam Restriction

In performing a radiographic examination, the radiographer should be aware of the anatomic area of interest and limit the x-ray field size to just beyond this area. Collimating to the appropriate field size is a basic method for protecting patients from unnecessary exposure.

BEAM RESTRICTION AND SCATTER RADIATION

In addition to decreasing the patient dose, beam-restricting devices reduce the amount of scatter radiation produced within the patient and reduce the amount of scatter to which the IR is exposed, thereby increasing radiographic contrast. The relationship between collimation (field size) and the quantity of scatter radiation

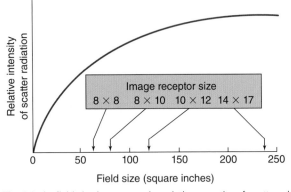

Fig. 8.3 As field size increases, the relative quantity of scattered radiation increases.

is illustrated in Fig. 8.3. As previously stated, collimation means decreasing the size of the projected x-ray field; hence, increasing collimation means decreasing x-ray field size, and decreasing collimation means increasing x-ray field size.

 IMPORTANT RELATIONSHIP

Collimation and Scatter Radiation

As collimation increases, the x-ray field size and quantity of scatter radiation decrease; as collimation decreases, the x-ray field size and quantity of scatter radiation increase.

Collimation and Contrast

Because collimation decreases the x-ray-beam field size, less scatter radiation is produced within the patient, and hence, less scatter radiation reaches the IR. As described in Chapter 4, this affects the radiographic contrast.

 IMPORTANT RELATIONSHIP

Collimation and Radiographic Contrast

> As collimation increases, the quantity of scatter radiation decreases and radiographic contrast increases; as collimation decreases, the quantity of scatter radiation increases, and radiographic contrast decreases.

Compensating for Collimation

Increasing the collimation decreases the volume of tissue irradiated, the amount of scatter radiation produced, the number of photons that strike the patient, and the number of x-ray photons that reach the IR to produce the raw image data. As a result, the exposure technique factors (kVp, milliamperage-seconds [mAs], or both) may need to be increased when increasing collimation to maintain exposure to the IR.

 IMPORTANT RELATIONSHIP

Collimation and Exposure to the Image Receptor

> As collimation increases, exposure to the IR decreases; as collimation decreases, exposure to the IR increases.

It has been recommended that significant collimation requires the mAs to be increased by 30% to 50% to compensate for the decrease in IR exposure. Postexposure electronic masking or cropping of the displayed digital image is a feature available at the radiographer's workstation. However, postexposure electronic masking should never replace preexposure collimation because it does not reduce scatter production, improve image contrast, or reduce patient radiation exposure. All anatomy that has been irradiated should be included for interpretation by the radiologist.

Important relationships regarding the restriction of the primary beam are summarized in Table 8.1.

! **RADIATION PROTECTION ALERT**

Postexposure Electronic Masking or Cropping

> Postexposure electronic masking or cropping the displayed image should never replace preexposure collimation because it does not reduce scatter production, reduce patient radiation exposure, or increase image contrast. All anatomy that has been irradiated should be included for interpretation by the radiologist.

TYPES OF BEAM-RESTRICTING DEVICES

Several types of beam-restricting devices, which differ in sophistication and utility, are available. Most beam-restricting devices are made of metal or a combination of metals that readily absorb x-rays.

Aperture Diaphragms

The simplest type of beam-restricting device is the aperture diaphragm. An aperture diaphragm is a flat piece of lead (diaphragm) that contains an opening (aperture). Commercially made aperture diaphragms are available (Fig. 8.4), or facilities can make their own for purposes specific to a radiographic unit. Aperture diaphragms are easy to use; they are placed directly below the x-ray tube window. An aperture diaphragm can be made by cutting

TABLE 8.1 Restricting the Primary Beam	
Increased Factor	**Result**
Collimation	Patient dose decreases
	Scatter radiation production decreases
	Radiographic contrast increases
	Exposure to the image receptor decreases
X-ray field size	Patient dose increases
	Scatter radiation production increases
	Radiographic contrast decreases
	Exposure to the image receptor increases

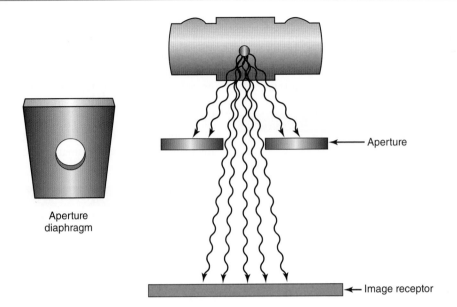

Fig. 8.4 Commercially made aperture diaphragm.

rubberized lead into the size needed to create the diaphragm and cutting a hole of the appropriate shape and size into the center to create the aperture.

Although the size and shape of the aperture can be changed, the aperture cannot be adjusted from the designed size, and therefore, the projected x-ray field size is not adjustable. In addition, because of the aperture's proximity to the radiation source (focal spot), a large area of unsharpness surrounds the radiographic image (Fig. 8.5). Although aperture diaphragms are still used in some applications, their use is not as widespread as other types of beam-restricting devices.

Cones and Cylinders

Cones and cylinders are shaped differently (Fig. 8.6), but they have many similar attributes. A cone or cylinder is essentially an aperture diaphragm that has an extended flange attached to it. The flange can vary in length and can be shaped as either a cone or a cylinder. The flange can also be made to telescope, increasing its total length. Like aperture diaphragms, cones and cylinders are easy to use but generally not in use today. They slide onto the tube, directly below the window. Cones and cylinders limit the unsharpness surrounding radiographic images more than aperture diaphragms do, with cylinders accomplishing this task slightly better than cones (Fig. 8.7). However, they are limited in terms of available sizes, and

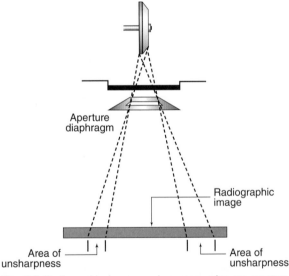

Fig. 8.5 Radiographic image unsharpness using an aperture diaphragm.

they are not interchangeable among tube housings. Cones have a disadvantage compared with cylinders: if the angle of the flange of the cone is greater than the angle of divergence of the primary beam, the base plate or aperture diaphragm of the cone is the only metal restricting the primary beam. Therefore cylinders generally were more useful than cones. Adjustable cylinders

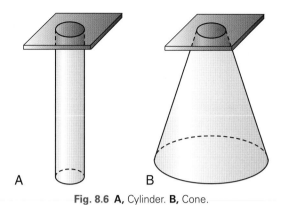

Fig. 8.6 **A,** Cylinder. **B,** Cone.

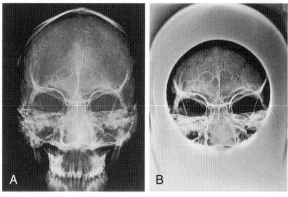

Fig. 8.8 Radiograph of the frontal and maxillary sinuses not using a cone (A) and using a cylinder extension (B). (From Mosby. Mosby's Radiographic Instructional Series: Radiographic Imaging. St. Louis: Mosby; 1998.)

are sometimes used for sinus images as the collimation is closer to the patient's skin surface. This helps reduce patient exposure and improves image quality since the beam restriction is closer to the patient's anatomy (see Fig. 8.8).

Collimators

The most sophisticated, useful, and accepted type of beam-restricting device for radiography today is the collimator, also known as variable aperture. Beam restriction accomplished with the use of a collimator is referred to as *collimation*. The terms collimation and *beam restriction* are used interchangeably.

A collimator has two or three sets of lead shutters (Fig. 8.9). Located immediately below the tube window, the entrance shutters limit the x-ray beam much as the

aperture diaphragm would. One or more sets of adjustable lead shutters are located 8 to 18 cm (3–7 inches) below the tube. These shutters consist of longitudinal and lateral leaves or blades, each with its own control. This design makes the collimator adjustable in terms of its ability to produce projected x-ray fields of varying sizes. The x-ray field shape produced by a collimator is always rectangular or square unless an aperture diaphragm, cone, or cylinder is slid in below the collimator. Collimators are equipped with a white light source and a mirror to project a light field onto the patient. This light is intended to accurately indicate where the primary

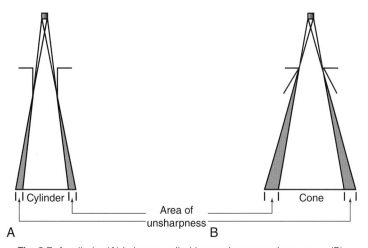

Fig. 8.7 A cylinder (A) is better at limiting unsharpness than a cone (B).

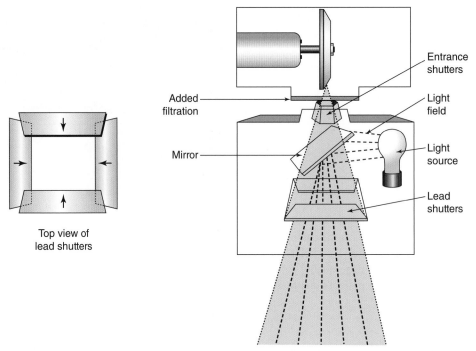

Top view of
lead shutters

Added filtration

Mirror

Entrance shutters

Light field

Light source

Lead shutters

Fig. 8.9 Collimators have two sets of lead shutters that are used to change the size and shape of the primary beam.

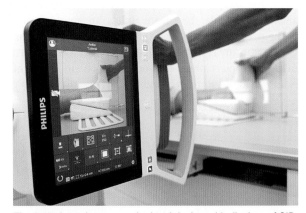

Fig. 8.10 A modern x-ray tube head design with displays of SID, x-ray field dimension, and video image of patient anatomy to be examined. *SID,* Source-to-image receptor distance. (© 2024 Koninklijke Philips N.V. All rights reserved.)

x-ray beam will be projected during exposure. In case of failure of this light, an x-ray field measurement guide (Fig. 8.10) is present on the front of the collimator. This guide indicates the projected field size on the basis of the adjusted size of the collimator opening at source-to-image receptor distances (SIDs). This guide helps to

ensure that the radiographer does not open the collimator to produce an x-ray field that is larger than the IR. Another problem that may occur is the lack of accuracy of the light field. The mirror that reflects the light down toward the patient or the light bulb itself could be slightly out of position, projecting a light field that inaccurately indicates where the primary beam will be projected. There is a means of testing the accuracy of this light field and the location of the center of the projected beam (Box 8.1).

A plastic template with crosshairs is affixed to the bottom of the collimator to indicate where the center of the primary beam (central ray) will be directed. This template is of great assistance to the radiographer in accurately centering the x-ray field to the patient.

Automatic Collimators

An **automatic collimator**, also called a **positive beam-limiting device**, automatically limits the size and shape of the primary beam to the size and shape of the IR. For a few years, automatic collimators were required by the US federal law on all new radiographic installations. This law has since been rescinded, and automatic collimators are no longer a requirement on any radiographic equipment. However, they are still widely used. Automatic collimators mechanically adjust the primary beam size and shape to the size and placement of the IR when the IR is placed in the Bucky tray, which is located just below the tabletop and behind the front of the upright unit. In newer digital radiography (DR) units with a single IR, automatic collimation may occur when the anatomic area to be imaged is selected. For example, if an anteroposterior (AP) shoulder is selected, the collimator may automatically adjust to a 20 × 30-cm (8 × 12-inch) x-ray field size, but if an AP lumbar spine is selected, the collimator will automatically adjust to a 25 × 35-cm (10 × 14-inch) x-ray field size.

Automatic collimation makes it difficult for the radiographer to increase the size of the primary beam to a field larger than that of the IR, which would result in increasing the patient's radiation exposure. **Positive beam-limiting devices** were seen as a way to protect patients from overexposure to radiation; however, it should be noted that automatic collimators have an override mechanism that allows the radiographer to disengage this feature.

RADIOGRAPHIC GRIDS

The radiographic grid was invented in 1913 by Gustave Bucky and continues to be the most effective means for limiting the amount of scatter radiation that reaches the IR. Approximately 0.625 cm (0.25 inch) thick and ranging from 20 × 25 cm (8 × 10 inches) to 43 × 43 cm

(17 × 17 inches), a grid is a device consisting of very thin lead strips with radiolucent interspaces intended to absorb scatter radiation emitted from the patient. Placed between the patient and the IR, grids are invaluable in the practice of radiography. They work well to improve radiographic contrast; however, they possess certain drawbacks. As discussed later in this chapter, using a grid requires additional mAs, resulting in a higher patient dose. Therefore grids are generally used only when the anatomic part is 10 cm (4 inches) or greater in thickness and more than 60 kVp is needed for the examination.

As scatter radiation leaves the patient, a significant amount is directed toward the IR. As previously stated, scatter radiation is detrimental to image quality because it adds unwanted exposure (fog) to the IR without adding any radiographic information. Scatter radiation decreases radiographic contrast. Ideally, grids would absorb, or clean up, all scattered photons directed toward the IR and would allow all transmitted photons exited from the patient to pass to the IR. Unfortunately, this does not happen (Fig. 8.11). When used properly, however, grids can greatly improve the subject contrast visualized on the radiographic image.

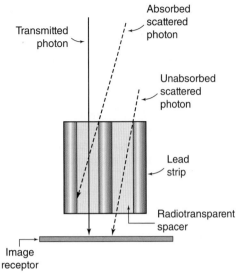

Fig. 8.11 Ideally, grids would absorb all scattered radiation and allow all transmitted photons to reach the image receptor (IR). In reality, however, some scattered photons pass through to the IR, and some transmitted photons are absorbed.

 IMPORTANT RELATIONSHIP

Scatter Radiation and Image Quality

Scatter radiation adds unwanted exposure (fog) to the IR and decreases image quality.

Grid Construction

Grids contain thin lead strips or lines that have a precise height, thickness, and space between them. Radiolucent interspace material separates the lead lines. Interspace material typically is made of aluminum or carbon fiber composite. Carbon fiber–type grids are considered "low-dose" grids as the interspace absorbs less primary radiation than aluminum. An aluminum front and back panel covers the lead lines and interspace material of the grid. Grid construction can be described by grid frequency and grid ratio. Grid frequency expresses the number of lead lines per unit length, in inches, centimeters, or both. Grid frequencies can range in value from 25 to 80 lines/cm (63–200 lines/inch). A typical value for grid frequency might be 40 lines/cm (100 lines/inch). Another way of describing grid construction is by its grid ratio. Grid ratio is defined as the ratio of the height of the lead strips to the distance between them (Fig. 8.12). Grid ratio can also be mathematically expressed as follows:

$$\text{Grid ratio} = h/D,$$

in which h is the height of the lead strips and D is the distance between them.

▶▶ **MATHEMATICAL APPLICATION**

Calculating Grid Ratio

What is the grid ratio when the lead strips are 2.4 mm high and separated by 0.2 mm?

$$\text{Grid ratio} = h/D$$
$$\text{Grid ratio} = \frac{2.4}{0.2} = 12 \text{ or } 12{:}1$$

Grid ratios range from 5:1 to 16:1. High-ratio grids remove, or clean up, more scatter radiation than lower-ratio grids having the same grid frequency, thereby further increasing displayed radiographic contrast.

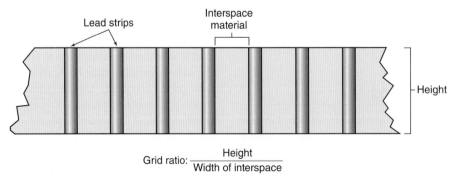

Fig. 8.12 Grid ratio is the ratio of the height of the lead strips to the distance between them.

There is a relationship among grid ratio, grid frequency, and the amount of lead content (measured in mass per unit area). Increasing the grid ratio for the same grid frequency increases the amount of lead content and therefore increases scatter absorption.

 IMPORTANT RELATIONSHIP
Grid Ratio and Radiographic Contrast

As the grid ratio increases for the same grid frequency, scatter cleanup improves and radiographic contrast increases; as the grid ratio decreases for the same grid frequency, scatter cleanup becomes less effective and radiographic contrast decreases.

Information about a grid's construction is contained on a label placed on the tube side of the grid. This label usually states the type of interspace material used, grid frequency, grid ratio, grid size, and information about the range of SIDs that can be used with the grid. The radiographer should read this information before using the grid because these factors influence grid performance, exposure technique selection, grid alignment, and image quality.

Grid Pattern

Grid pattern refers to the linear pattern of the lead lines of a grid. Two types of grid patterns exist: linear and crossed or crosshatched. A linear grid has lead lines that run in only one direction (Fig. 8.13). Linear grids are the most popular grid pattern because they allow angulation of the x-ray tube along the length of the lead lines. A crossed grid or crosshatched grid has lead lines that run at right angles to one another (Fig. 8.14). Crossed grids remove more scattered photons than linear grids because they contain more lead strips, oriented in two directions. However, applications are limited with a crossed grid because the x-ray tube cannot be angled in any direction without producing grid cutoff (i.e., absorption of the transmitted x-rays). Grid cutoff is undesirable and is discussed later in this chapter.

Grid Focus

Grid focus refers to the orientation of the lead lines relative to one another. A parallel grid or nonfocused grid has lead lines that run parallel to one another (Fig. 8.15). Parallel grids are used primarily in fluoroscopy and mobile imaging. A focused grid has lead lines that are angled, or canted, to approximately match the angle of

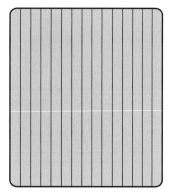
Fig. 8.13 Linear grid pattern.

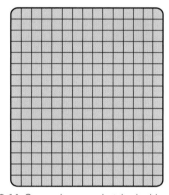
Fig. 8.14 Crossed or crosshatched grid pattern.

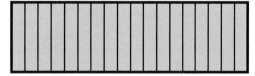
Fig. 8.15 Parallel, or nonfocused, type of grid.

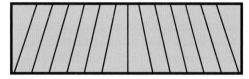
Fig. 8.16 Focused type of grid.

divergence of the primary beam (Fig. 8.16). The advantage of focused grids compared with parallel grids is that focused grids allow more transmitted photons to reach the IR. As seen in Fig. 8.17, transmitted photons are more likely to pass through a focused grid to reach the IR than they are to pass through a parallel grid.

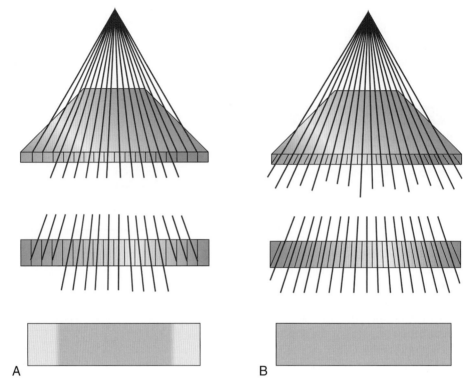

Fig. 8.17 Comparison of transmitted photons passing through a parallel grid (A) and a focused grid (B).

IMPORTANT RELATIONSHIP

Focused Versus Parallel Grids

Focused grids have lead lines that are angled to approximately match the divergence of the primary beam. Thus focused grids allow more transmitted photons to reach the IR than parallel grids.

As seen in Fig. 8.18, if imaginary lines were drawn from each of the lead lines in a linearly focused grid, these lines would meet to form an imaginary point called the **convergent** or **focal point**. If points were connected along the length of the grid, they would form an imaginary line called the **convergent line**. Both the convergent line and the convergent point are important because they determine the focal distance of a focused grid. The **focal distance** (sometimes referred to as *grid radius*) is the distance between the grid and the convergent line or point, and it is important because it is used to determine the focal range of a focused grid. The **focal range** is the recommended range of SIDs that can be

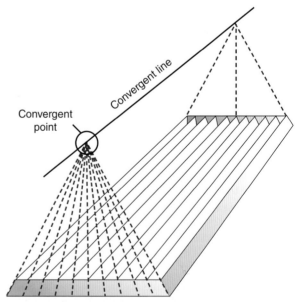

Fig. 8.18 Imaginary lines drawn above a linear focused grid from each lead strip meet to form a convergent point; the points form a convergent line.

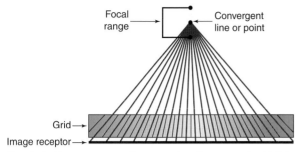

Fig. 8.19 The convergent line or point of a focused grid falls within a focal range.

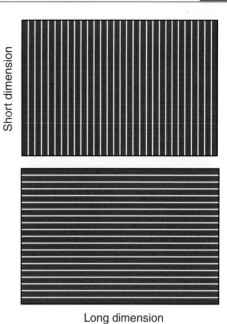

Fig. 8.20 A long-dimension grid has lead strips running parallel to the long axis of the grid. A short-dimension grid has lead strips running perpendicular to the long axis of the grid. (From Johnston JN, Fauber TL. Essentials of Radiographic Physics and Imaging. 3rd ed. St. Louis: Mosby; 2020.)

used with a focused grid. The convergent line or point always falls within the focal range (Fig. 8.19). For example, a common focal range is 90 to 105 cm (36–42 inches), with a focal distance of 100 cm (40 inches). Another common focal range is 165 to 185 cm (66–74 inches), with a focal distance of 180 cm (72 inches). Because the lead lines in a parallel grid are not angled, they have a focal range extending from a minimum SID to infinity.

Types of Grids

Grids are available for use by the radiographer in several forms and can be stationary or moving. Stationary, nonmoving grids include the wafer grid, grid cassette, and grid cap. A wafer grid matches the size of the cassette and is used by placing it on top of the IR. Wafer grids typically are taped to the IR to prevent them from sliding during the radiographic procedure. A grid cassette is an IR that has a grid permanently mounted on its front surface. A grid cap or encasement contains a permanently mounted grid and allows the IR to slide in behind it; this is useful because the grid is secure, and many IRs can be interchanged for radiation exposures.

Stationary and Reciprocating Grids

When grids are stationary, it is possible to examine them closely and see the grid lines on the radiographic image. Slightly moving the grid during the x-ray exposure blurs the grid lines (motion unsharpness), rendering them less visible.

Moving or reciprocating grids are part of the Bucky, which has historically been referred to as the *Potter-Bucky diaphragm*. Located directly below the radiographic tabletop, the grid is found just above the tray that holds the IR. In some systems, the IR and the grid are built into the table design and there is no Bucky tray. The grid moves along the long axis of the table with the IR. Grid motion is electrically controlled by the x-ray exposure switch. The grid moves slightly back and forth in a lateral direction over the IR during the entire exposure. These grids typically have dimensions of 43 × 43 cm (17 × 17 inches) so that a 35 × 43-cm (14 × 17-inch) IR can be or is positioned under the grid either lengthwise or crosswise, depending on the examination requirements.

Long-Dimension Versus Short-Dimension Grids

Linear grids can be constructed with either long dimension or short dimension. A long-dimension linear grid has lead strips running parallel to its long axis, whereas a short-dimension linear grid has lead strips running perpendicular to its long axis (Fig. 8.20). For example, whereas a 35 × 43-cm (14 × 17-inch) long-dimension grid has 43-cm (17-inch)-long lead strips, a short-dimension grid has 35-cm (14-inch)-long lead strips. A short-dimension grid may be useful for examinations when it is difficult to correctly center or angle the central ray for the long-dimension grid (e.g., imaging a decubitus or stretcher chest in the crosswise IR direction).

Grid Performance

The purpose of using grids in radiography is to reduce scatter radiation reaching the IR to increase image contrast. In addition to improving contrast by cleaning up scatter, grids reduce the total amount of x-rays reaching the IR. The better the grid is at absorbing scattered photons, such as with a higher-ratio grid, the fewer the photons reach the IR. To compensate for this reduction, additional mAs must be used to maintain exposure to the IR. The grid conversion factor (GCF), or Bucky factor, can be used to determine the required adjustment in mAs when changing from using a grid to nongrid (or vice versa) or for changing to grids with different grid ratios.

The GCF can be mathematically expressed as follows:

$$GCF = \frac{mAs\ with\ the\ grid}{mAs\ without\ the\ grid}$$

 IMPORTANT RELATIONSHIP

Grid Ratio and Exposure to Image Receptor

As the grid ratio increases, exposure to the IR decreases; as the grid ratio decreases, exposure to the IR increases.

Table 8.2 presents specific grid ratios and grid conversion factors. When a grid is added to the IR, mAs must be increased by the factor indicated to maintain the same number of x-ray photons reaching the IR. This calculation requires multiplication by the GCF for the particular grid ratio.

Likewise, if a radiographer chooses not to use a grid during a procedure but knows the appropriate mAs only for when a grid is used, the mAs must be decreased by the GCF. This calculation requires division by the GCF for the particular grid ratio.

TABLE 8.2 **Grid Conversion Factor (GCF)/Bucky Factor**	
Grid Ratio	**GCF/Bucky Factor**
No grid	1
5:1	2
6:1	3
8:1	4
12:1	5
16:1	6

 MATHEMATICAL APPLICATION

Adding a Grid

If a radiographer produced a shoulder image with non-grid exposure using 3 mAs and then wanted to use a 12:1 ratio grid, what mAs should be used to produce the same exposure to the IR?

Nongrid exposure = 3 mAs
GCF (for 12:1 grid) = 5 (from Table 8.2)

$$GCF = \frac{mAs\ with\ the\ grid}{mAs\ without\ the\ grid}$$

$$5 = \frac{mAs\ with\ the\ grid}{3}$$

$$\frac{5}{1} = \frac{X}{3};\ X = 15$$

$$15 = mAs\ with\ the\ grid$$

When adding a 12:1 ratio grid, mAs must be increased by a factor of 5 (in this case to 15 mAs).

MATHEMATICAL APPLICATION

Removing a Grid

If a radiographer produced a knee image using an 8:1 ratio grid and 10 mAs and on the next exposure wanted to use nongrid exposure, what mAs should be used to produce the same exposure to the IR?

Grid exposure = 10 mAs
GCF (for 8:1 grid) = 4 (from Table 8.2)

$$GCF = \frac{mAs\ with\ the\ grid}{mAs\ without\ the\ grid}$$

$$4 = \frac{10\ mAs}{mAs\ without\ the\ grid}$$

$$\frac{4}{1} = \frac{10}{X};\ 4X = 10;\ X = \frac{10}{4}$$

$$2.5 = mAs\ without\ the\ grid$$

When removing an 8:1 ratio grid, mAs must be decreased by a factor of 4 (in this case to 2.5 mAs).

The GCF is also useful when changing between grids with different grid ratios. When changing from one grid ratio to another, the following formula should be used to adjust the mAs:

$$\frac{mAs_1}{mAs_2} = \frac{GCF_1}{GCF_2}$$

MATHEMATICAL APPLICATION

Decreasing the Grid Ratio

If a radiographer used 40 mAs with a 12:1 ratio grid, what mAs should be used with a 6:1 ratio grid to produce the same exposure to the IR?

Exposure 1: 40 mAs, 12:1 grid, GCF = 5

$$\frac{mAs_1}{mAs_2} = \frac{GCF_1}{GCF_2}$$

Exposure 2: _____ mAs, 6:1 grid, GCF = 3

$$\frac{40}{mAs_2} = \frac{5}{3}$$

5X = 120; X = 120/5; X = 24
mAs_2 = 24

Decreasing the grid ratio requires less mAs.

 MATHEMATICAL APPLICATION

Increasing the Grid Ratio

If a radiographer performed a routine mobile pelvic examination using 40 mAs with an 8:1 ratio grid, what mAs should be used if a 12:1 ratio grid is substituted?

Exposure 1: 40 mAs, 8:1 grid, GCF = 4
Exposure 2: _____ mAs, 12:1 grid, GCF = 5

$$\frac{mAs_1}{mAs_2} = \frac{GCF_1}{GCF_2}$$

$$\frac{40}{mAs_2} = \frac{4}{5}$$

4X = 200; X = 200/4; X = 50
mAs_2 = 50

Increasing the grid ratio requires additional mAs.

The increase in mAs required to maintain the exposure to the IR results in an increase in patient dose. This increase is significant, as the GCF numbers indicate. It is important to remember that patient dose is increased by the following factors:

- Using a grid compared with not using a grid
- Using a higher-ratio grid

 IMPORTANT RELATIONSHIP

Grid Ratio and Patient Dose

As the grid ratio increases, patient dose increases because of the increase in mAs; as the grid ratio decreases, patient dose decreases because of the decrease in mAs.

! RADIATION PROTECTION ALERT

Grid Selection

Decisions regarding the use of a grid and grid ratio should be made by balancing image quality and patient protection. To minimize patient exposure, grids should be used only when appropriate, and the grid ratio selected should be the lowest capable of providing sufficient contrast improvement. In examinations in which the anatomic part does not produce excessive scatter, a grid may not be necessary because the computer can vary contrast in the displayed image.

Grid Cutoff

In addition to the disadvantage of increased patient dose associated with grid use, another disadvantage is the possibility of grid cutoff. Grid cutoff refers to a decrease in the number of transmitted photons that reach the IR because of some misalignment of the grid. The primary radiographic effect of grid cutoff is a further reduction in the number of photons reaching the IR. Grid cutoff may require the radiographer to repeat the radiographic image, increasing patient dose yet again. Grid ratio has a significant impact on grid cutoff, with higher grid ratios resulting in more potential cutoff.

Types of Grid Cutoff Errors

Grid cutoff can occur because of four types of errors in grid use. To reduce or eliminate grid cutoff, the radiographer must have a thorough understanding of the importance of proper grid alignment in relation to the IR and x-ray tube.

Upside-down focused. Upside-down focused grid cutoff occurs when a focused grid is placed upside down on the IR, resulting in the grid lines going opposite the angle of divergence of the x-ray beam resulting in a significant loss of exposure along the edges of the image (Fig. 8.21). Photons easily pass through the center of the grid because the lead lines are perpendicular to the IR surface. Lead lines that are more peripheral to the center have steeper angles and absorb the transmitted photons. Upside-down focused grid error is easily avoided because every focused grid should have a label indicating the tube side. This side of the grid should always face the tube, away from the IR.

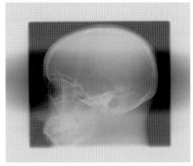

Fig. 8.21 Radiographic image produced with an upside-down focused grid.

The grid being angled (Fig. 8.22). Off-level grid cutoff can often occur with mobile radiographic studies or horizontal beam examinations and is visualized as a loss of exposure across the entire IR. This type of grid cutoff is the only type that occurs with both focused and parallel grids.

IMPORTANT RELATIONSHIP

Off-Level Error and Grid Cutoff

Angling the x-ray tube across the grid lines or angling the grid itself during exposure produces an overall decrease in exposure across the entire IR.

IMPORTANT RELATIONSHIP

Upside-Down Focused Grids and Grid Cutoff

Placing a focused grid upside down on the IR causes the edges of the IR to be significantly underexposed.

Off-level. Off-level grid cutoff results when the x-ray beam is angled across the lead strips. It is the most common type of cutoff and can occur from either the tube or

Off-center. Also called *lateral decentering*, off-center grid cutoff occurs when the central ray of the x-ray beam is not aligned from side to side with the center of a focused grid. Because of the arrangement of the lead lines of the focused grid, the divergence of the primary beam does not match the angle of these lead strips when not centered (Fig. 8.23). Off-center grid cutoff may cause an overall loss of exposure across the entire IR.

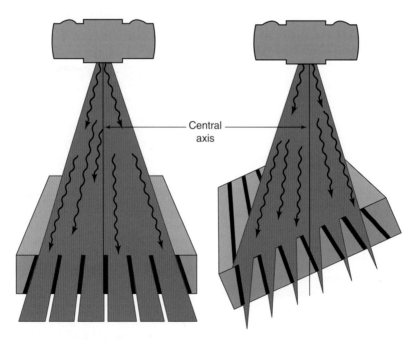

Central axis

Proper position   Off-level

Fig. 8.22 An off-level grid can cause grid cutoff.

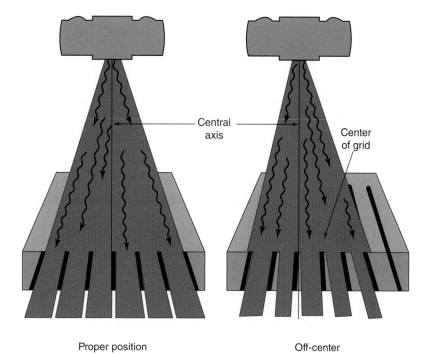

Fig. 8.23 Centering to one side of a focused grid can cause off-center grid cutoff.

IMPORTANT RELATIONSHIP

Off-Center Error and Grid Cutoff

If the center of the x-ray beam is not aligned from side to side with the center of a focused grid, grid cutoff can occur as a loss of exposure across the entire IR.

Off-focus. Off-focus grid cutoff occurs when using an SID outside the recommended focal range. Grid cutoff occurs if the SID is less than or greater than the focal range and results in a loss of exposure at the periphery of the IR (Fig. 8.24).

IMPORTANT RELATIONSHIP

Off-Focus Error and Grid Cutoff

Using an SID outside the focal range creates a loss of exposure at the periphery of the IR.

With modern digital IRs, exposure techniques have been reduced significantly and because of this there is less margin of exposure error for grid cutoff. Proper grid alignment is more important than ever because there is

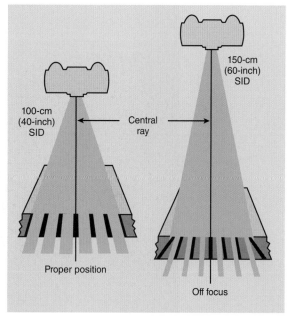

Fig. 8.24 Grid cutoff from using an SID outside the recommended focal range. *SID,* Source-to-image receptor distance. (Bushong, SC. *Radiologic Science for Technologists: Physics, Biology, and Protection.* 11th ed. St. Louis: Mosby; 2017.)

less exposure to compensate for any degree of grid cutoff. Grid alignment errors may be difficult to identify because the computer will adjust for exposure errors to the IR. However, adjusting the brightness during computer processing may not overcome a grid alignment error and still produce a poor-quality image (Fig. 8.25). When using a grid, the radiographer should pay close attention to the alignment of the grid to the x-ray tube and IR.

Table 8.3 summarizes important relationships regarding the use of radiographic grids.

Moiré Effect

The moiré effect or zebra pattern is an artifact that can occur when a stationary grid is used during computed radiography (CR) imaging (Fig. 8.26). If the grid frequency is similar to the laser scanning frequency or scans parallel to the grid strips during CR image processing, a zebra pattern can result in the digital image. The use of a higher grid frequency or a moving grid with CR imaging eliminates this type of grid error. Advancements in postprocessing grid artifact correction or suppression software have also been used to reduce digital image artifacts caused by using a stationary grid. In addition, if a grid cassette is placed in a Bucky, imaging the double grids creates a zebra pattern on the radiograph.

Grid Usage

The radiographer needs to consider several factors when deciding the type of grid, if any, to be used for an

TABLE 8.3	**Radiographic Grids**
Increased Factor	**Result**
Grid ratio[a]	Contrast increases
	Patient dose increases
	The likelihood of grid cutoff increases

[a]Milliamperage-seconds adjusted to maintain exposure to the image receptor.

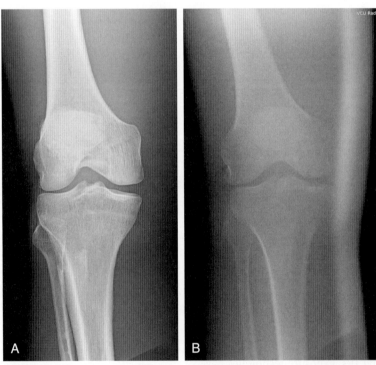

Fig. 8.25 Grid cutoff. **A,** Image created with proper alignment of CR image receptor and no grid cutoff. **B,** Image created with off-level grid cutoff. The overall brightness was maintained, but the image quality is poor. *CR,* Computed radiography. (From Johnston JN, Fauber TL. Essentials of Radiographic Physics and Imaging. 3rd ed. St. Louis: Elsevier; 2020.)

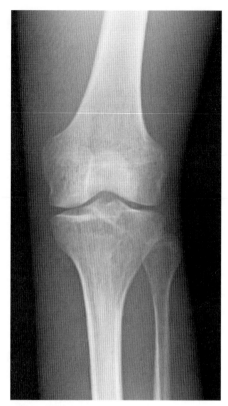

Fig. 8.26 Moiré effect. Radiographic image demonstrating the zebra pattern as a result of the moiré effect. (Courtesy Andrew Woodward.)

examination. Although quite efficient at preventing scatter radiation from reaching the IR, grids are not appropriate for all examinations. When appropriate, selection of a grid involves consideration of contrast improvement, patient dose, and the likelihood of grid cutoff. Radiographers typically choose between parallel and focused grids, high- and low-ratio grids, grids with different focal ranges, and whether to use a grid at all.

As indicated earlier, the choice of whether to use a grid is based on the kVp necessary for the examination and the thickness of the anatomic part being examined. Generally, parts 10 cm (4 inches) or larger, together with kVp values higher than 60, produce enough scatter to necessitate the use of a grid. The next question is which grid to use. There is no single best grid for all situations. A 16:1 focused grid provides excellent contrast improvement, but the patient's dose is high, and the radiographer must ensure that the grid and x-ray tube are perfectly aligned to prevent grid cutoff. The 5:1 parallel grid does

a mediocre job of scatter cleanup, especially at kVp values greater than 80. However, the patient dose is significantly lower, and the radiographer need not be concerned with the cutoff caused by being off-center, the SID used, or having the grid upside down. Selection between grids with different focal ranges depends on the radiographic examination. Supine abdomen studies should use a grid that includes 100 cm (40 inches) in the focal range; upright chest studies should have grids that include 180 cm (72 inches). In general, most radiographic rooms use an 8:1, 10:1, or 12:1 focused grid, which provides a compromise between contrast improvement and patient dose. Stationary grids, for mobile examinations, may have a lower ratio, be a parallel type, or both to allow the radiographer greater positioning latitude.

Grids differ from one another in performance, especially in the areas of grid ratio and focal distance. Before using a grid, the radiographer must determine the grid ratio so that the appropriate exposure factors can be selected. Also, the radiographer must be aware of the focal range of focused grids so that an appropriate SID is selected.

Box 8.2 lists the attributes of grids typically used in radiography. Box 8.3 summarizes grid errors and their radiographic effects. Box 8.4 provides information on quality control checks for grid uniformity and alignment.

Radiation Protection

Limiting the size of the x-ray field to the anatomic area of interest will decrease scatter production and reduce patient exposure. Although the mAs may be increased to compensate for decreasing the size of the x-ray field, the tissues located closest to the edge of the collimated x-ray beam or outside the collimated x-ray beam will receive the least amount of radiation exposure. Tissues that lie inside the collimated edge of the x-ray beam will receive the greatest amount of radiation exposure. Collimating

BOX 8.2 **Typical Grid**
• Is linear instead of crossed
• Is focused instead of parallel
• Is of mid–grid ratio (8:1–10:1)
• Has a focal range that includes an SID of 100 cm (40 inches) or 180 cm (72 inches)

SID, Source-to-image receptor distance.

BOX 8.3   Grid Cutoff Errors and Their Radiographic Effects

Grid Error	Radiographic Effect
Upside-down focused grid: placing a focused grid upside down on the IR	Significant underexposure to the lateral edges of the IR
Off-level error: angling the x-ray tube across the grid lines or angling the grid itself during exposure	Decrease in radiation exposure to the entire IR
Off-center error: the center of the x-ray beam is not aligned from side to side with the center of a focused grid	Decrease in radiation exposure to the entire IR
Off-focus error: using an SID outside the focal range	A loss of exposure at the periphery of the IR

IR, Image receptor; *SID*, source-to-image receptor distance.

BOX 8.4   Quality Control Check: Grid Uniformity and Alignment

- Nonuniformity of a grid (lack of uniform lead strips) may create artifacts on the image. Grid uniformity can be easily evaluated by imaging a grid and measuring pixel brightness throughout the image. Pixel brightness level readings should be within ±0.20 for proper uniformity.
- Misalignment of a focused grid (off-center) can reduce exposure to the IR as a result of grid cutoff. A grid alignment tool made of radiopaque material with cut-out holes in a line can be imaged to evaluate correct alignment of the grid with the x-ray field.

IR, Image receptor.

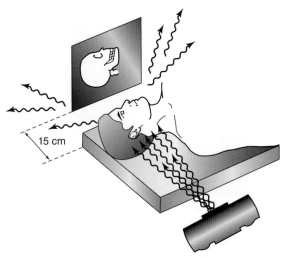

Fig. 8.27 The air gap technique used in magnification radiography of the lateral skull.

to the anatomic area of interest is an important radiation protection practice that should be routinely performed.

The use of grids requires an increase in mAs to maintain exposure to the IR. As a result, patient radiation exposure is increased when using grids. The higher the grid ratio, the greater the mAs needed to maintain exposure to the IR, and therefore, patient radiation exposure is increased. Limiting the use of grids or using a grid with a lower grid ratio decreases the radiation exposure to the patient.

AIR GAP TECHNIQUE

Although the radiographer may use the grid most often to prevent scatter from reaching the IR, the grid is not the only available tool. The **air gap technique**, although limited in its usefulness, provides another method for limiting the scatter reaching the IR. The air gap technique is based on the simple concept that much of the scatter will miss the IR if there is increased distance between the patient and the IR (increased object-to-image receptor distance [OID]) (Fig. 8.27). The greater the gap, the greater the reduction in scatter reaching the IR. Like when using a grid, contrast is increased, the number of photons reaching the IR is reduced because less scatter reaches the IR, and the mAs must be increased to compensate. There may be slightly less exposure because a grid absorbs some of the transmitted photons (grid cutoff), but the air gap technique does not.

The air gap technique is limited in its usefulness because the necessary OID results in decreased spatial resolution. To overcome this increase in unsharpness, an increase in SID is required, which may not always be feasible. Lateral cervical spine positioning creates a natural increase in OID because of the positions of the shoulders.

SCATTER CONTROL AND DIGITAL IMAGING

Computer processing during digital imaging typically produces an image with appropriate brightness. If the amount of x-ray exposure reaching the IR is low, computer processing functions to produce the appropriate brightness, which may result in an image with increased quantum noise. This can occur with all forms of grid cutoff or if the mAs is not increased to compensate for adding a grid or changing to a higher-ratio grid. Excessive noise in a digital image is one of the primary reasons for repeating the image.

If the digital IR receives too much exposure, computer processing produces appropriate brightness; however, image contrast may be decreased because of excessive scatter. This may occur when a grid is removed, and mAs is not decreased or by not making adjustments in mAs when a change is made to a lower-ratio grid.

Grid errors during digital imaging can easily be masked by computer processing. The radiographer should evaluate the exposure indicator value along with the overall quality of the digital image to determine whether any exposure errors exist.

Scatter correction software continues to be developed to improve digital image quality, especially for mobile and trauma imaging where the use of a stationary grid may not be practical. Scatter correction software, applied during computer processing, can also be used in combination with low grid ratios to improve image quality. Continued advancements in grid development and software processing technology will overcome many challenges of imaging with and without grids.

Several manufacturers have developed software for grid replacement that produces a visible image with higher contrast when no grid has been employed. These software algorithms are used as a postprocessing feature and intended to lessen the reliance on grids for routine use. This software will not replace grids completely, particularly for thicker body parts in the extreme. Additionally, software enhancements have been developed to hide or visibly remove the grid lines from the final image using "grid suppression" software.

Generally, it is understood that with DR there is less scatter created since the exposure mAs levels are lower because of the increase in dose efficiency of digital IRs. That being the case, the trend is to use grids less often and with lower grid ratios. The most popular grids used currently have grid ratios no greater than 10:1 for Bucky exposures and 5:1 or 6:1 for mobile examinations.

SHIELDING ACCESSORIES

Efforts to control the amount of scatter radiation produced within the patient and reaching the IR are important considerations during radiography. Restricting the size of the x-ray beam to the anatomic area of interest reduces the radiation exposure to the patient and improves image quality. There are situations in which it is beneficial to use shielding devices to absorb the scatter radiation exiting the patient by placing a lead shield on the x-ray table close to the collimated edge of the area of interest. This practice absorbs scatter exiting the patient that could degrade image quality if it strikes the IR. The lateral lumbar spine projection and the lateral (L5–S1) spot are projections in which a significant amount of scatter exits the patient. Placing a lead shield behind the patient's lower back absorbs the scatter and reduces the amount striking the IR (Fig. 8.28). Accurate placement

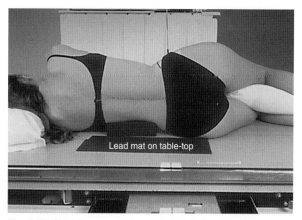

Fig. 8.28 Shielding accessory: lead shield placed to absorb scatter radiation from the patient. (From Bontrager KL, Lampignano JP. Textbook of Radiographic Positioning and Related Anatomy. 7th ed. St. Louis: Mosby; 2010.)

of the lead shield is important so it does not impact the processing of the digital image. It is important to note that placing a lead shield on the table to limit the scatter radiation reaching the IR does not reduce the exposure to the patient.

Because the patient is the greatest source of scatter radiation, all persons remaining in the radiographic room during an exposure must wear a lead apron. This, together with standing as far from the patient as possible, decreases the amount of exposure to scatter radiation.

It is the radiographer's responsibility to reduce the amount of scatter radiation produced and reaching the IR. Reducing the amount of scatter produced through beam restriction and the amount reaching the IR by using a grid, avoiding grid cutoff errors, and making appropriate exposure adjustments as needed help to produce good-quality radiographic images. However, computer algorithms have decreased the need for grids and higher grid ratios, but not entirely. This will likely be the case for many years to come as long as patients and radiation produce scatter that needs to be controlled.

CHAPTER SUMMARY

- Scatter radiation, the result of Compton interactions, is detrimental to radiographic image quality. Excessive scatter results in additional unwanted exposure (fog) and reduces image quality.
- The effect of scatter radiation can be reduced by limiting the amount produced and by absorbing the scatter before it reaches the IR.
- The amount of scatter produced increases as the volume of irradiated tissue increases, and the proportion and energy of scatter exiting the patient increase as kVp increases.
- Beam restriction limits the area exposed to radiation, the patient dose, and the amount of scatter produced in the patient. Aperture diaphragms, cones and cylinders, and collimators are types of beam restrictors.
- Radiographic grids are devices placed between the patient and the IR to absorb scatter radiation. Consisting of a series of lead strips and radiolucent interspaces, grids allow transmitted radiation to pass through while scatter radiation is absorbed.
- Grid designs include linear parallel, focused parallel, crossed, short dimension, and long dimension, each with advantages and disadvantages.
- The use of a grid in a radiographic examination results in fewer photons reaching the IR. The grid conversion (or Bucky) factor is used to calculate the change in exposure (mAs) needed when grids are used.

- Adding a grid requires an increase in mAs to maintain exposure to the IR, therefore increasing radiation exposure to the patient.
- Grid alignment errors, producing grid cutoff, include using an upside-down focused grid and errors caused by off-level, off-center, and off-focus equipment alignment.
- The use and type of a grid depends on the thickness of the part, kVp, patient dose, contrast improvement, and likelihood of grid errors.
- Grid errors during digital imaging can easily be masked by computer processing.
- Grid artifact correction or suppression and scatter correction software are technological advancements that can overcome the challenges of imaging with and without a grid.
- The air gap technique is another method, although seldom used, for reducing the amount of scatter reaching the IR.
- Placing a lead shield behind the patient's lower back when performing a lateral lumbar spine absorbs the scatter and reduces the amount striking the IR.
- Because the patient is the greatest source of scatter radiation, all persons remaining in the radiographic room during an exposure must wear a lead apron.

REVIEW QUESTIONS

1. The projected shape of the unrestricted primary beam is _____.
   A. square
   B. rectangular
   C. circular
   D. elliptical

2. One purpose of beam-restricting devices is to _____ by changing the size and shape of the primary beam.
   A. increase patient dose
   B. decrease scatter radiation produced
   C. increase exposure to the IR
   D. decrease image contrast

3. The most effective type of beam-restricting device is the _____.
   A. cone
   B. aperture diaphragm
   C. cylinder
   D. collimator

4. Of the beam-restricting devices listed in question 3, which two are most similar to one another?
   A. A and B
   B. A and C
   C. B and C
   D. B and D

5. The purpose of automatic collimation is to ensure that _____.
   A. the quantity of scatter production is minimal
   B. the field size does not exceed the IR size
   C. maximal spatial resolution and contrast are achieved
   D. exposure to the IR is maintained

6. When making a significant increase in collimation, _____.
   A. mAs should be increased
   B. kVp should be increased
   C. mAs should be decreased
   D. kVp should be decreased

7. Which one of the following increases as collimation increases?
   A. Patient exposure
   B. Scatter production
   C. Fog
   D. Contrast

8. Which of the following statements are true for positive beam-limiting devices?
   A. They automatically limit the size and shape of the primary beam to IR.
   B. They are required on all new radiographic installations.
   C. In newer DR units, may automatically restrict the beam to anatomic area selected.
   D. A and B only.
   E. A and C only.

9. The purpose of a grid in radiography is to _____.
   A. increase exposure to the IR
   B. increase image contrast
   C. decrease patient dose
   D. increase spatial resolution

10. Grid ratio is defined as the ratio of the _____.
    A. height of the lead strips to the distance between them
    B. width of the lead strips to their height
    C. number of lead strips to their width
    D. width of the lead strips to the width of the interspace material

11. Compared with parallel grids, focused grids _____.
    A. have a greater grid frequency and lead content
    B. can be used with either side facing the tube
    C. have a wider range of grid ratios and frequencies
    D. allow more transmitted photons to reach the IR

12. With which one of the following grids would a convergent line be formed if imaginary lines from its grid lines were drawn in space above it?
    A. Linear focused
    B. Crossed focused
    C. Linear parallel
    D. Crossed parallel

13. If 10 mAs is used to produce a particular level of exposure to the IR without a grid, what value of mAs would be needed to produce that same level of exposure using a 12:1 grid?
    A. 30
    B. 40
    C. 50
    D. 60

14. With exposure technique compensation, which of the following would result in the greatest radiation exposure to the patient?
    A. 35 × 43-cm x-ray field size
    B. Air gap technique
    C. Cylinder beam restrictor
    D. 12:1 grid ratio

15. Off-focus grid cutoff occurs by using an SID that is not _____.
    A. within the focal range of the grid
    B. equal to the focal distance of the grid
    C. at the level of the convergent line of the grid
    D. at the level of the convergent point of the grid

16. The type of motion most often used for moving grids today is _____.
    A. longitudinal
    B. reciprocating
    C. circular
    D. single stroke

17. A grid should be used whenever the anatomic part size exceeds _____.
    A. 3 cm
    B. 6 cm
    C. 10 cm
    D. 12 cm

18. With radiographic exposures that do not use a grid, which of the following is not an advantage of scatter correction software?
    A. Reduced image noise
    B. Improved image contrast
    C. Reduced patient radiation exposure
    D. Improved spatial resolution

19. The air gap technique uses an increased _____ instead of a grid.
    A. kVp
    B. mAs
    C. SID
    D. OID

20. _____ improves the visible appearance of a radiographic image without the use of a grid.
    A. Decreased collimation
    B. Grid replacement software
    C. Increased SID
    D. Decreased OID

21. Following exposure technique adjustment, which of the following would NOT decrease patient radiation exposure using a DR receptor?
    A. Increasing kVp and decreasing mAs
    B. Positive beam limitation
    C. Switching from a 10:1 grid to a 8:1 grid
    D. Using a crosshatched grid

Exposure Technique Selection

CHAPTER OUTLINE

OBJECTIVES

After completing this chapter, the reader will be able to perform the following:

1. Define all the key terms in this chapter.
2. State all the important relationships in this chapter.
3. State the purpose of automatic exposure control (AEC) in radiography.
4. Differentiate among the types of radiation detectors used in AEC systems.
5. Recognize how detector size and configuration affect the response of an AEC device.
6. Explain how alignment and positioning affect the response of an AEC device.
7. Discuss patient and exposure technique factors and their effects on the response of an AEC device.

8. Analyze poor-quality images produced using AEC and identify possible causes.
9. Describe the patient radiation protection issues associated with AEC.
10. State the importance of calibration of the AEC system to the type of image receptor used.
11. Define anatomically programmed techniques.
12. Differentiate between the types of exposure technique charts.
13. State exposure technique modifications for the following considerations: pediatric, geriatric, and bariatric patients and varying projections and positions, soft tissue, casts and splints, contrast media, and pathological conditions.

KEY TERMS

anatomically programmed
  technique

automatic exposure control
  (AEC)

backup time

body mass index (BMI)

calipers

comparative anatomy

contrast medium

density controls

detectors

exposure adjustment

exposure technique charts

extrapolated

fixed kVp/variable mAs technique
  chart

ionization or ion chamber

mAs readout

minimum response time

optimal kVp

phototimers

variable kVp/fixed mAs technique
  chart

The radiographer is responsible for selecting exposure factor techniques to produce quality radiographic images for a wide variety of equipment and patients. There are many possible combinations of kilovoltage peak (kVp), milliamperage (mA), source-to-image-receptor distance (SID), exposure time, image receptors (IRs), and grid ratios. When patients of various sizes and with various pathological conditions are considered, the selection of proper exposure factors becomes a formidable task. Tools are available to assist the radiographer in selecting appropriate exposure techniques such as automatic exposure control (AEC) devices, anatomically programmed techniques, and exposure technique charts. Knowledge about the performance of these tools and their operation assists radiographers in producing quality radiographic images.

AUTOMATIC EXPOSURE CONTROL

An automatic exposure control (AEC) system is a tool available on most modern radiographic units to assist the radiographer in determining the amount of radiation exposure to produce a quality image. AEC is a system used to consistently control the amount of radiation reaching the IR by terminating the length of exposure. AEC systems also are called *automatic exposure devices,* and sometimes they are erroneously referred to as *phototiming.* When using AEC systems, the radiographer must still use individual discretion to select an appropriate kVp, mA, IR, and grid. However, the AEC device determines the exposure time (and total exposure) that is used.

IMPORTANT RELATIONSHIP

Principle of AEC Operation

Once a predetermined amount of radiation is transmitted through a patient, the x-ray exposure is terminated. This determines the exposure time and therefore the total amount of radiation exposure to the IR.

AEC systems are excellent at producing consistent levels of exposure to the IR when used properly; however, radiographers must also be aware of the limitations of using an AEC system in patient positioning and centering, detector size and selection, collimation, and IR variation.

AEC Radiation Detectors

All AEC devices work by the same principle of operation: radiation is transmitted through the patient, which creates ionizations in a sensing material which is then converted into an electrical signal, terminating the exposure time; this occurs when a predetermined amount of radiation has been detected, as indicated by the charge of the electrical signal produced. Service personnel calibrate the predetermined level of radiation to meet the departmental standards of image quality.

The difference in AEC systems lies in the type of device that is used to convert radiation into electricity. Two types of AEC systems have been used in the past: phototimers and ionization chambers. Phototimers represent the first generation of AEC systems used in radiography, and it is from this type of system that the term *phototiming* has evolved. Phototiming specifically refers to the use of an AEC device that uses photomultiplier tubes or photodiodes, even though these systems are uncommon today. Therefore the use of the term phototiming is usually incorrect. The more common type of AEC system uses ionization chambers or solid-state detectors. Regardless of the specific type of AEC system used, almost all systems use a set of three radiation-measuring detectors, arranged in a specific manner (Fig. 9.1). The radiographer selects the configuration of these devices, determining which one (or more) of the three measures radiation exposure reaching the IR. These devices are variously referred to as *sensors*, *chambers*, *cells*, or *detectors*. These radiation-measuring devices are referred to here for the remainder of the discussion as detectors. In this chapter, AEC detectors are differentiated from flat-panel detector type IRs.

IMPORTANT RELATIONSHIP

Radiation-Measuring Devices

Detectors are the AEC devices that measure the amount of radiation transmitted through the patient (exit or remnant). The radiographer selects the combination of the detectors to use.

Phototimers

Phototimers used a fluorescent (light-producing) screen and a device that converts light into electricity. A photodiode is a solid-state device that converts visible light energy into electrical energy. Phototimer AEC devices were considered as exit-type devices because the detectors are positioned behind the IR (Fig. 9.2) so that radiation must exit the IR before it is measured by the detectors. Light paddles, coated with a fluorescent material, served as the detectors; radiation interacted with these paddles, producing visible light. This light was then transmitted to remote photomultiplier tubes or photodiodes that convert it into electricity. The timer is tripped, and the radiographic exposure was terminated when a sufficient charge had been received. This electrical charge was in proportion to the radiation to which the light paddles had been exposed. Phototimers have largely been replaced with ionization chamber or solid-state systems. In these designs, remnant radiation from the patient is received into a sensing area that create ionizations and electron pairs. The ionizations created are proportional to the x-ray exposure that creates them, and the ion pairs create an electrical current that leaves the sensing area as an amplified signal. This electrical signal ultimately sends a message to the x-ray generator to end the exposure.

Ionization Chamber Systems

An ionization or ion chamber is a hollow cell that contains air and is connected to the timer circuit via an

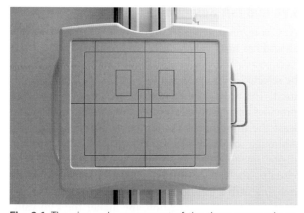

Fig. 9.1 The size and arrangement of the three automatic exposure control (AEC) detectors are clear on this upright chest unit. (From Johnston JN, Fauber TL. *Essentials of Radiographic Physics and Imaging.* 3rd ed. St. Louis: Mosby; 2020.)

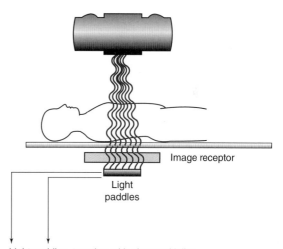

Light paddles, together with photomultiplier tubes, measure radiation exposure after it passes through the image receptor.

Fig. 9.2 The phototimer automatic exposure control (AEC) system has light paddles (detectors) located directly below the image receptor (IR). This is an exit-type device in that the x-rays must exit the IR before they are measured by the detectors.

electrical wire. Ionization chamber AEC devices are entrance-type devices because the detectors are positioned in front of the IR (Fig. 9.3) so that radiation can interact with the detectors just before interacting with the IR. When the ionization chamber is exposed to radiation from a radiographic exposure, the air inside the chamber becomes ionized, creating an electrical charge. This charge travels along the wire to the timer circuit. The timer is tripped, and the radiographic exposure is terminated when a sufficient charge has been received. This electrical charge is in proportion to the radiation to which the ionization chamber has been exposed. Most AEC systems today use ionization chambers or solid-state devices.

 IMPORTANT RELATIONSHIP

Function of the Ionization Chamber

The ionization chamber interacts with exit radiation before it reaches the IR. Air in the chamber is ionized, an electrical charge proportional to the amount of radiation is created, and this charge travels to the timer circuit where the exposure is terminated.

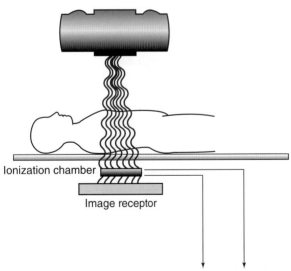

Ionization chamber measures radiation exposure before it reaches the image receptor.

Fig. 9.3 The ionization chamber automatic exposure control (AEC) system has the detectors located directly in front of the image receptor (IR). This system is termed *entrance type* because the x-ray exposure is measured just before entering the IR.

mAs Readout

When a radiographic study is performed using an AEC device, the total amount of radiation (milliamperage-seconds [mAs]) required to produce the appropriate exposure to the IR is determined by the system. Many radiographic units include an mAs readout display, where the actual amount of mAs used for that image is displayed immediately after the exposure, sometimes for only a few seconds. It is critical for the radiographer to take note of this information when it is available. Knowledge of the mAs readout has numerous advantages. It allows the radiographer to become more familiar with manual exposure technique factors. If the image is unacceptable, knowing the mAs readout provides a basis from which the radiographer can make exposure adjustments by switching to a manual technique. There may be procedures with different positions where AEC and the manual technique are combined because of difficulty with accurate centering. For example, knowing the mAs readout for the anteroposterior (AP) lumbar spine gives the radiographer an option to switch to manual techniques for the oblique exposures, making technique adjustments based on reliable mAs information.

 IMPORTANT RELATIONSHIP

AEC and mAs Readout

If the radiographic unit has an mAs readout display, the radiographer should take note of the reading after an exposure is made. This information can be invaluable.

kVp and mA Selections

AEC controls only the quantity of radiation reaching the IR and has no effect on other image characteristics, such as contrast. The kVp for a particular examination should be selected without regard to whether an AEC device is used. The radiographer must select the kVp level that provides an appropriate level of subject contrast and is at least the minimum kVp needed to penetrate the part. Although contrast can be computer manipulated in digital imaging, the kVp should still be selected to best visualize the area of interest. High kVp is used for chest imaging with a grid to best visualize the widely varying tissues (Fig. 9.4). In addition, the higher the kVp value used, the shorter is the exposure time needed by the AEC device. Because high kVp radiation is more penetrating (reducing the total amount of x-ray exposure to

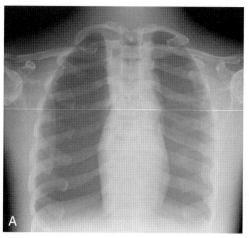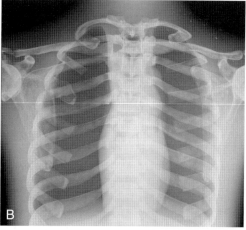

Fig. 9.4 Kilovoltage. **A,** Radiographic image created using a high kilovoltage peak (kVp) (109) and the outer two automatic exposure control (AEC) detectors. The image displays low subject contrast typical for chest imaging. **B,** Radiographic image created using a low kVp (60) and the outer two AEC detectors. The image displays high subject contrast not typical for chest imaging. The milliamperage-seconds (mAs) readout indicated significantly more radiation than **A** as a result of using a low kVp. (From Johnston JN, Fauber TL. *Essentials of Radiographic Physics and Imaging.* 3rd ed. St. Louis: Elsevier; 2020.)

the patient because more x-ray photons exit the patient) and the detectors are measuring the quantity of radiation, the preset amount of radiation exposure is reached sooner with a higher kVp.

◤ IMPORTANT RELATIONSHIP

kVp and AEC Response

The radiographer must set the kVp as needed to ensure adequate penetration and enhance the subject contrast for the part examined. The kVp selected determines the length of exposure time when using AEC. A low kVp requires more exposure time to reach the predetermined amount of exposure. A high kVp decreases the exposure time to reach the predetermined amount of exposure and reduces the overall radiation exposure to the patient.

❗ RADIATION PROTECTION ALERT

Kilovoltage Selection

Using a higher kVp with AEC decreases the exposure time and the overall mAs needed to produce a diagnostic image, significantly reducing patient exposure. The kVp selected for an examination should display the desired subject contrast for the part examined while being as high as possible to minimize the patient's radiation exposure.

When radiographers use a control panel that allows the mA and time to be set independently, they should select the mA without regard to whether an AEC device is used. The mA selected has an inverse effect on the exposure time needed by the AEC device, as it does when using a manual exposure technique to maintain exposure to the IR. Therefore, if radiographers want to decrease the exposure time for a particular examination, they may easily do so by increasing the mA value. For a given procedure, increasing the mA on the control panel decreases the exposure time, and decreasing the mA selected on the control panel increases the exposure time.

◤ IMPORTANT RELATIONSHIP

mA and AEC Response

If the radiographer can set the mA when using AEC, it will inversely affect the time of exposure for a given procedure. Increasing the mA decreases the exposure time to reach the predetermined amount of exposure. Decreasing the mA increases the exposure time to reach the predetermined amount of exposure.

Minimum Response Time

The term minimum response time refers to the shortest exposure time that the system can produce. Minimum response time (1 ms with modern AEC systems) is usually longer with AEC systems than with other types of radiographic timers (i.e., other types of radiographic timers usually are able to produce shorter exposure times than AEC devices). This can be a problem with some segments of the patient population, such as pediatric or uncooperative patients. Typically, the radiographer increases the mA so that the time of exposure terminates more quickly. If the minimum response time is longer than the amount of time needed to terminate the preset exposure, it results in an increased amount of radiation reaching the IR. With pediatric patients and other patients who cannot or will not cooperate with the radiographer by holding still or holding their breath during the exposure, AEC devices may not be the technology of choice.

Backup Time

Backup time refers to the maximum length of time for which the x-ray exposure will continue when using an AEC system. The backup time may be set by the radiographer or automatically controlled by the radiographic unit. It may be set as backup exposure time or as backup mAs (the product of mA and exposure time). The backup time acts as a safety mechanism when an AEC system fails or the equipment is not used properly. In either case, the backup time protects the patient from receiving unnecessary exposure and protects the x-ray tube from reaching or exceeding its heat-loading capacity. If the backup time is automatically controlled, it should terminate at a maximum of 600 mAs when equipment is operated at or above 50 kVp.

 IMPORTANT RELATIONSHIP

Function of Backup Time

Backup time, the maximum exposure time allowed during an AEC examination, serves as a safety mechanism when AEC is not used properly or is not functioning properly.

The backup time might be reached as a result of operator oversight when an AEC examination, such as a chest x-ray, is conducted at the upright unit and the radiographer has set the control panel for a table unit. The table detectors are forced to wait for an excessively long time to measure enough radiation to terminate the exposure. The backup time is reached, and the exposure

is terminated, limiting patient exposure and preventing the tube from overloading. However, newer x-ray units with AEC include a sensor in the receptor tray for the IR and do not allow an exposure to activate if the table unit detectors are selected but the x-ray tube is centered to the upright unit.

When controlled by the radiographer, the backup time should be set high enough to exceed the exposure needed but low enough to protect the patient from excessive exposure in case of a problem. Setting the backup time at 150% to 200% of the expected exposure time is appropriate.

 IMPORTANT RELATIONSHIP

Setting Backup Time

The backup time should be set to 150% to 200% of the expected exposure time. This allows the properly used AEC system to appropriately terminate the exposure but protects the patient and tube from excessive exposure if a problem occurs.

! RADIATION PROTECTION ALERT

Monitoring Backup Time

To minimize patient exposure, the backup time should be neither too long nor too short. Backup time that is too short results in the exposure being stopped prematurely, and the image may need to be repeated because of poor quality. Backup time that is too long results in the patient receiving unnecessary radiation if a problem occurs and the exposure does not end until the backup time is reached. In addition, the image may have to be repeated because of poor quality.

Similar to using a manual technique, overexposure may not be visually apparent when using the AEC device because the computer will adjust the displayed brightness. It is therefore important for the radiographer to monitor the exposure indicator along with image quality to determine whether over- or underexposure has occurred.

Exposure Adjustment

AEC devices are equipped with a mechanism (exposure adjustment) that allows the radiographer to adjust the amount of preset radiation detection values (also known as density controls). These are generally in the form of selections on the control panel that are numbered −2, −1, +1, +2, and +3. The actual numbers presented on exposure adjustment vary, but each selection changes exposure time by some predetermined amount or increment expressed as a percentage. A common increment is 25%, meaning that the predetermined exposure level needed to terminate the timer can be either increased or decreased from normal in one increment (+25% or −25%) or two increments (+50% or −50%).

A diagnostic quality image (Fig. 9.5A) was produced using 81 kVp and the center detector with 0 exposure adjustment, Fig. 9.5B was produced using 81 kVp and the center detector with +3 exposure adjustment, and Fig. 9.5C was produced using 81 kVp and the center detector with −3 exposure adjustment. Although the displayed brightness was adjusted by the computer, the actual mAs applied and exposure indicator for each of the images varied greatly and reflected the exposure to the IR.

Manufacturers usually provide information for their equipment on how these exposure adjustments should be used. Common sense and practical experience should also serve as guidelines for the radiographer. Routinely using plus or minus exposure adjustments to produce an acceptable image indicates that a problem exists, possibly a problem with the AEC calibration.

Alignment and Positioning Considerations
Detector Selection

Selection of the detectors to be used for a specific examination is critical when using an AEC system. AEC systems with multiple detectors typically allow the radiographer to select any combination of one, two, or three detectors. Radiographic equipment can also be purchased with five AEC detectors (Fig. 9.6), which provide greater flexibility in imaging a wide variety of patients. The selected detectors actively measure radiation during exposure, and the electrical signals are averaged. Typically, the detector that receives the greatest amount of exposure has the greatest impact on the total exposure.

Measuring radiation that passes through the anatomic area of interest is important. The general guideline is to select the detectors that would be superimposed by the anatomic structures that are of greatest interest and need to be visualized on the displayed image. Failure to select the proper detector(s) could result in either underexposure or overexposure to the IR. In the case of a posteroanterior (PA) chest radiograph, the area of radiographic interest includes the lungs and heart; therefore one or two outside detectors should be selected to place the detectors directly beneath the critical anatomic area.

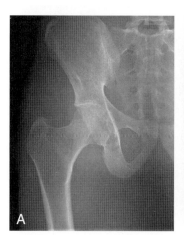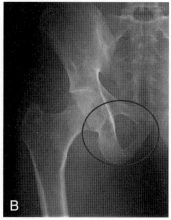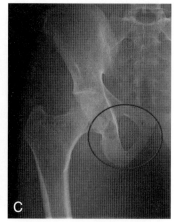

Fig. 9.5 Exposure adjustment. **A,** Radiographic image of the hip using 81 kVp, the center automatic exposure control (AEC) detector, and 0 exposure adjustment. **B,** Radiographic image of the hip using 81 kVp, the center AEC detector, and +3 exposure adjustment. The displayed image demonstrates less quantum noise than image **A**. **C,** Radiographic image of the hip using 81 kVp, the center AEC detector, and −3 exposure adjustment. The displayed image demonstrates more quantum noise than **B**. The mAs readout for **B** and **C** reflect the exposure adjustment accordingly. (From Johnston JN, Fauber TL. *Essentials of Radiographic Physics and Imaging.* 3rd ed. St. Louis: Elsevier; 2020.)

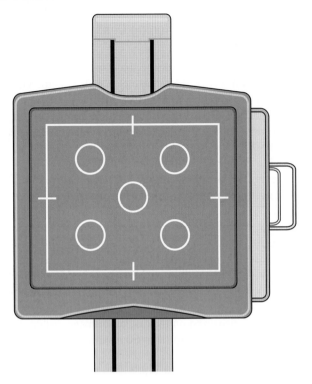

Fig. 9.6 Multiple detectors. Illustration of radiographic equipment with five automatic exposure control (AEC) detectors.

If the center detector was mistakenly selected, the anatomy superimposing this detector includes the thoracic spine. If the exposure is made, the resultant image shows sufficient exposure in the spine, with the lungs overexposed (Fig. 9.7). Although displayed brightness was adjusted by the computer, the actual mAs applied and exposure indicator reflect the image overexposure. It is important for radiographers to evaluate image quality, the applied mAs, and the exposure indicator when using the AEC device. AEC device manufacturers provide recommendations for which detectors to use for specific examinations. Recommendations for detector combination can also be found in many radiographic procedure textbooks.

Many radiographic units have AEC devices in both a table receptor tray and an upright receptor holder. If more than one receptor per radiographic unit uses AEC, the radiographer must be certain to select the correct receptor before making an exposure. Failure to do so may result in the patient and IR being exposed to excessive radiation. If the backup time is reached, the exposure is prematurely terminated, and a repeat radiographic study may need to be done, increasing patient dose.

A similar problem can occur in some systems when not using an image receptor holder, such as with

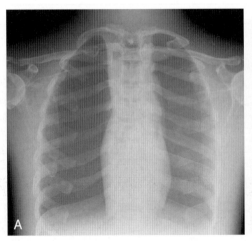
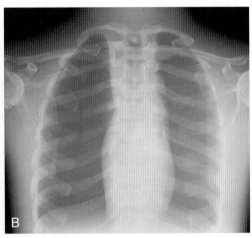

Fig. 9.7 Detector selection. **A,** Radiographic image displayed using the outer two automatic exposure control (AEC) detectors appropriate for chest imaging. **B,** Radiographic image displayed when the center detector was inappropriately selected for a chest image, placing the thoracic spine directly over the detector. The resulting chest image has increased radiation exposure in the area of the spine, and therefore the lungs are overexposed. Although the displayed brightness in the area of interest was computer adjusted, the mAs readout reflected the overexposure of the image receptor (IR) for chest image. (From Johnston JN, Fauber TL. *Essentials of Radiographic Physics and Imaging.* 3rd ed. St. Louis: Elsevier; 2020.)

cross-table, tabletop or stretcher, or wheelchair studies. If the AEC system is activated with these types of examinations, an unusually long exposure results because the detectors are not being exposed to radiation. Again, the backup time will likely be reached, and the patient's dose will be excessive. Modern radiographic units are designed so that an exposure does not occur if the AEC device has been selected and there is no IR detected in the receptor tray.

 IMPORTANT RELATIONSHIP

Detector Selection

> The combination of detectors affects the amount of exposure reaching the IR. If the area of radiographic interest is not directly over the selected detectors, that area will likely be overexposed or underexposed.

Patient Centering

Proper centering of the part being examined is crucial when using an AEC system. The anatomic area of interest must be properly centered over the detectors that the radiographer has selected; improper centering of the part over the selected detectors may underexpose or overexpose the IR. For example, when an AEC device is used for a thoracic spine image, if the central ray (CR) is positioned over the right lung and the center detector is selected (as appropriate), the soft tissue and ribs superimpose the detector rather than the spine. In this case, the soft tissue and ribs demonstrate sufficient exposure, but the spine itself is underexposed (Fig. 9.8).

IMPORTANT RELATIONSHIP

Patient Centering

> Accurate centering of the area of interest over the detectors is critical to ensure proper exposure to the IR. If the area of interest is not properly centered to the detectors, overexposure or underexposure may occur.

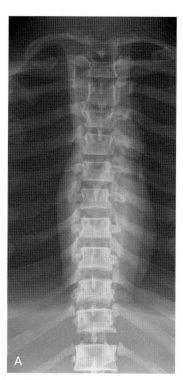 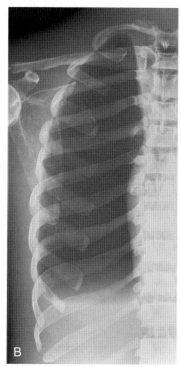

Fig. 9.8 Centering. **A,** The center detector was selected for this thoracic spine and the central ray (CR) midpoint to the thoracic spine. **B,** The CR was centered over the right lung field. The resulting image demonstrates appropriate brightness levels in the right lung and ribs, but the thoracic vertebral bodies are underexposed. (From Johnston JN, Fauber TL. *Essentials of Radiographic Physics and Imaging.* 3rd ed. St. Louis: Elsevier; 2020.)

When the anatomy of interest is not centered directly over the detector, the image is underexposed or overexposed, possibly requiring the image to be repeated and the patient to receive more radiation than necessary.

If the digital IR is underexposed or overexposed, the computer adjusts the exposure error, but the image quality displayed, patient exposure, or both are compromised. Underexposure may result in the visibility of quantum noise, and overexposure increases patient exposure and may decrease the subject contrast displayed. It is important for radiographers to evaluate image quality, the applied mAs, and the exposure indicator when using the AEC device. Errors in selecting the appropriate combination of AEC detectors, detector size, or positioning errors may not be visually apparent because of computer adjustment of the displayed image brightness.

Detector Size

The size and shape of the detectors manufactured within an AEC system is fixed and cannot be adjusted. Therefore it is important for the radiographer to determine whether AEC should be used during the radiographic procedure. The radiographer must first determine whether the patient's anatomic area of interest can adequately cover the detector combination. For example, if the patient for a procedure is very small, such as a toddler, their chest may not adequately cover the outer two detectors. In this case, the patient's chest is smaller than the dimensions of the selected detectors. If a portion of the detector is directly exposed to the primary beam, the radiation exposure level necessary to terminate the exposure is reached almost immediately, resulting in underexposure of the area of interest.

It is critical for the radiographer to determine whether the anatomic area of interest can adequately superimpose the dimension of the detector combination. If the detector combination is larger in size than the area of interest, the use of a manual exposure technique would be necessitated.

> ## ! RADIATION PROTECTION ALERT
>
> ### *Errors in AEC Use*
>
> It is important for radiographers to evaluate image quality, the applied mAs, and the exposure indicator when using the AEC device. Errors in selecting the appropriate combination of AEC detectors, detector size, or positioning errors may not be visually apparent because of computer adjustment.

Compensating Issues
Patient Considerations

The AEC system is designed to compensate for changes in patient thickness. If the area of interest is thicker because of an increase in the patient's size, the exposure time will lengthen to reach the preset exposure to the detectors. AEC systems that do not adequately compensate for changes in patient thickness may need to be recalibrated.

Some patients may require greater technical consideration when AEC is used for radiographic procedures. For example, abdominal examinations using AEC can be compromised if a patient has an excessive amount of bowel gas. If a detector is superimposed over an area of the abdomen with excessive gas, the timer will prematurely terminate the exposure, resulting in underexposure to the IR. Likewise, destructive pathological conditions can cause underexposure of the area of radiographic interest. The presence of positive contrast media, an additive pathological condition, or a prosthetic device (metal) superimposing the detector can cause excessive exposure.

If the anatomic area directly over the detector does not represent the anatomic area of interest, inappropriate exposure to the IR may result. This can happen when the anatomic area over the detector contains a foreign object, a pocket of air, or contrast media. The radiographer must consider these circumstances individually and determine how to best image the patient or part. Using the exposure adjustment controls may work in some cases, but in others, it may be necessary to recenter the patient or part. Sometimes the best solution is a manual technique determined through use of a technique chart. AEC is not a replacement for a knowledgeable radiographer using critical thinking skills.

> ## ! RADIATION PROTECTION ALERT
>
> ### *Patient Variability*
>
> Factors related to the patient affect the time of exposure reaching the IR and ultimately the image quality; such factors include pathology, contrast media, foreign objects, and pockets of gas. Increases or decreases in patient thickness result in changes in the time of exposure if the AEC system is functioning properly. It is up to the radiographer to determine whether a manual exposure technique is a better choice than the AEC device.

Collimation

The size of the x-ray field is a factor when AEC systems are used because the additional scatter radiation produced by failure to accurately restrict the beam may cause the detector to prematurely terminate the exposure. The detector is unable to distinguish transmitted radiation from scattered radiation and, as always, ends the exposure when a preset amount of exposure has been reached. Because the detector is measuring both types of radiation exiting the patient, the timer is turned off too soon when scatter is excessive, resulting in underexposure of the area of interest.

In addition, if the x-ray field size is collimated too closely, the detector does not initially receive sufficient exposure and may prolong the exposure time, which could result in overexposure. The radiographer should open the collimator to the extent that the part being examined is appropriately imaged but not so much as to cause the AEC device to terminate the exposure before the area being imaged is properly exposed.

IMPORTANT RELATIONSHIP

Collimation and AEC Response

Excessive or insufficient collimation may affect the amount of exposure reaching the IR. Insufficient collimation may result in excessive scatter reaching the detectors, causing the exposure time to terminate too quickly. Excessive collimation may result in an extremely long exposure time.

Image Receptor Variations

Different types of IRs cannot be interchanged easily after an AEC device is calibrated to terminate exposures at a preset level. When calibration is performed, it is done for a specific type of IR and its sensitivity to the radiation exposure.

IMPORTANT RELATIONSHIP

Type of IR and AEC Response

The AEC system is calibrated based on the type of IR used. If an IR of a different type is used, the detectors will not sense the difference, and the exposure time will terminate at the preset value, which may jeopardize image quality.

The AEC device cannot sense when the radiographer uses a different type of IR and instead produces an exposure based on the system for which it was calibrated, resulting in either too much or too little exposure for that IR.

Calibration

As with any radiographic unit, it is imperative that systematic equipment testing be performed to ensure proper system performance. Calibration and quality control testing are essential procedures to maintain the proper functioning of the AEC system (Box 9.1).

For an AEC device to function properly, the radiographic unit, including the type of IR, and the AEC device must be calibrated to meet departmental standards. When a radiographic unit with AEC is first installed, the AEC device is calibrated (and at intervals thereafter). The purpose of this calibration is to ensure that consistent and appropriate exposures to the IR are produced.

Failure to maintain regular calibration of the unit results in a lack of consistent and reproducible exposures to the detectors and could affect image quality. This situation ultimately leads to overexposure of the patient, poor efficiency of the imaging department, and the possibility of improper interpretation of radiographic images.

The radiographer must use AEC accurately, regardless of the type of IR used. Failure to do so can result in overexposure of the patient to ionizing radiation or production of a poor-quality image. It cannot be overstated

---

BOX 9.1 Quality Control Check: AEC

- The AEC device should provide consistent exposures to the IR for variations in technique factors, patient thicknesses, and detector selection. Several aspects of the AEC performance can be monitored by imaging a homogeneous patient-equivalent phantom plus additional thickness plates.
- Consistency of exposures with varying mA, kVp, part thicknesses, and detector selection can each be evaluated individually and in combination by imaging a patient-equivalent phantom and measuring the resultant milligray (mGy) exposure and pixel brightness levels displayed. Reproducibility of exposures for a given set of exposure factors and selected detector should result in mGy readings within 5% and pixel brightness levels for areas within the displayed image should be within 30%.

AEC, Automatic exposure control; *IR,* imaging receptor; *kVp,* kilovoltage peak; *mA,* milliamperage.

that when using digital IRs, the radiographer must be very conscientious about excessive radiation exposure to the patient. If a high amount of radiation reaches the digital IR, the displayed image may appear diagnostic while the patient receives unnecessary exposure. During computer processing, displayed brightness can be adjusted after underexposure; however, there may be an increase in the visibility of quantum noise. The radiographer must monitor the exposure indicator as a means of detecting AEC malfunctions for digital IRs.

The response of the AEC device when changing exposure variables and their effect on exposure time and displayed brightness in the area of interest are presented in Table 9.1.

ANATOMICALLY PROGRAMMED TECHNIQUE

Anatomic programming, or anatomically programmed technique, refers to a radiographic system that allows the radiographer to choose a particular selection on the control panel that represents an anatomic area for which a preprogrammed set of exposure factors are displayed and can be selected. The appearance of these controls varies depending on the unit (Fig. 9.9), but the operation of all anatomically programmed systems is based on the same principle. Anatomically programmed techniques are controlled by an integrated circuit or computer chip that has been programmed with exposure factors for different projections and positions of different anatomic parts. After an anatomic part and projection or position has been selected, the radiographer can adjust the exposure factors that are displayed.

Anatomically programmed technique systems and AEC are not related in their functions, other than as systems for making exposures. However, these two different systems are commonly combined in radiographic units because of their similar dependence on integrated computer circuitry and often are used in conjunction with one another. A radiographer can use an anatomically programmed technique to select a projection or position for a specific anatomic part and view the kVp, mA, and exposure time for a manual technique. When anatomically programmed techniques are used in conjunction with AEC on some radiographic units, the system not only selects and displays manual exposure factors but also selects and displays the AEC detectors to be used for a specific radiographic examination. For

example, pressing the "Lungs PA" choice results in selection of 120 kVp, the upright unit, and the two outside AEC detectors. As with AEC, the anatomically programmed technique is a system that automates some of the work of radiography. However, the individual judgment and discretion of the radiographer is still required to use the anatomically programmed technique system correctly for the production of diagnostic quality images (see Box 9.2).

> ## ⚠ RADIATION PROTECTION ALERT
>
> ### Anatomically Programmed Technique and Patient Exposure
>
> When using a preprogrammed set of exposure factors, the radiographer must evaluate the appropriateness of the selected exposure technique factors. Adjustment of the preprogrammed exposure factors may be necessary for that patient or procedure.

EXPOSURE TECHNIQUE CHARTS

Exposure technique charts are useful tools that assist the radiographer in selecting a manual exposure technique or when using AEC, regardless of the type of IR. Exposure technique charts are pre-established guidelines used by the radiographer to select standardized, manual, or AEC exposure factors for each type of radiographic examination. Technique charts standardize the selection of exposure factors for the typical patient so that the quality of radiographic images is consistent. Additional information, such as collimation, AEC detector selection, and grid use, can be included in the technique chart.

For each radiographic procedure, the radiographer consults the technique chart for the recommended exposure variables—kVp, mAs, type of IR, grid, and SID. Based on the thickness of the anatomic part to be imaged, the radiographer selects the exposure factors presented in the technique chart. For example, if a patient is scheduled for a routine abdominal examination, the radiographer positions the patient and aligns the central ray to the patient and IR, measures the abdomen for a manual technique, and consults the chart for the predetermined standardized exposure variables.

Because many factors have an impact on the selection of appropriate exposure factors, technique charts are instrumental in the production of consistent quality

TABLE 9.1 Digital Imaging and Automatic Exposure Control

An upright PA chest examination performed using the following factors produces a diagnostic image:

Flat-panel detector	AEC with two outer detectors
120 kVp	Upright Bucky
400 mA	0 (normal) exposure adjustment

Assuming all other factors remain the same, unless indicated, how would the following changes affect the response of the AEC device and image quality?

Change	Effect on Exposure Time	Effect on Displayed Brightness in Area of Interest	Explanation
CR IR	No effect	No effect	The AEC is calibrated to the flat-panel detector. The exposure ends when the exposure is sufficient for the IR, which is suboptimal for the CR image receptor. The computer maintains the brightness, but quantum noise is apparent because of underexposure of the imaging plate.
Center detector selected	Increased	No effect	Because the thoracic spine lies over the center detector, the IR receives more exposure than is needed. The mAs and exposure indicator will reflect an increase in exposure to the image receptor. The computer maintains the brightness, but the image contrast is decreased because of excessive scatter, and the patient is overexposed.
70 kVp	Increased	No effect	The length of exposure to the IR will be increased, resulting in an increase in the actual mAs to maintain the exposure to the IR. However, the displayed subject contrast is increased because of the lower kVp.
100 mA	Increased	No effect	The length of exposure is increased to maintain exposure to the IR.
−2 exposure adjustment	Decreased	No effect	Changing the exposure adjustment selection changes the setting of the AEC, so it turns off the exposure much sooner. The mAs and exposure indicator will reflect a decrease in exposure to the IR. The computer maintains the brightness, but quantum noise is apparent because of underexposure of the IR.
Patient has a cardiac pacemaker positioned over the detector	Increased	No effect	The detector that is behind the pacemaker takes a long time to turn off the exposure because the radiation must pass through the pacemaker. The mAs and exposure indicator will reflect an increase in exposure to the IR. The computer maintains the brightness, but the image contrast is decreased because of excessive scatter, and the patient is overexposed.

AEC, Automatic exposure control; *CR,* computed radiography; *IR,* imaging receptor; *kVp,* kilovoltage peak; *mA,* milliamperage; *mAs,* milliamperage-second; *PA,* posteroanterior.

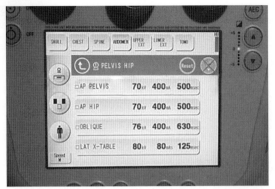

Fig. 9.9 Anatomically programmed technique selections are displayed on this console (pelvis hip in this image). The radiographer can choose from anatomic areas and positions/projections. Each selection displays the preprogrammed technical factors that the radiographer can decide to use or adjust. (From Frank, E, Long, B, Ehrlich, RA. *Radiography Essentials for Limited Practice*. 6th ed. St. Louis: Elsevier Inc.; 2021.)

radiographic images, reduction in repeat radiographic studies, and reduction in patient exposure. The proper development and use of technique charts are keys to the selection of appropriate exposure factors.

IMPORTANT RELATIONSHIP

Exposure Technique Charts and Radiographic Quality

Exposure technique charts are important for digital imaging because digital systems have a wide dynamic range and can compensate for exposure technique errors. Technique charts should be developed and used with all types of radiographic imaging systems to optimize for radiological protection. Meaning the radiation dose should be appropriate to the imaging procedure and avoid unnecessary exposure to the patient while producing quality images for diagnostic interpretation.

Conditions

A technique chart presents the exposure factors that are to be used for a specific examination on the basis of the type of radiographic equipment. Technique charts help to ensure that consistent image quality is achieved throughout the entire radiology department; they also decrease the number of repeat radiographic studies needed and therefore decrease patient exposure.

Technique charts do not replace the critical thinking skills required of the radiographer. The radiographer must continue to use individual judgment and discretion in properly selecting exposure factors for each patient and type of examination. The primary task of the radiographer is to produce diagnostic quality images while delivering the least amount of radiation exposure. Technique charts are designed for an average or typical patient and do not account for unusual circumstances. Patient variability in terms of body habitus or physical condition or the presence of a pathological condition requires the radiographer to problem solve when selecting exposure factors. These atypical conditions require accurate patient assessment and appropriate exposure technique adjustment by the radiographer.

A technique chart should be established for each x-ray tube, even if a single generator is used for more than one tube. For example, if a radiographic room has two x-ray tubes, one for a radiographic table and one for an upright unit, each tube should have its own technique chart because of possible inherent differences in the radiation output produced by each tube. Furthermore, a mobile radiographic unit must also have its own technique chart.

For technique charts to be effective tools in producing images of consistent quality, departmental standards for displayed image quality should be established. In addition, the standardization of exposure factors and the use of accessory devices are needed. For example, an average adult knee can be adequately imaged with or without the use of a grid. Although both images might be acceptable, departmental standards may specify that the knee be imaged with the use of a grid. These types of decisions should be made before technique chart development takes place so that the departmental standards can be clarified. Technique charts are then constructed using these standards, to which radiographers should adhere.

For technique charts to be effective, the radiographic system should be operating properly. A good quality control program for all radiographic equipment ensures monitoring of any variability in the performance of the equipment.

Accurate measurement of part thickness is important for the effective use of technique charts. The measured part thickness determines the selected kVp and mAs values for the radiographic examination. If the part is measured inaccurately, incorrect exposure factors may be selected. Measurement of part thickness must be standardized throughout the radiology department.

Calipers are devices that measure part thickness and may be readily accessible in every radiographic room (Fig. 9.10). In addition, the technique chart should specify the exact location for measuring part thickness. Part measurement may be performed at the location of the central ray midpoint or the thickest portion of the area to be radiographed. Errors in part thickness measurement are common mistakes made when one is consulting technique charts.

Because the range of exposures needed to produce a quality digital image is wider (wide exposure latitude), precise measurement of the anatomic part is not as critical. Although the technique charts discussed in this chapter use patient measurement to determine the exposure factors to be selected, categorizing the typical patient according to size (small, medium, large, and extra-large) may be sufficient when using digital IRs.

Types of Technique Charts

Technique charts can vary widely in terms of their design, but they share some common characteristics. The primary exposure factors of kVp and mAs and common accessory devices used, such as IRs of various

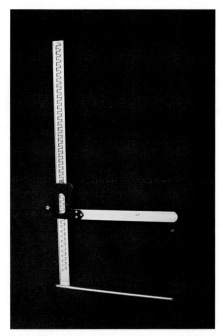

Fig. 9.10 A caliper is used to measure part thickness. (From Johnston JN, Fauber TL. *Essentials of Radiographic Physics and Imaging*. 3rd ed. St. Louis: Mosby; 2020.)

types and grid ratios, are included regardless of the type of technique chart used. Two primary types of exposure technique charts exist: fixed kVp/variable mAs and variable kVp/fixed mAs. Each type of chart has different characteristics, and both have advantages and disadvantages. Although variable kVp/fixed mAs–type technique charts have limited value in digital imaging, differentiating between the design of these types of technique charts provides useful information.

Variable kVp/Fixed mAs Technique Chart

The variable kVp/fixed mAs technique chart is based on the concept that kVp can be increased as the anatomic part size increases. Specifically, the baseline kVp is increased by 2 for every 1 cm (0.4 inch) increase in part thickness, whereas mAs is maintained (Table 9.2). The baseline kVp is the original kVp value predetermined for the anatomic area to be imaged. The baseline kVp is then adjusted for changes in part thickness.

If this type of technique chart were used today, accurate measurement of part thickness would be important. Part thickness must be accurately measured to ensure that the 2-kVp adjustment is appropriately applied. The radiographer consults the technique chart and prepares the exposure factors specified for the type of radiographic examination (i.e., mAs, SID, grid use, and type of IR). The anatomic part is accurately measured, and the

kVp is appropriately adjusted. For example, a standard exposure technique for a patient's knee measuring 10 cm (4 inches) is 63 kVp at 8 mAs, flat-panel IR, and the use of a 10:1 table Bucky grid. A patient with a knee measuring 15 cm (6 inches) would require a change only in the kVp from 63 to 73 (2-kVp change for every 1-cm [~0.5-inch] change in part thickness).

 IMPORTANT RELATIONSHIP

Variable kVp/Fixed mAs Technique Chart

The variable kVp chart adjusts the kVp for changes in part thickness while maintaining a fixed mAs (2-kVp change for every 1-cm [~0.5-inch] change in part thickness).

Determination of the baseline kilovoltage for each anatomic area was not standardized. Historically, various methods have been used to determine the baseline kVp value. The goal is to determine a kVp value that adequately penetrates the anatomic part when using a 2-kVp adjustment for every 1-cm (~0.5-inch) change in tissue thickness. The baseline kVp value can be experimentally determined with the use of radiographic phantoms (patient-equivalent devices).

Developing a variable kVp technique chart that can be used effectively throughout the kilovoltage range has proved to be problematic. In addition, technological advances in digital IRs have challenged the applicability of the variable kVp–/fixed mAs–type technique chart.

In general, changing the kVp values for variations in part thickness may be ineffective throughout the entire range of radiographic examinations. A variable kVp/fixed mAs chart may be most effective with pediatric patients or when small extremities, such as hands, toes, and feet, are being imaged. At low kVp levels, small changes in kVp may be more effective than changing the mAs.

This type of chart has the advantage of being easy to formulate because making kVp changes to compensate for different part sizes is simple. However, because kVp is variable, subject contrast may also vary, and these types of charts tend to be less accurate for part-size extremes. In addition, adequate penetration of the part is not assured, and digital receptors may not operate as designed at lower kVp levels.

Fixed kVp/Variable mAs Technique Chart

The fixed kVp/variable mAs technique chart (Table 9.3) uses the concept of selecting an optimal kVp value that is

TABLE 9.2   Variable kVp/Fixed mAs Technique Chart

Anatomic part: knee	IR: flat-panel detector
Projection: AP	Tabletop/Bucky: Bucky
Measuring point: midpatella	Grid ratio: 10:1
SID: 100 cm (40 inches)	Focal spot size: small

cm	kVp	mAs
10	63	8
11	65	8
12	67	8
13	69	8
14	71	8
15	73	8
16	75	8
17	77	8
18	79	8

AP, Anteroposterior; *IR,* image receptor; *kVp,* kilovoltage peak; *mAs,* milliamperage-seconds; *SID,* source-to-image-receptor distance.

TABLE 9.3 Fixed kVp/Variable mAs Technique Chart

Anatomic part: knee	IR: flat-panel detector
Projection: AP	Tabletop/Bucky: Bucky
Measuring point: midpatella	Grid ratio: 10:1
SID: 100 cm (40 inches)	Focal spot size: small

cm	kVp	mAs
10–13	73	4
14–17	73	8
18–21	73	16

AP, Anteroposterior; *IR*, image receptor; *kVp*, kilovoltage peak; *mAs*, milliamperage-seconds; *SID*, source-to-image-receptor distance.

required for the radiographic examination and adjusting the mAs for variations in part thickness. Optimal kVp can be described as the kVp value that is high enough to ensure penetration of the part and is at the preferred energy of the image receptor sensitivity but not too high to diminish displayed subject contrast. For this type of chart, the optimal kVp value for each part is indicated and mAs is varied as a function of part thickness.

⚡ IMPORTANT RELATIONSHIP

Fixed kVp/Variable mAs Technique Chart

The fixed kVp/variable mAs technique chart identifies optimal kVp values and alters the mAs for variations in part thickness (every 4- to 5-cm [1.6- to 2-inch] change in part thickness, the mAs should be adjusted by a factor of 2).

Optimal kVp values required for each anatomic area have not been standardized. Although charts identifying common kVp values for different anatomic areas can be found, experienced radiographers tend to develop their own optimal kVp values. The goal is to determine the kVp that penetrates the part without compromising subject contrast; however, digital computer postprocessing provides the opportunity to vary the image contrast displayed. Specifying the optimal kVp value used in a fixed kVp/variable mAs technique chart encourages all radiographers to adhere to the departmental standards.

After optimal kVp values are established, fixed kVp/variable mAs technique charts alter the mAs for variations in the thickness of the anatomic part. Because x-rays are attenuated exponentially, a general guideline

is that for every 4- to 5-cm (1.6- to 2-inch) change in part thickness, the mAs should be adjusted by a factor of 2. Using the previous example for a patient's knee measuring 10 cm (4 inches) and an optimal kVp, the exposure technique would be 73 kVp at 4 mAs, flat-panel IR with a 10:1 table Bucky grid. A patient with a knee measuring 15 cm (6 inches) would require a change only in the mAs from 4 to 8 (a 5-cm [2-inch] increase in part thickness requires a doubling of the mAs).

Accurate measurement of the anatomic part is important but is less critical compared with the precision needed with variable kVp charts. An advantage of fixed kVp/variable mAs technique charts is that patient groups can be formed for around 4- to 5-cm (1.6- to 2-inch) changes. Alternatively, patients can be grouped by size (e.g., small, medium, large, extra-large) or actual weight ranges in pounds (e.g., 45–59 kg [100–130 pounds]), and therefore measuring the thickness would not be required. In addition, using consistently higher "optimal" kVp ranges with digital imaging systems can reduce the variability among exposure techniques for the same or similar anatomic region.

The fixed kVp/variable mAs technique chart has the advantages of easier use, more consistency in the production of quality images, greater assurance of adequate penetration of all anatomic parts, uniform displayed subject contrast, and increased accuracy with extreme variation in the size of the anatomic part.

Exposure Technique Chart Development

Radiographers can develop effective technique charts that assist in exposure technique selection. The steps involved in technique chart development are similar, regardless of the design of the technique chart. The primary tools needed are radiographic phantoms, calipers for accurate measurement, and a calculator. After diagnostic images are produced using these phantoms, exposure techniques can be extrapolated (mathematically estimated) for imaging other similar anatomic areas.

A critical component in technique chart development is to determine the minimal kVp value that adequately penetrates the anatomic part being radiographed. One available method is to use the concept of comparative anatomy, which can assist the radiographer in determining minimal kVp values. This concept states that different parts of the same size can be imaged by use of the same exposure factors, provided that the minimal kVp value needed to penetrate the part is used in each case. For example, a radiographer knows what exposure factors to use with a particular radiographic unit for a knee that measures 10 cm (4 inches) for the AP projection, but now needs to image a shoulder; the radiographer measures the shoulder for the AP projection and determines that it measures 10 cm (4 inches). The radiographer does not have a technique for a shoulder for this radiographic unit. The concept of comparative anatomy states that the shoulder in this case can be successfully radiographed using the same technique that the radiographer has used for the 10-cm (4-inch) knee as long as the minimal kVp to penetrate the part has been used for the shoulder or knee.

The stages for development of exposure technique charts are similar, regardless of the type of chart (Box 9.3). Patient-equivalent phantoms for sample anatomic areas provide a means for establishing standardized exposure factors. Using the concept of comparative anatomy assists the radiographer in extrapolating exposure techniques for similar anatomic areas. The exposure technique chart created can also include a range of acceptable exposure

indicators expected for the anatomic part imaged. After the initial development of an exposure technique chart, the chart must be tested for accuracy and revised if necessary.

Poor radiographic quality may result when the exposure technique chart is not used properly. Radiographers need to problem solve by evaluating the numerous exposure variables that could have contributed to a poor-quality image before assuming that the chart is ineffective.

A commitment by management and staff to use exposure technique charts is critical to the consistent production of quality images. Well-developed technique charts are of little use if radiographers choose not to consult them.

IMPORTANT RELATIONSHIP
Exposure Technique Charts

> A commitment by management and staff to use exposure technique charts is critical to the consistent production of quality radiographic images. Well-developed technique charts are of little use if radiographers choose not to consult them.

SPECIAL CONSIDERATIONS

Appropriate exposure factor selection and its modification for variability in the patient are critical to the production of a quality image. The radiographer must be able to recognize a multitude of patient and equipment variables and have a thorough understanding of how these variables affect the resulting image to make adjustments to produce a quality radiographic image.

Pediatric Patients

Pediatric patients are a technical challenge for radiographers for many reasons. Because of their smaller size, they require lower kVp and mAs values than adults.

Pediatric chest radiography requires the radiographer to choose fast exposure times to stop diaphragm motion in patients who cannot or will not voluntarily suspend their breathing. A fast exposure time may eliminate the possibility of using AEC systems for pediatric chest radiography. Owing to their small size, pediatric patients may not adequately cover AEC detectors, and therefore, a manual exposure technique should be used.

Exposure factors used for the adult skull can be used for pediatric patients aged 6 years and older, because the

---

BOX 9.3   **How to Develop an Exposure Technique Chart**

- Select a kVp value appropriate to the anatomic area to be imaged. Determine the mAs value that produces the desired exposure to the IR.
- Using a patient-equivalent phantom, produce several images by varying the kVp and mAs values. Use the general rules for exposure technique adjustment (i.e., the 15% rule). Exposures to the IR should be similar.
- Evaluate the quality of the images and eliminate those deemed unacceptable.
- Of the remaining acceptable images, select those having a kVp value appropriate for the type of technique chart desired and according to departmental standards.
- Provide a range of acceptable exposure indicators (per departmental standards) expected for the anatomic part imaged.
- Extrapolate the exposure techniques (variable kVp or variable mAs) for changes in part thickness.
- Use the concept of comparative anatomy to develop technique charts for similar anatomic areas.
- Test the technique chart for accuracy and revise if needed.

IR, Imaging receptor; *kVp,* kilovoltage peak; *mAs,* milliamperage-seconds.

bone density of these children has developed to an adult level. However, exposure factors must be modified for patients younger than 6 years. It is recommended for the radiographer to decrease the kVp by at least 15% to compensate for this lack of bone density. In addition, one should limit the use of grids whenever possible. Radiographic examination of all other parts of pediatric patients' anatomy requires an adjustment in exposure techniques.

Because pediatric patients are more sensitive to ionizing radiation and have a longer life span than adults, it is even more critical to monitor the exposure indicator during digital imaging in an effort to minimize unnecessary radiation exposure.

Geriatric Patients

Aging patients may experience physical changes such as limitations in hearing, vision, and balance. Additionally, their skin is thinner and more easily torn or bruised. Psychological changes in the mental state of geriatric patients may impact their ability to follow instructions during imaging procedures. Radiographers should be prepared to provide enhanced patient care in terms of additional time for imaging procedures; sensitivity to patient comfort by using a table pad, positioning sponges, and blankets for warmth; and attention to the safety of geriatric patients during transport on and off the table and positioning during the procedure.

Exposure techniques may need to be decreased for patients who appear thin and frail. Tissues may be lower in subject contrast and therefore require decreased kVp, which results in higher subject contrast. To eliminate motion, it is recommended for the radiographer to accordingly adjust the mA and exposure time.

Bariatric Patients

Body mass index (BMI) is a person's weight in kilograms divided by the square of height in meters. A high BMI (>30) can be an indicator of obesity. Imaging patients who are categorized as obese are more commonplace in radiology. Bariatric surgery is becoming more routine, and therefore imaging procedures may be needed both before and after surgery. Bariatric patients bring unique challenges in terms of their weight and body diameter.

Important issues to consider when imaging bariatric patients include the table weight limit and the size (aperture) diameter of fluoroscopic imaging equipment. Bariatric patients need an increase in both kVp and

mAs values to produce diagnostic images. In addition, the use of a grid is important to reduce the scatter radiation from reaching the IR, which would decrease displayed image contrast. Depending on the imaging procedure performed, bariatric patients may need to be imaged in quadrants owing to the size limitation of the IR.

Projections and Positions

Different radiographic projections and patient positions of the same anatomic part often require modification of exposure factors. For example, an oblique position of the lumbar spine requires more exposure than an AP projection because of an increase in the amount of tissue through which the primary beam must pass. However, an oblique ankle image requires slightly less exposure than the AP for comparable exposure to the IR.

General guidelines, based on variations in radiographic projection or patient position, can be followed to change exposure factors. Compared with an AP projection, an increase or a decrease in the amount of tissue should determine any changes in exposure factors for oblique and lateral patient positions.

Casts and Splints

Casts and splints can be produced from materials that attenuate x-rays differently. Selecting appropriate exposure factors can be challenging because of the wide variety of materials used for these devices. The radiographer should pay close attention to both the type of material and how the cast or splint is used.

Casts

Casts can be made of either fiberglass or plaster. Fiberglass generally requires no change in exposure factors from the values used for the same anatomic part without a cast.

Plaster presents a problem in terms of exposure factors. Plaster casts require an increase in exposure factors compared with that needed to image the same part without a cast. However, the method and amount of increase in exposure have not been standardized.

Exposure factor adjustments for cast materials may be based on the part thickness using a technique chart. For example, if an AP ankle measured through the CR is 10 cm (4 inches) without the cast and 20 cm (8 inches) with the cast, the radiographer simply increases the exposure technique to that of an ankle measuring 20 cm (8 inches) to obtain an acceptable image.

Splints

Splints present less of a challenge for the determination of appropriate exposure factors than casts. Inflatable (air) and fiberglass splints do not require any increase in exposure. Wood, aluminum, and solid plastic splints may require that exposure factors be increased but only if they are in the path of the primary beam. For example, if two pieces of wood are bound to the sides of a lower leg, no increase in exposure is necessary for an AP projection because the splint is not in the path of the primary beam and does not interfere with the radiographic image. Using the same example, if a lateral projection is produced, the splint is in the path of the primary beam and interferes with the imaging of the part. An increase in the exposure technique is required to produce a properly exposed radiographic image.

Pathologic Conditions

Pathological conditions that can alter the absorption characteristics of the anatomic part being examined are divided into two categories: additive and destructive. Additive diseases are pathologies that increase the absorption characteristics of the part, making the part more difficult to penetrate. Destructive processes are diseases or conditions that decrease the absorption characteristics of the part, making the part less difficult to penetrate. As an example, patients with compromised cardiac health can develop conditions such as pulmonary edema or congestive heart failure (CHF). These conditions result in the normally aerated lung tissues filling with fluids and naturally increase the tissue opacity of the lungs. This is an additive condition and may warrant an increase in exposure technique. Similarly, a significant lung lobe collapse (atelectasis) causes a tissue consolidation in the lungs, increasing its tissue opacity and decreasing the degree of lung aeration. An increase in exposure may be required, depending upon the degree of the lung tissue collapse.

In the abdomen, a condition known as ascites results in the large collection of fluid in the abdominal cavity. This fluid tends to accumulate in the central region of the abdomen making it more opaque in tissue makeup and often an increase in kVp and mAs is needed to achieve better image quality with less quantum noise. Additionally, patients who have developed a severe bowel obstruction may have large collections of bowel gas in loops of intestines. The large gas collection makes the abdomen easier to penetrate and less exposure may be required. Occasionally, these patients can also develop ascites in addition to the bowel obstruction making technique selection quite challenging.

In the skeletal system, a bone disorder known as osteopetrosis creates very dense bones that appear quite opaque on images. Although the bones are more dense in tissue makeup, they are structurally very weak, brittle, and prone to fracture. This would be an additive condition and require increased exposure. Bones that have lost mineralization and bone mass exhibit osteoporosis and are less dense in tissue makeup. This is a destructive condition and requires a reduction in exposure. Table 9.4 lists additive and destructive diseases. Generally, it is necessary to increase the kVp when imaging parts that have been affected by additive diseases and to decrease the kVp when imaging parts affected by destructive diseases.

TABLE 9.4 Common Additive and Destructive Diseases and Conditions by Anatomic Area

Additive Conditions	Destructive Conditions
Abdomen	
Aortic aneurysm	Bowel obstruction
Ascites	Free air
Cirrhosis	
Hypertrophy of some organs (e.g., splenomegaly)	
Chest	
Atelectasis	Emphysema
Congestive heart failure	Pneumothorax
Malignancy	
Pleural effusion	
Pneumonia	
Skeleton	
Hydrocephalus	Gout
Metastases (osteoblastic)	Metastases (osteolytic)
Osteochondroma (exostoses)	Multiple myeloma
Paget's disease (late stage)	Paget's disease (early stage)
Osteoporosis	
Nonspecific Sites	
Abscess	Atrophy
Edema	Emaciation
Sclerosis	Malnutrition

However, it is not necessary to compensate for all additive and destructive diseases. It is often desirable to image diseases with exposure factors that would normally be used for a specific anatomic part so that the effect of that disease on that part can be clearly visualized.

When it is necessary or desirable to compensate for additive or destructive diseases or conditions, it is best to make changes in the kVp. Changing the kVp is fundamentally correct because the kVp affects the penetrating ability of the primary beam, and it is the penetrability of the anatomic part that is affected by these specific diseases and conditions. It is impossible to state an exact amount or percentage by which the kVp should be changed, because the state or severity of the disease or condition differs with each patient; however, a minimum change of 15% in kVp is recommended. There are some instances in which a change in mAs may be more appropriate to the type of pathological condition. For example, if the anatomic area has a significant increase in gas, such as in bowel obstruction, a large decrease in mAs is best.

Soft Tissue

Objects such as small pieces of wood, glass, or swallowed bones are difficult to radiographically visualize using the normal exposure factors for a specific anatomic part. Several situations in which a soft tissue technique (decreased mAs) may be needed are visualization of the larynx in a young child with croup, possible foreign body obstruction in the throat, and foreign body location in the extremities (Fig. 9.11). However, digital imaging systems allow visualization of soft tissues without changing the exposure technique.

Contrast Media

A contrast medium (also called *contrast agent*) is used when imaging anatomic tissues that have low subject contrast. A contrast medium is a substance that can be instilled into the body by injection or ingestion. The type of contrast medium used changes the absorption characteristics of the area of interest by either increasing or decreasing the attenuation of the x-ray beam. Positive contrast agents, such as barium (atomic #56) and iodine (atomic #53), have a high atomic number and absorb more x-rays (increase attenuation) than the surrounding tissue (Fig. 9.12). Negative contrast agents, such as air (atomic #8), decrease the attenuation of the x-ray beam and transmit more radiation than the surrounding tissue (Fig. 9.13). Positive contrast agents

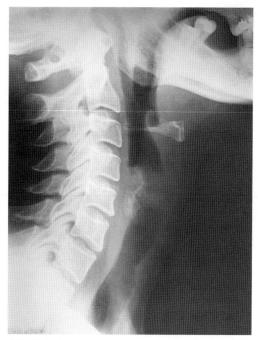

Fig. 9.11 Soft tissue imaging. Lateral soft tissue neck image. (From Frank E. *Merrill's Atlas of Radiographic Positioning and Procedures.* 12th ed. St. Louis: Mosby; 2012.)

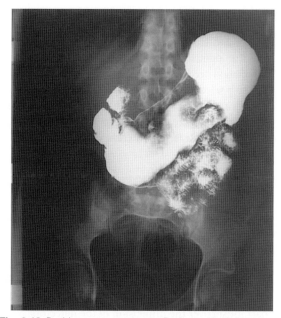

Fig. 9.12 Positive contrast agents. Radiographic image showing increased brightness on the displayed image because of the increase in x-ray beam attenuation by use of a positive contrast agent.

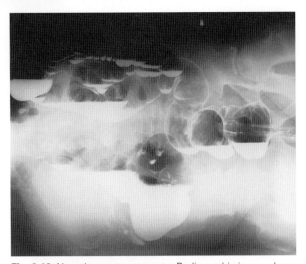

Fig. 9.13 Negative contrast agents. Radiographic image showing decreased brightness on the displayed image because of the decrease in x-ray beam attenuation by use of a negative contrast agent.

are radiopaque and produce more brightness on the displayed image than the adjacent tissues; negative contrast agents are radiolucent and produce less brightness on the displayed image than the adjacent tissues.

Although negative contrast agents decrease the attenuation characteristics of the part being examined, their use does not require a change in exposure factors. Negative contrast agents can also be used in conjunction with positive contrast agents. Positive contrast media studies require an increase in exposure factors compared with imaging the same part without a positive contrast medium. The use of a contrast agent is an effective method of increasing the displayed subject contrast when imaging areas of low subject contrast.

The quality of the radiographic image depends on a multitude of variables. Knowledge of these variables and their radiographic effect assists the radiographer in selecting exposure techniques to produce quality radiographic images.

CHAPTER SUMMARY

- AEC systems are designed to produce sufficient radiation exposure to the IR to produce a quality image.
- AEC uses detectors (typically ionization or solid-state type) that measure the amount of radiation exiting the patient and terminate the exposure when it reaches a preset amount; this amount corresponds to the amount of radiation needed to produce diagnostic image quality.
- The kVp selected must penetrate the part and produce the desired subject contrast displayed on the image. Increasing or decreasing the kVp causes the exposure time to be decreased or increased accordingly when using AEC.
- Changing the mA, when available, causes the exposure time to be decreased or increased accordingly when using AEC.
- The mAs readout displayed after the AEC exposure informs the radiographer of the total radiation exposure used for the procedure.
- For AEC to work accurately, the x-ray beam must be centered precisely to the anatomic area of interest, the correct detectors must be selected, and the anatomic part must cover the dimension of the detectors.
- Other AEC features that can be manipulated include exposure adjustment controls that allow increased or decreased exposure to the IR and the backup time

- (or mAs) provides a safety mechanism that prevents the exposure from exceeding a set amount.
- Limitations of AEC systems include that they typically allow only one type of IR and that the minimum response time may be longer than the exposure needed.
- Anatomically programmed technique is another exposure system that allows the selection of a specific body part and position, resulting in display of preprogrammed exposure factors. These may include AEC information.
- Quality control is important in monitoring the performance of the AEC system. Reproducibility of exposures for a given set of exposure factors and selected detector should result in milliroentgen (mR) readings within 5% and pixel brightness levels for areas within the displayed image should be within 30%.
- Exposure technique charts standardize the selection of exposure factors for a typical patient so that the quality of radiographic images is consistent.
- The variable kVp/fixed mAs technique chart is based on the concept that kVp can be increased as the anatomic part size increases. The baseline kVp is adjusted for changes in part thickness.

- The fixed kVp/variable mAs technique chart uses the concept of selecting an optimal kVp value that is required for the radiographic examination and adjusting the mAs for variations in part thickness.

- Exposure factors may need to be modified for pediatric, geriatric, and bariatric patients and varying projections and positions, casts and splints, pathological conditions, soft tissue, and contrast media.

REVIEW QUESTIONS

1. AEC devices work by measuring _____.
   A. radiation leaving the tube
   B. radiation that exits the patient
   C. radiation that is absorbed by the patient
   D. attenuation of primary radiation by the patient

2. How many detectors are typically found in an AEC system?
   A. One
   B. Two
   C. Three
   D. Four

3. Minimum response time refers to _____.
   A. the proper exposure time needed for an optimal exposure when an AEC device is used
   B. exposure time minus the amount of time the AEC detectors spend measuring the radiation
   C. the difference in exposure times between AEC systems and electronic timers
   D. the shortest exposure time possible when an AEC device is used

4. Which statement regarding the use of AEC during digital imaging is true?
   A. Adjusting the mA and kVp values affect image brightness.
   B. The AEC does not need to be calibrated to a digital image receptor.
   C. If the backup time is reached, image brightness is increased.
   D. Changing the exposure adjustment control to −2 affects the exposure to the IR.

5. The purpose of the backup timer is to _____.
   A. ensure a diagnostic exposure each time AEC is used
   B. produce consistent levels of exposure on all images
   C. determine the exposure time that is used
   D. limit unnecessary x-ray exposure

6. What detector(s) should be selected for a right AP shoulder when the patient is supine on the x-ray table?
   A. Right detector only
   B. Center detector only
   C. Right and left detectors only
   D. Right, center, and left detectors

7. The purpose of anatomically programmed techniques is to _____.
   A. present the radiographer with a preselected set of exposure factors
   B. override AEC when the radiographer has made a mistake in its use
   C. determine which AEC detectors should be used for a specific examination
   D. prevent overexposure and underexposure of images, which sometimes happen when AEC is used

8. Which statement concerning both AEC and anatomically programmed techniques is true?
   A. The skilled use of both requires less knowledge of exposure factors on the part of the radiographer.
   B. The use of both requires the radiographer to be less responsible for accurate centering of the anatomic part.
   C. The individual judgment and discretion of the radiographer is still necessary when using these systems.
   D. The tasks involved with practicing radiography generally are made more difficult with these systems.

9. When using AEC with digital imaging systems, assuming all other factors are correct, selecting the center detector on a PA chest image results in _____.
   A. decreased exposure in the lung area
   B. increased exposure in the lung area
   C. appropriate exposure in the lung area
   D. increased quantum noise in the image

10. When using AEC with digital imaging systems, assuming all other factors are correct, selecting the −2 exposure adjustment on a PA chest image results in _____.
    A. increased quantum noise
    B. increased brightness in the lung area
    C. appropriate brightness in the lung area
    D. A and C

11. Which of the following special considerations may require an increase in mAs?
    A. contrast media
    B. bariatric patient
    C. plaster cast
    D. all of the above

12. What type of exposure technique system uses a fixed mAs regardless of part thickness?
    A. Fixed kVp
    B. Variable kVp
    C. Manual
    D. AEC

13. A primary goal of an exposure technique chart is to _____.
    A. extend the life of the x-ray tube
    B. improve the radiographer's accuracy
    C. produce quality images consistently
    D. increase the patient workflow

14. Which of the following is an important condition required for technique charts to be effective?
    A. Equipment must be calibrated to perform properly.
    B. One technique chart should be used for all radiographic units.

C. All technologists should use the same mAs setting.
    D. The chart should not be revised once it has been used.

15. Instilling a negative contrast agent in the gastrointestinal tract has what effect in the area of interest on the displayed image?
    A. Increased brightness
    B. Decreased contrast
    C. Decreased brightness
    D. No effect

16. A patient diagnosed with congestive heart failure would be considered a(n)_____ condition.
    A. common
    B. destructive
    C. rare
    D. additive

Dynamic Imaging: Fluoroscopy

CHAPTER OUTLINE

OBJECTIVES

After completing this chapter, the reader will be able to perform the following:

1. Define all the key terms in this chapter.
2. State all the important relationships in this chapter.
3. Differentiate between fluoroscopic and radiographic imaging.
4. Recognize the unique features of an image-intensified fluoroscopic unit and explain how the image is created and viewed.
5. Explain the process of brightness gain and the conversion factor during image intensification.
6. Define *automatic brightness* control and state its function.
7. Explain how using the magnification mode affects image quality and patient exposure.
8. Identify common types of image degradation resulting from image-intensified fluoroscopy.
9. Describe the charge-coupled device (CCD) and how it converts the output phosphor image for viewing on a display monitor.
10. Differentiate between image-intensified and flat-panel fluoroscopic technologies.
11. Identify the unique design features of flat-panel detector fluoroscopy and their effect on image quality and patient exposure.
12. Differentiate between continuous and pulsed fluoroscopy and their impacts on patient radiation dose.
13. Recognize the fluoroscopic features that impact image quality and patient radiation exposure.
14. Identify specialized fluoroscopic units and their use in radiology.
15. State radiation safety procedures used to reduce exposure to the patient and personnel.
16. Recognize the need for quality control on fluoroscopic units.

KEY TERMS

accelerating anode
air kerma
automatic brightness control (ABC)

automatic exposure rate control (AERC)
brightness gain
charge-coupled device (CCD)

complementary metal oxide semiconductor (CMOS)
continuous fluoroscopy
conversion factor

The previous chapters discussed radiographic imaging for producing static (stationary) images of anatomic tissues. However, imaging of the functioning or motion (dynamics) of anatomic structures is needed for evaluation and is accomplished by fluoroscopy.

Fluoroscopy allows imaging of the movement of internal structures. It differs from radiographic imaging by its use of a continuous or pulsed beam of x-rays to create images of moving internal structures that can be viewed on a monitor. Internal structures, such as vascular or gastrointestinal systems, can be visualized in their normal state of motion with the aid of special liquid or gas substances (contrast media) that are either injected or instilled.

Traditional fluoroscopic units are designed with the x-ray tube underneath the tabletop and the image receptor (IR), such as an image-intensifier tube or digital detector, above the patient (Fig. 10.1). During fluoroscopy the image receptor is regarded as a primary protective barrier and must be coincident with the central ray (CR) of the x-ray beam to enable exposure for all situations. Radiology rooms can be designed solely for radiography or fluoroscopy but can also combine the two systems for radiography and fluoroscopy. These designs are commonly referred to as radiographic/fluoroscopic (R/F) systems, and the newer systems are using flat-panel fluoroscopic detector technology. Traditional R/F units require the operator or radiographer to perform the procedures tableside.

This chapter discusses the components of traditional image-intensified and digital fluoroscopic units, viewing and recording systems, and important fluoroscopic features in use today.

IMAGE INTENSIFICATION

In image-intensified fluoroscopy, the milliamperage (mA) used during imaging is considerably lower (0.5–5 mA) than that in the radiographic mode, which is operated at a

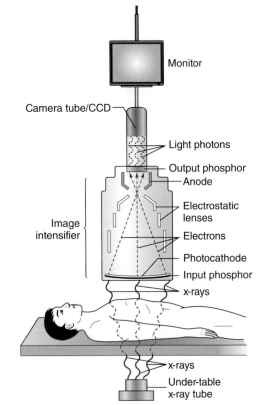

Fig. 10.1 Fluoroscopic image-intensified system used for dynamic imaging of internal structures. *CCD*, Charge-coupled device.

higher mA of 50 to 1200 mA. A low mA provides for the increased time the image intensifier is operated. Because the time of exposure is lengthened, the control panel includes a timer that buzzes audibly when 5 minutes of x-ray fluoroscopic time has been used. Another important feature of a fluoroscopic unit is the dead-man switch. The continuous x-ray beam is activated by either a hand switch on the unit or a foot pedal that must be continuously depressed for the x-rays to be produced. Releasing the pressure applied to the pedal or switch terminates the radiation exposure.

The image intensifier is an electronic vacuum tube that converts the remnant (exit) x-ray beam to light, then to electrons, then back to light, increasing the light intensity in the process. The entire intensifier tube is approximately 50 cm (20 inches) in length and 15 to 58 cm (6–23 inches) in diameter (diameter depends on the manufacturer and intended use). Image intensification (Fig. 10.2) is the process in which the exit radiation from the anatomic area of interest interacts with the input phosphor for conversion to visible light. The input phosphor is made of cesium iodide and is bonded to the curved surface of the intensifier tube itself. Cesium iodide absorbs the remnant x-ray photon energy and emits light in response, proportional to the percentage of x-ray absorption. Thousands of light photons are created from just one x-ray photon. The light intensities are equal to the intensities of the exit radiation and are converted to electrons by a photocathode (photoemission). The photocathode is made of cesium and antimony compounds. These metals emit electrons in response to light stimulus in a process called photoemission. The ratio of light to electron emission is not one to one.

It takes many light photons to result in the emission of one electron. The photocathode is bonded directly to the input phosphor using a very thin adhesive layer and both have a curved shape which is critical to its design. This concave shape ensures that all the electrons emitted from the photocathode travel the same distance to the output phosphor. As a result, the image brightness is maintained throughout the fluoroscopic image. The electrons are focused by electrostatic focusing lenses and accelerated toward an anode. The electrostatic focusing lenses are not really lenses at all but are negatively charged circular plates along the length of the image-intensifier tube. These negatively charged plates repel the electron stream, focusing it toward the small output phosphor. To set the electron stream in motion at a constant velocity, an accelerating anode is located at the neck of the image intensifier near the output phosphor. This accelerating anode maintains a constant potential of approximately 25 kVp.

These high-energy electrons result in hundreds of light photons being emitted from the output phosphor. The output phosphor is made of silver-activated zinc cadmium sulfide and is much smaller than the input phosphor. It is located at the opposite end of the image-intensifier tube, just beyond the accelerating anode. The output phosphor absorbs electrons and emits light in response. The result of this process is an increase in image brightness (Fig. 10.2).

The image light intensities from the output phosphor are converted to an electronic video signal and sent to a display monitor for viewing. Fig. 10.3 is an example of a typical radiographic and image-intensified fluoroscopic unit. Static radiographic images are recorded from a charge-coupled device (CCD) camera that is connected to the output phosphor. This lessens the need for overhead images taken radiographically.

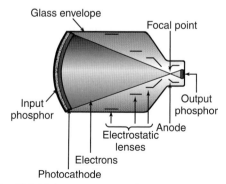

Fig. 10.2 Major components of an image intensifier.

IMPORTANT RELATIONSHIP

Image-Intensified Fluoroscopy

Dynamic imaging of internal anatomic structures can be accomplished with the use of an image intensifier. The exit radiation is absorbed by the input phosphor, converted to electrons, sent to the output phosphor, released as visible light, and converted to an electronic signal that is digitized and processed by a computer and sent to the display monitor.

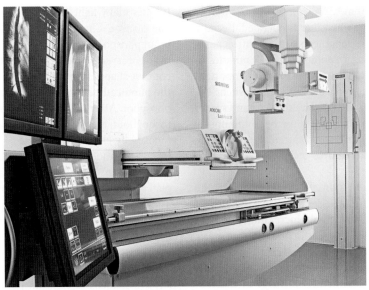

Fig. 10.3 A typical radiographic and image-intensified fluoroscopic unit. (From Johnston JN, Fauber TL. *Essentials of Radiographic Physics and Imaging.* 3rd ed. St. Louis: Mosby; 2020.)

Brightness Gain

A brighter image is a result of high-energy electrons striking a small output phosphor. Accelerating the electrons increases the light intensities at the output phosphor (**flux gain**). The reduction in the size of the output phosphor image compared with that of the input phosphor image also increases the light intensities (**minification gain**). **Brightness gain** is the product of both flux gain and minification gain and results in a brighter image on the output phosphor.

 IMPORTANT RELATIONSHIP

Brightness Gain

A brighter image is created on the output phosphor when accelerated electrons strike a smaller output phosphor.

Although the term *brightness gain* continues to be used, it is now a common practice to express this increase in brightness with the term *conversion factor*. **Conversion factor** is an expression of the luminance at the output phosphor divided by the input exposure rate. The SI unit of luminance is the candela per square meter (cd/m^2) and the input exposure rate is milligray per second (mGy_a/s). The conversion factor is $cd/m^2 \div mGy_a/s$. The numeric conversion factor value is roughly equal to 1% of the brightness gain value. For example, a brightness gain of 20,000 would have a conversion factor of 200. The higher the conversion factor or brightness gain value, the greater the efficiency of the image intensifier. See Box 10.1 for brightness gain and conversion factor formulas.

Automatic Brightness Control

The radiographer must also be familiar with **automatic brightness control (ABC)**, a function of the fluoroscopic unit that maintains the overall appearance of the fluoroscopic image (contrast and brightness) by automatically adjusting the kilovoltage peak (kVp), mA, or both. ABC (also known as automatic brightness stabilization [ABS]) generally operates by monitoring the current through the image intensifier or the output phosphor intensity and adjusting the exposure factors if the monitored value falls below preset levels. The fluoroscopic unit allows the operator to select a desired brightness level, and this level is subsequently maintained by ABC. ABC is slightly slow in its response to changes in patient tissue thickness and tissue density as the fluoroscopy tower is moved about over the patient; this is visible to the radiographer as a lag in the image brightness on the monitor as the tower is moved.

BOX 10.1 Brightness Gain and Conversion Factor Formulas

$$\text{Brightness gain} = \text{Minification gain} \times \text{Flux gain}$$

$$\text{Flux gain} = \frac{\text{Number of output light photons}}{\text{Number of input x-ray photons}}$$

$$\text{Minification gain} = \left(\frac{d_i}{d_o}\right)^2$$

d_i = input phosphor diameter; d_o = output phosphor diameter

$$\text{Conversion factor} = \frac{\text{Output phosphor illumination (cd/m}^2)}{\text{Input exposure rate (mGy}_a/s)}$$

Example:
Input phosphor = 20 cm
Output phosphor = 3 cm
Flux gain = 400

$$\frac{20^2}{3^2} \times 400 = 44.4 \times 400 = 17,760 \text{ brightness gain}$$

Conversion factor = 177.6 (17,760 × 0.01 [1% of brightness gain])

Magnification Mode

Another function of most image intensifiers is the multifield mode or magnification mode. When operated in magnification mode, the voltage to the electrostatic focusing lenses is increased. This increase tightens the diameter of the electron stream, and the focal point is shifted farther from the output phosphor (Fig. 10.4). The effect is that only the electrons from the central area of the input phosphor interact with the output phosphor and contribute to the image, giving the appearance of magnification. For example, a 30/23/15-cm (12/9/6-inch) trifocus image intensifier can be operated in any of these three modes. When operated in the 23-cm (9-inch) mode, only the electrons from the central 23 cm (9 inch) of the input phosphor interact with the output phosphor; the electrons about the periphery miss and do not contribute to the image. The same is true for the 15-cm (6-inch) mode. The degree of magnification (magnification factor [MF]) may be found by dividing the full-size input diameter by the selected input diameter. For example, MF = 30 ÷ 15 = 2× magnification.

This magnification improves the operator's ability to see small structures (spatial resolution, discussed shortly) but at the expense of increasing the patient dose. Remnant x-ray photons are converted to light and then to electrons and are focused on the output phosphor. If fewer electrons are incident on the output phosphor, the output intensity decreases. To compensate,

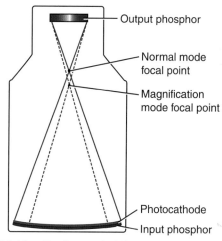

Fig. 10.4 Magnification mode. When the image intensifier is operated in magnification mode, the voltage to the electrostatic focusing lenses is increased. This increase tightens the diameter of the electron stream, and the focal point is shifted farther from the output phosphor, resulting in a magnified image. (From Johnston JN, Fauber TL. *Essentials of Radiographic Physics and Imaging*. 3rd ed. St. Louis: Mosby; 2020.)

more x-ray photons are needed at the beginning of the process to produce more light, resulting in more electrons striking the output end of the image intensifier. ABC automatically increases x-ray exposure to achieve this. Again, with an increase in x-rays used, comes an increase in patient dose.

⚡ IMPORTANT RELATIONSHIP

Magnification Mode and Patient Dose

> Operating the image intensifier in one of the magnification modes increases the operator's ability to see small structures but at the price of increasing the radiation dose to the patient.

Magnification modes improve spatial resolution, which refers to the smallest structure that may be detected in an image. Spatial resolution is measured in line pairs per millimeter (lp/mm), and typical fluoroscopic systems have spatial resolution capabilities of 1 to 2 lp/mm but greatly depend on the rest of the imaging chain (i.e., the viewing and recording systems).

Distortion is also an issue with image-intensified fluoroscopy. In radiography, distortion is a misrepresentation of the true size or shape of an object. In the case of fluoroscopy, shape distortion can be a problem. In fluoroscopy, distortion is a result of inaccurate control or focusing of the electrons released at the periphery of the photocathode and the curved shape of the photocathode. The combined result is an unequal magnification (distortion) of the image, creating what is called a "pincushion appearance" (Fig. 10.5). This problem also causes a loss of brightness around the periphery of the image (peripheral falloff), which is referred to as *vignetting*.

One last factor to consider with image intensifiers is noise. Image noise results when insufficient information is present to create the image. In the case of fluoroscopy, this lack of image-forming information ultimately goes back to an insufficient quantity of x-rays. If too few x-rays exit the patient and expose the input phosphor, not enough light will be produced, decreasing the number of electrons released by the photocathode to interact with the output phosphor. This results in a "grainy" or "noisy" image (Fig. 10.6). Although other factors in the fluoroscopic chain may contribute to noise, the solution generally comes back to increasing the mA (quantity of radiation). For image-intensified fluoroscopy, this is a small increase in mA because these systems operate at 2 to 5 mA. Because older image intensifier units are operated as continuous fluoroscopy, to minimize radiation dose, the operator should intermittently pulse the x-ray beam by activating the exposure switch on and off rapidly.

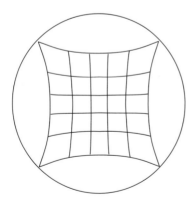

Image displaying
"pincushion" distortion

Fig. 10.5 Pincushion distortion. Appearance of the pincushion effect. The *circle* represents the television monitor display, and the *grid* represents the effect on the image. (From Johnston JN, Fauber TL. *Essentials of Radiographic Physics and Imaging*. 3rd ed. St. Louis: Mosby; 2020.)

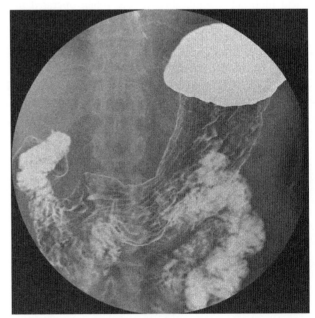

Fig. 10.6 Quantum noise. If too few x-rays exit the patient and expose the input phosphor, not enough light will be produced, decreasing the number of electrons released by the photocathode to interact with the output phosphor. A "grainy" or "noisy" image results. (From Bontrager K, Lampignano J. *Textbook of Radiographic Positioning and Related Anatomy*. 7th ed. St. Louis: Mosby; 2010.)

Charge-Coupled Device

To view the image from the output phosphor on a display monitor, it must first be converted to an electrical signal and then digitized for image processing and display. The method for achieving this is similar to the camera on a smartphone and uses charge couple device (CCD) electronics. As a solid-state device, the CCD is fiberoptically coupled to the output phosphor of the image intensifier, and light from the output phosphor is converted to an electrical signal. Before the use of

CCD electronics, television camera tubes (Vidicon and Plumbicon) converted the light from the output phosphor into a video (electric) signal. CCD electronics rapidly replaced camera tubes and are used on image-intensified units still in operation today. A CCD is a light-sensitive semiconducting device that generates an electrical charge when stimulated by light and stores this charge in a capacitor (Fig. 10.7A,B). The charge is proportional to the light intensity and is stored in rows of pixels. A CCD consists of a series of semiconductor

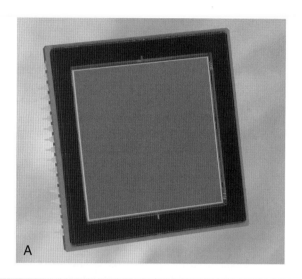

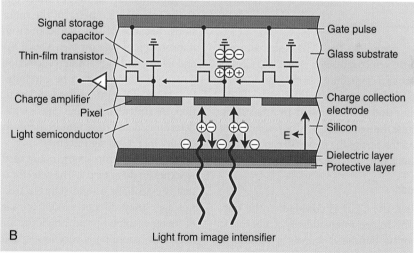

Fig. 10.7 A, The charge-coupled device (CCD). **B,** The CCD is a light-sensitive semiconducting device that generates an electrical charge when stimulated by light and stores this charge in a capacitor until the charge is sent as an electronic signal to the display monitor. (From Johnston JN, Fauber TL. *Essentials of Radiographic Physics and Imaging.* 3rd ed. St. Louis: Elsevier; 2020.)

capacitors, with each capacitor representing a pixel. Each pixel is composed of photosensitive material that dislodges electrons when stimulated by light photons.

To digitize the charge from this device, the electrodes between each pixel, called *row gates*, are charged in sequence, moving the signal down the row, where it is transferred into the capacitors. From the capacitors, the charge is sent as an electronic signal to the display monitor. In this way, each pixel is individually "read" and sent to a display monitor.

A key advantage of CCD technology is the fact that it creates an analog signal that is instantly digitized at the point of image capture from the output phosphor of the image intensifier. This digital signal is processed by a computer and the image quality is improved because the CCD is more sensitive to a wider range of light intensities and does not create any geometric distortion of images. The CCD is more light sensitive (higher detective quantum efficiency [DQE]) and exhibits less noise and no spatial distortion. It also has a higher spatial resolution and requires less radiation in the system, reducing patient dose.

 IMPORTANT RELATIONSHIP

Charge-Coupled Device

The CCD is a device that converts the light image from the intensifier's output phosphor to an electronic signal that is digitized and can be reconstructed on the display monitor.

Serving a similar purpose as the CCD is the complementary metal oxide semiconductor (CMOS). CMOS devices are made up of a crystalline silicon matrix. Each detector element (DEL) has its own amplifier, photodiode, and storage capacitor and is surrounded by transistors. They do not have quite the light sensitivity or resolution of CCDs, but they use a fraction of the power to run, are very inexpensive to manufacture, and are improving.

Coupling of Devices

As discussed earlier, the CCD is coupled to the output phosphor of the image intensifier by a fiberoptic bundle. The fiberoptic bundle is simply a bundle of very thin optical glass filaments. This system is very durable and simple in design and very efficient in light capture from the output phosphor to the input surface of the CCD. The electronic signal from the CCD will be converted by the display monitor (discussed later) into a visible image.

DIGITAL FLUOROSCOPY

Digital fluoroscopy has evolved over time with modern systems now employing CCD and flat-panel technology with liquid crystal display (LCD) monitors. When in digital form, the image can be postprocessed and stored in that format or archived in a sophisticated computer storage system. The introduction of flat-panel technology has replaced the conventional image intensifier. This is the case with both fixed and mobile fluoroscopic systems.

Flat-panel detectors (FPD), often referred to as panels, are very popular in general fluoroscopy (Fig. 10.8). They are much lighter and more compact than intensifiers, produce a digital signal directly (no need for a CCD), and because it is a digital system producing a digital signal (without the electronic components of the old image-intensified system), there is less electronic noise. Detector arrays are currently available in field-of-view (FOV) sizes of 25×25 to 43×43 cm (10×10 to 17×17 inches).

The excellent image quality of fluoroscopic FPD panels has made them a standard of care with clinicians, and a very large percentage of institutions now use them for all fluoroscopic studies. With image intensifiers, major image quality drawbacks centered around the inherent design of its curved input surface and phosphor as well as the internal geometry of the intensifier tube dimensions. Because of this, clinicians were often faced with fluoroscopic image problems such as blooming, peripheral falloff, and vignetting (pincushioning). Additionally, patient anatomy had to be carefully positioned within the center of the intensifier window for optimum resolution. As intensifier tubes aged with use, their quality deteriorated and dose requirements for acceptable image quality increased significantly.

With FPD fluoroscopy, many of these image quality weaknesses do not exist. The detector is a flat input surface that is essentially a solid-state electronic device and does not age. They do not exhibit pin-cushioning or falloff of image resolution and brightness on its edges and the degree of blooming is very low, enabling the operator to view a much greater dynamic range of tissue visibility and contrast resolution.

FPD fluoroscopy is very dose efficient when compared to image intensifiers due to the high DQE of the

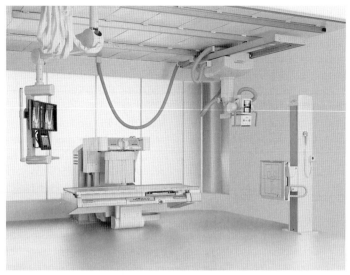

Fig. 10.8 Digital fluoroscopy using flat-panel detector technology. (Courtesy Siemens Healthcare, Malvern, PA.)

scintillator, which may be cesium iodide or gadolinium oxysulfide, in its indirect design and thin-film transistor (TFT) technology. Fluoro doses can be reduced as much as 50% compared to intensified fluoroscopy and because the panel is rectangular or square in shape, often it can be rotated for interventional studies to better match the orientation of patient anatomy. Fluoroscopic image brightness is maintained using Automatic Exposure Rate Control (AERC) circuits that vary in real time, fluoro mA, kVp, pulse width, and beam filtration during fluoroscopy. This feature is quicker in response than image intensifiers and ensures optimum image quality more reliably with demanding interventional procedures.

Spatial resolution with flat-panel detectors is better than with image intensifiers and currently is approximately 2.5 to 3.2 lp/mm compared to 1 to 2 lp/mm with intensifiers. They also exhibit increased contrast resolution and greater dynamic response to subtle tissues, often not seen with image intensifiers. These features are very important to clinicians as their applications continue to gain in popularity.

Flat-Panel Detector Fluoroscopy

The flat-panel detector used for fluoroscopic applications is the indirect-capture detector (discussed in Chapter 5). As discussed in Chapter 5, the scintillator of this system uses cesium iodide or gadolinium oxysulfide as the phosphor. The photodetector is amorphous silicon, which is a liquid that can be painted onto a substrate (foundation or

 IMPORTANT RELATIONSHIP

Digital Fluoroscopic Systems

The use of flat-panel detectors in place of an image intensifier offers several advantages, such as a reduction in the size, bulk, and weight of the fluoroscopic tower; allowing for easier manipulation of the tower; and greater access to the patient during the examination. The flat-panel detectors also replace other recording devices, and, because they operate in radiographic mode, in many cases, additional radiographic images are not needed. The images, both dynamic and static, can also be readily archived with the patient record.

underlying layer) and is the material that makes flat-panel detectors possible. The other component is a thin-film-transistor (TFT) array. TFTs are electronic components layered onto a glass substrate that includes a readout, charge collector, and light-sensitive elements. The panel is configured into a network of detector elements (DELs) covered by the scintillator plate with each DEL containing a photodetector [sensing area] and a TFT). With this system, x-ray energy is absorbed by the scintillator and converted to light energy. This light is then absorbed by the photodetectors and converted to electrical charges, which are in turn captured and transmitted by the TFT array, converted from an analog to digital signal for image processing, and then to a display monitor for viewing.

Although the cesium iodide amorphous silicon indirect-capture detector is essentially the same as that for digital radiography (DR), there are a few differences for use as a dynamic digital detector in digital fluoroscopy applications. In general, dynamic versions of these detectors must respond in rapid sequences to create a dynamic image. Current dynamic versions are capable of up to 60 frames per second (fps). To accomplish this, rapid readout speeds (how the active matrix processes the image data) are necessary.

The panel design is a two-dimensional (2D) rectilinear array of DELs that can be electronically processed line by line in a fraction of a second. Furthermore, for fluoroscopic applications, very-low-noise flat-panel detector systems are needed. Fluoroscopy generally operates at a low-dose output; hence, any operational noise degrades the fluoroscopic image, making noise a greater factor in detectors used for this application. Application-specific integrated circuits (ASICs) are used to minimize noise and amplify signal from the active matrix. These circuits are particularly important in fluoroscopic applications because they minimize noise, maximize readout speed, and allow for switching from low-dose to high-dose inputs (for static imaging). Another consideration with the low-dose fluoroscopic applications is the need to maintain a large fill factor (the area of each DEL that is sensitive to x-ray detection materials). With general radiography that uses a larger mA output, this is generally not a problem, but it becomes a problem with fluoroscopic applications because of the lower radiation doses used in fluoroscopic imaging, particularly with indirect-capture detectors. Other features such as a light-emitting diode array "backlighting system" have also been incorporated to erase the detector between frames to prevent "ghosting" caused by any residual exposure charge from the previous frame.

◤ IMPORTANT RELATIONSHIP

Flat-Panel Detectors in Fluoroscopy

Flat-panel detectors used in fluoroscopy require rapid readout speeds for dynamic imaging. Current dynamic versions are capable of up to 60 frames per second. Application-specific integrated circuits (ASICs) minimize noise, maximize readout speed, and allow for switching from low-dose to high-dose inputs (for static imaging).

There are two styles of general digital R/F systems that focus on the position of the x-ray tube relative to the patient. One design positions the x-ray tube under the patient with the FPD above the patient (Fig. 10.8). This system facilitates table-side fluoroscopy and requires an additional x-ray tube for radiography, as well as a radiographic detector in the table tray and upright holder. These systems are typically more expensive because of the additional detectors and x-ray tube. The other design positions the x-ray tube above the patient with the FPD under the tabletop (Fig. 10.9). In this system, the detector performs both radiography and fluoroscopy as does the x-ray tube. The source-to-image receptor distance (SID) is variable from 100 to 180 cm (40 to 72 inches) and the table will tilt upright and Trendelenburg position. This feature allows for routine chest and cervical spine radiography as well as upright studies. This design is very similar to the remote-controlled fluoroscopic systems that have been in the marketplace for several years. All radiographic and fluoroscopic controls are remotely located behind the lead-lined control booth and the radiologist performs fluoroscopy using these controls and communicates with the patient by way of an intercom speaker and microphone. Some radiologists prefer this approach since it allows for fluoroscopy with full lead protection in the control booth.

A key feature of this design also is its economics in that a single FPD is used for all work, including fluoroscopy. Some systems also offer a remote control console on a wheeled pedestal that can be positioned at a safe distance from the patient during fluoroscopy to lower operator exposure.

Both system designs offer full functionality for both general fluoroscopic and radiographic examinations. A key distinction, however, deals with the scatter radiation area coming from the patient during fluoroscopy. During fluoroscopy, the patient is the primary source of radiation exposure to fluoroscopic personnel.

With the x-ray tube above the patient, the most intense scatter radiation to the operator is directed above the waist to include the upper trunk, neck, and head (Fig. 10.10A). Although the upper trunk and chest are protected by a lead apron, often the thyroid gland and eyes are not protected.

With the x-ray tube beneath the patient, the scatter area to the operator is below the chest and toward the floor (Fig. 10.10B). This operator anatomy is typically protected by a fluoroscopic lead apron, to just below the knees. These two designs are popular, and it is important that fluoroscopic staff understand the scatter radiation areas coming from the patient with each design, as a radiation safety practice.

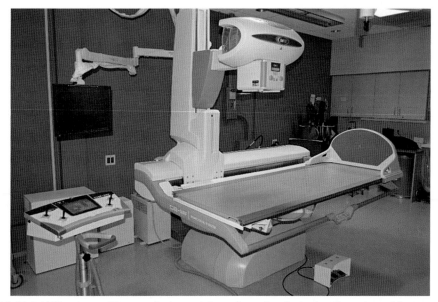

Fig. 10.9 Digital R/F system with x-ray tube located above the patient for both radiography and fluoroscopy. The image receptor is located just under the tabletop. The R/F unit includes a moveable remote control console. (Courtesy Randy Griswold.

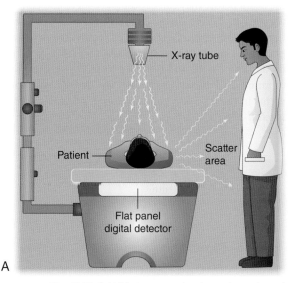

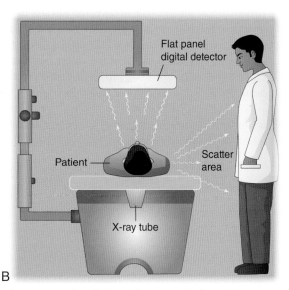

Fig. 10.10 A, With the x-ray tube above the patient, the most intense scatter radiation to the operator is directed above the waist to include the upper trunk, neck, and head. **B,** With the x-ray tube beneath the patient, the scatter area to the operator is below the chest and toward the floor. Note: Distance between the digital detector and patient (OID) in B is for illustration only.

IMPORTANT RELATIONSHIP

Scatter Radiation

During fluoroscopy, the patient is the primary source of radiation exposure to fluoroscopic personnel. With the x-ray tube above the patient, the most intense scatter radiation to the operator is directed above the waist to include the upper trunk, neck, and head. With the x-ray tube beneath the patient, the scatter area to the operator is below the chest and toward the floor.

FLUOROSCOPIC FEATURES

Modern fluoroscopic equipment offers several features that impact the quality of the fluoroscopic image and radiation dose to the patient. There are several controls and settings, both on the control console and tower, that allow adjustment of the radiation output and image quality. The consideration for selecting kVp is the same as for general radiography. Using higher kVp settings (appropriate for the examination) results in a higher energy beam and lower patient dose.

Collimation of the fluoroscopic beam reduces the field size exposing the patient. Fully open, the unit exposes the patient to a beam adequate to cover the full size of the image intensifier or detector. With the newest units, lines appear on the last image hold (LIH) displayed on the monitor, indicating the position of the collimator plates. This allows the collimator to be further adjusted without exposing the patient to additional radiation (virtual collimation). The collimator should be adjusted to eliminate all anatomic structures not necessary to the examination

being performed. Collimation changes the field of view (FOV) displayed, but it does not magnify the image (Fig. 10.11). By reducing the area of tissue being exposed, the overall patient dose is reduced.

The option to include the grid is also a control feature. The grid reduces the amount of scatter reaching the detector surface and improves image quality. But because it also removes some useful radiation from the remnant beam, mA (quantity of radiation) must be increased to maintain overall exposure to the detector. In general, its use increases radiation dose to the patient. The decision to use it should be based on the examination and the anatomic area's capacity to produce scatter radiation. The abdomen, for example, produces more scatter radiation, and the grid should be selected; however, the extremities or pediatric patients may not require its use.

Modern fluoroscopic units also allow for the selection and interchangeability of added filtration thickness or material. The operation of this control may entail the substitution of filters of different thicknesses or switching of filtration material. The typical material used for beam filtration is aluminum, which has an atomic number ideally suited to removing low-energy x-ray photons. It is important to remove these low-energy photons from the beam before they can expose the patient and contribute only to patient dose. This filtration acts to increase the average energy of the beam by removing low-energy photons. Higher atomic materials such as copper are used in some units and may be selected when additional filtration and beam hardening are desired. Advancements in the type and combination of materials used in *spectral filtration* are incorporated into the design of

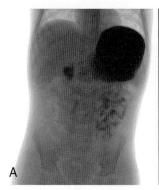 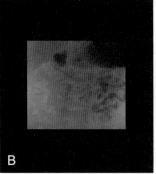

Fig. 10.11 Collimation and field of view (FOV). **A,** Full FOV image without collimation. **B,** Smaller FOV with increased collimation. Note the anatomy visualized is not magnified. (From Johnston JN, Fauber TL. *Essentials of Radiographic Physics and Imaging.* 3rd ed. St. Louis: Elsevier; 2020.)

modern fluoroscopic equipment and assist in reducing patient skin dose while maintaining quality fluoroscopic images.

Anatomic programs are also available on modern fluoroscopic units. These programs are preset fluoroscopic examination settings established and programmed into the unit at the time of manufacture or at the time of installation as dictated by the facility. Each preset brings up a predetermined set of exposure factors, filter thickness and type, and so on, just as they do on radiographic units. Along this same line are the default settings on the unit. These defaults are intended to be "ideal" or "standard" values for minimizing dose and maximizing image quality. They are not hard and fast rules of operation and should be changed depending on circumstances and the examination to be performed. The operator should evaluate the default settings when they appear on the control panel to ensure they match the examination and patient (e.g., size, pediatric versus adult, pathology, anatomy of interest).

 IMPORTANT RELATIONSHIP

Fluoroscopic Features

Use of virtual collimation during LIH, preset anatomic programs, and added filtration reduces the patient dose. Conversely, use of a grid increases the patient dose.

Automatic Exposure Rate Control

Like ABC used in older image-intensified units, automatic exposure rate control (AERC) serves a similar function in modern fluoroscopy. AERC automatically adjusts the tube current (mA), voltage (kVp), filtration, and pulse width to maintain radiation exposure to the flat-panel detector. A variety of variables during a fluoroscopic examination can result in changes in the radiation exposure reaching the FPD. Changes in patient thickness, tissue attenuation, object-to-image receptor distance (OID), collimation, and FOV may require an increase or decrease in the radiation reaching the detector.

Pulsed Fluoroscopy

An operational feature of modern fluoroscopy units is pulsed fluoroscopy, using a pulsed beam technology to reduce radiation output necessary for the fluoroscopic image and patient radiation dose. This is simply a design of the unit that rapidly turns the x-ray beam on and off during operation. This operation introduces important mA pulse characteristics to optimize fluoroscopic image quality at reduced patient dosages. These include pulse height (mA), pulse width, pulse interval, and pulse rate.

Pulse rate refers to how many pulses occur per second of operation. Think of this as how many exposures occur per second. Pulse width refers to the length of each pulse, and pulse height is the level of mA per pulse. Pulse interval is the time in milliseconds (ms) between successive mA pulses. Think of pulse width as how long each exposure lasts and pulse interval as the "x-ray-off time" between pulses. The operator can select pulse rates generally from 1 to 30 pulses per second. Pulse widths are generally less than 6 ms for pediatrics and less than 10 ms for adults. Because the pulse widths are much lower than 33 ms when compared with image-intensified fluoroscopy, the mA used is typically higher (50–1200) to maintain enough exposure to the detector for image quality (maintaining the needed signal-to-noise ratio [SNR] or contrast-to-noise ratio [CNR]). If the unit is operated at 30 pulses per second, the radiation dose is no different than continuous fluoroscopy, yet image quality is improved due to reduced motion artifacts. However, if operated at pulse rates below 30, a radiation dose reduction is realized (Fig. 10.12). It is important to remember that selected pulse rates should correlate with the dynamic motion characteristics of the area being studied. Fast-moving anatomy such as the heart and chest structures requires a faster pulse rate than the slow-moving structures of an orthopedic fracture repair in surgery.

 IMPORTANT RELATIONSHIP

Pulsed Fluoroscopy

Operating the fluoroscope in a pulsed mode reduces the number of images each second, decreases the patient dose, and should match the dynamic motion of patient anatomy.

 MIND IMAGE

Pulsed Fluoroscopy

A pulsating shower head can be invigorating and great for showering. The shower head pulses the water at a pulse rate and intensity. This is similar to pulsed fluoroscopy. Both are designed to conserve and improve the intensity of the beam, whether water or x-rays.

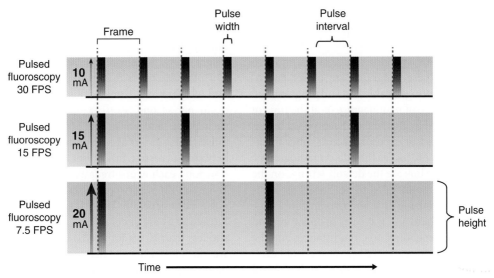

Fig. 10.12 Pulsed fluoroscopy can vary the number of images (frames per second *[FPS]*). Decreasing the FPS will increase the pulse interval and typically the milliamperage *(mA)* to provide sufficient x-ray exposure for a quality fluoroscopic image. (From Abrahams, RB, Sensakovic, WF, Huda, W. *Imaging Physics: Case Review Series*. St. Louis: Elsevier, Inc.; 2020.)

Dose Rates

Most fluoroscopic units today allow for the selection of dose rates. The dose rate setting may be labeled as low, medium, or high (or icons may be used to imply the same). These settings change the dose generally by a percentage such as 50% (medium is 50% of high, and low is 50% of medium). These selections control the radiation dose rate at the detector, and automatic changes in the filter may occur along with changes in the pulse rate.

As with radiography, the operator should select the dose rate depending on the examination to be performed. For example, differentiation of soft tissue structures with lower subject contrast requires a higher dose rate, and barium studies (higher subject contrast) require a comparatively lower dose rate.

 IMPORTANT RELATIONSHIP

Pulsed Fluoroscopy and Dose Rates

Using pulsed fluoroscopy along with lower dose rates appropriate to the procedure reduces the patient radiation dose.

Dose Monitoring

Air kerma (**k**inetic **e**nergy **r**eleased in **ma**tter) specifies the intensity of x-rays at a given point in air at a known distance from the focal spot or source of x-rays, and the cumulative or total air kerma is monitored during the fluoroscopic procedure. Other dose displays such as dose area product (DAP) and kerma area product (KAP) provide indicators of patient radiation risk and should be documented in the patient's record. DAP meters (measure exposure in air followed by a computation to estimate the absorbed dose to the patient) are required on all new fluoroscopes in the United States and internationally. KAP is the same as DAP and is the product of the total air kerma and the area of the x-ray beam at the entrance of the patient. Units of DAP and KAP are expressed in micro or milligray (Gy) per area squared but can vary by manufacturer (Box 10.2). A cumulative dose (more recently referred to as *reference dose*) may also be displayed in Gy that estimates the patient's skin dose for the fluoroscopic procedure. These radiation dose units (DAP or KAP and reference dose) should be monitored during the procedure and the operator notified if an agreed-upon *radiation or dose threshold* has been reached. The radiographer may be

BOX 10.2 Dose Monitoring

Air kerma: Kinetic energy released in mass and specifies the intensity of x-rays at a given point in air at a known distance from the source of x-rays.

Kerma area product (KAP), also known as dose area product (DAP), is the product of cumulative air kerma and the area of the x-ray beam at the entrance of the patient.

Dose monitoring units may vary by manufacturer:

$$1\,\mu Gy\text{-}m^2 = 1\,cGy\text{-}cm^2 = 10\,mGy\text{-}cm$$

1 centi = 10 milli = 10,000 micro   1 centimeter squared (cm^2) = 0.0001 m^2

Cumulative air kerma (reference dose) is measured in Gy and provides an estimate about the total patient skin dose for the fluoroscopic procedure.

---

responsible for monitoring and documenting these radiation dose units in the patient's medical record. In addition to dose displays, the total amount of fluoro time for the procedure should be documented in the patient's record. An important quality control check on the fluoro unit is the fluoroscopic exposure rate that measures the intensity of the x-ray beam and should not exceed approximately 88 mGy/min or 10 R/min in the United States.

Frame Averaging

Frame averaging is an operation that reduces the overall patient dose and image noise by averaging multiple video image frames together (Fig. 10.13). Because the combining of frames reduces noise, less radiation is needed to maintain image quality; however, spatial resolution is decreased. Frame averaging is user-selectable and is a video process that combines successive video frames in rapid succession for display on a monitor.

Video images on a monitor consist of individual video frames that are each 33 ms in duration and are being seen at a frame rate of 30 frames per second (fps). To the human eye this pulse rate of 30 fps is seen as a continuous video image on the screen, when in fact it is scintillating (pulsating visible light) at 30 fps. With frame averaging, the video system combines successive frames in rapid succession for display. For example, you can select a frame averaging rate of 6 fps for display. The system will take six video frames and combine them into one frame for display and do so for each set of six frames coming in at 30 fps. By frame averaging, the observable video noise is less apparent, and the image looks less noisy to the observer. An important point to remember with frame averaging is that averaging more

frames per unit of time decreases temporal resolution (TR) and increases the likelihood of "image smearing" as dynamic images are being acquired. Decreasing the frame averaging rate (from 6 to 3 as an example) improves TR and is preferred for fast-moving anatomical structures such as the heart and blood vessels. For slower-moving anatomy, frame averaging is very effective at reducing noise and uses less radiation.

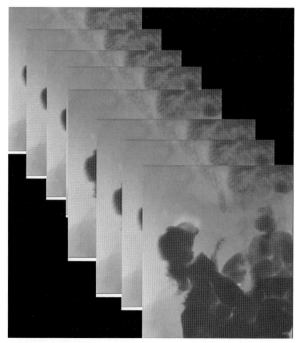

Fig. 10.13 Frame averaging is a video process of combining successive frames for display.

IMPORTANT RELATIONSHIP

Frame Averaging

Frame averaging is an operation that averages multiple video image frames together in rapid succession for display and reduces overall patient dose and image noise.

Pixel Binning

During fluoroscopy, the DELs can work individually or as combined DELs through a process known as **pixel binning**. During digital fluoroscopy x-ray exposures are pulsed exposures at selected pulse rates. This is necessary as each DEL, as a charge collection unit, must be read out following each x-ray exposure and the DEL "zeroed out" from residual charge. Additionally, the DEL must be recharged again in preparation for the next pulse of x-ray exposure, a step known as refreshing. This whole process takes a few milliseconds to complete for each fluoroscopic frame. Pulsing the fluoroscopic exposures enables this process and pixel binning reduces the total number of DEL units that are working during this fast fluoroscopic framing sequence. The pulsed frame rates are variable and can be as fast as

30 frames per second (fps). To avoid fluoroscopic image "flicker," frame rates of at least 20 fps are required.

Additional advantages of pixel binning deal with the file size of the fluoroscopic imaging sequence and the signal-to-noise ratio (SNR). As an array of DELs with micron dimensions, the total number of DELs is very large and when you consider each of these DELs working independently at fast frame rates the total data file size can be monumental. For example, a 40 × 40-cm (16 × 16-inch) field of view (FOV) can consist of 4 million DELs, each with a 200-micron dimension. The file size for one image is 8 MB and if the frame rate is 30 fps, the file size data rate increases to 240 MB/s. For a fluoroscopic acquisition that may run for only 10 seconds, the file size expands to 2.35 GB. Pixel binning is a practical approach to the huge file sizes created with digital fluoroscopy.

Pixel binning requires that individual DELs work as combined units. Binning combinations can be 2 × 2, 3 × 3, or 4 × 4 (Fig. 10.14), and as the effective DEL size increases there is some loss of image resolution. By combining DELs, the collective SNR increases, and visible noise is reduced. Binning combinations are generally controlled by the fluoroscopic equipment settings based on fluoroscopic examination requirements and pixel binning does require a small increase in dose.

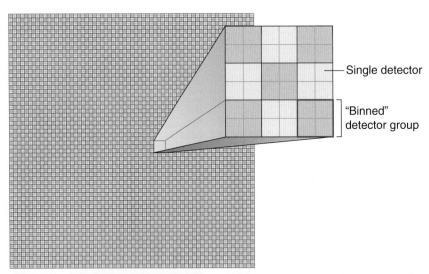

Fig. 10.14 Detector elements can work individually or in combined units through a process referred to as pixel binning. Illustration demonstrates a 2 × 2 binning group. (From Abrahams, RB, Sensakovic, WF, Huda, W. *Imaging Physics: Case Review Series*. St. Louis: Elsevier, Inc.; 2020.)

Pixel Binning

During fluoroscopy, the DELs can work individually or as combined DELs through pixel binning. Pixel binning reduces the total number of DEL units that are working during fast fluoroscopic framing sequence, increases the collective SNR, reduces visible noise, and is a practical approach to the huge file sizes created with digital fluoroscopy.

Magnification

Electronic magnification is the selection of a smaller FOV. When a smaller FOV is selected, an area smaller than the size of the detector is exposed by the x-ray beam, but the area is enlarged to fill the display monitor area magnifying the anatomic structures (Fig. 10.15). Like intensified fluoroscopy, flat-panel detectors provide several different magnification modes. However, the spatial resolution of flat-panel detectors is the same for some FOV options, and the patient radiation dose is not significantly increased provided binning (the process of grouping and averaging adjacent DELs to reduce noise) is not used. For some FOVs, binning reduces the spatial resolution; however, for a smaller FOV, spatial resolution is increased, and noise is decreased as the radiation exposure rate is increased slightly to decrease noise levels. However, the increase in radiation dose is less compared with magnification during image-intensified fluoroscopy. Selecting the magnification mode automatically adjusts the x-ray beam collimation to match the displayed tissue image and avoids irradiating tissue that does not appear in the image. The largest FOV should be used whenever possible to reduce patient radiation dose along with increased collimation to reduce irradiation of unnecessary patient tissues.

Display Monitor

Advancements in monitors have improved the quality of the displayed fluoroscopic image. These improved display monitors are currently used with both image-intensified units and digital fluoroscopic units (Fig. 10.16).

Liquid crystal display monitors are standard display options and offer superior resolution and brightness over conventional television (cathode ray tube [CRT]) monitors. LCD monitors are made up of several layers (Fig. 10.17). The heart of the LCD is the liquid crystal layer sandwiched between polarizing layers that contain nematic liquid crystals. These crystals are typically rod shaped, are semiliquid, and can change the direction of light (unpolarized electromagnetic radiation [EMR] waves traveling in two planes) that passes through them. The crystals exist in an unorganized "twisted" state. When an electric current is applied, they organize or "untwist." In the untwisted state, they organize into configurations that block or allow light to pass through depending on the polarizing filters. The polarized layers on each side are oriented perpendicular to one other, meaning that light that may be able to pass through one would be at the wrong orientation to pass through the other. When electric current is applied to the liquid crystal layer, the "untwisting" changes the orientation of light passing through (polarizing the EMR waves to travel in one

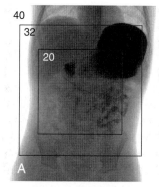
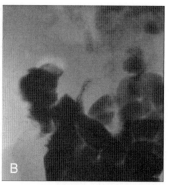

Fig. 10.15 Electronic magnification. **A,** Full field-of-view (FOV) image. **B,** Electronic magnification mode results in a magnified image displayed. (From Johnston JN, Fauber TL. *Essentials of Radiographic Physics and Imaging.* 3rd ed. St. Louis: Elsevier; 2020.)

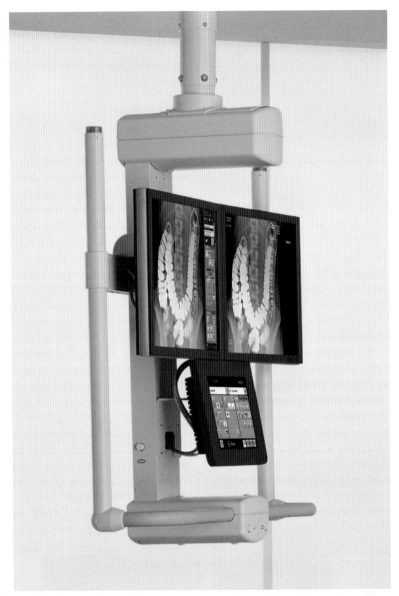

Fig. 10.16 Display monitor. Modern high-resolution liquid crystal display (LCD) monitor with a touch screen display. (Courtesy Siemens Healthcare, Malvern, PA.)

plane) the back layer and allows it to pass through the front. A TFT panel is located behind the liquid crystal layer. The number of TFTs is equal to the number of pixels displayed. The TFTs control the current to each pixel and switch it on or off by causing the liquid crystals to twist or untwist. A monochromatic LCD monitor displays the light as shades of gray. A color LCD monitor has a color filter layer added to display shades of color. The intensity of light is controlled by the current to the crystals, which is controlled by the TFTs. This in turn determines the shade of gray if monochromatic or the shade of color if using a color monitor. LCD monitors are expressed in megapixels (MP) and radiologists typically interpret images using 5 MP displays or greater.

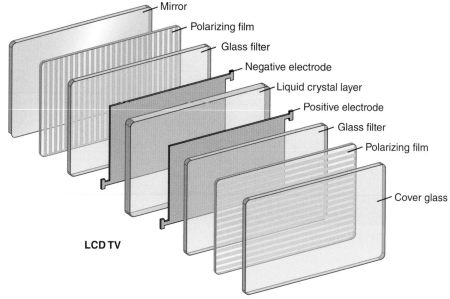

Mirror
Polarizing film
Glass filter
Negative electrode
Liquid crystal layer
Positive electrode
Glass filter
Polarizing film
Cover glass

LCD TV

Fig. 10.17 Liquid crystal display *(LCD)* monitor. LCD monitors are composed of several layers. (From Johnston JN, Fauber TL. *Essentials of Radiographic Physics and Imaging.* 3rd ed. St. Louis: Mosby; 2020.)

Image Recording

A sequence of digital radiographic images can be recorded per second with flat-panel detector fluoroscopy, which reduces the need for follow-up radiographic images. These radiographic images have improved quality (less noise) than fluoroscopic images; however, patient radiation exposure is significantly increased. Switching from fluoroscopy to the radiographic mode is very fast and controlled by the fluoroscopic system controls. Use of features such as LIH or last frame hold along with fluoro loop save saves single images or a fluoro sequence loop to memory (based on the equipment's memory capacity). Saved fluoro images have increased noise but significantly less exposure to the patient. These fluoroscopic images can be postprocessed and maintained in the patient's permanent record.

SPECIALIZED FLUOROSCOPIC UNITS

Mobile C-arm units have fluoroscopic capabilities that are typically used in the operating suite or emergency department when imaging is necessary during nonroutine procedures. Display monitors are also included, offering both static and dynamic imaging during the procedure. Because it is a fluoroscopic system, many of the features of a fixed fluoroscopic unit are also made available with a C-arm. A C-arm unit is designed with an x-ray tube and image intensifier or digital detector attached in a C configuration (Figs. 10.18 and 10.19). As a result, the unit can be positioned in a variety of planes, enabling viewing from different perspectives. Generally, three sets of locks are provided to move and hold the C-arm in place. One set moves the entire "C" toward or away from the base (the equivalent of moving a table side to side). Another set allows the "C" to pivot about its axis (the equivalent of angling a general radiographic tube head assembly). The last set allows the "C" to slide along its arc (the equivalent of moving the patient from anteroposterior or posteroanterior positions to oblique to lateral positions without having to move the patient).

Generally, the x-ray tube should be positioned under the patient and the image receptor above the patient. Positioning the C-arm in this manner during the imaging procedure reduces the radiation exposure to the operator. Because the C-arm uses fluoroscopy, standard radiation exposure techniques and safety practices used during fluoroscopy in the radiology department must also be adhered to during operation of a C-arm unit. The radiographer should also pay attention to the distance between the patient and the x-ray tube as well as to the total fluoroscopy time. In this situation, fluoroscopy is

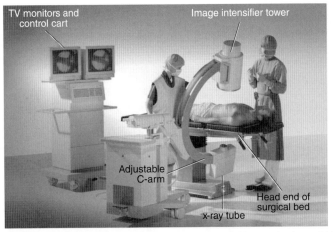

Fig. 10.18 A mobile C-arm unit. (Courtesy Philips Healthcare, Andover, MA.)

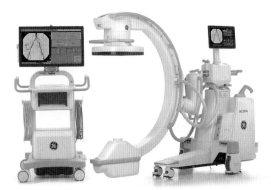

Fig. 10.19 OEC Elite CFD C-arm unit. (Courtesy GE Healthcare © General Electric Company.)

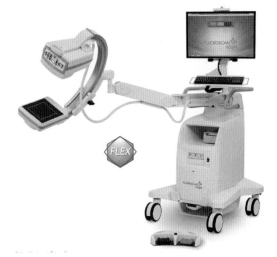

Fig. 10.20 Mini C-arm unit. (Courtesy Hologic, Inc.)

being used in an "uncontrolled" environment, and it is the radiographer's responsibility to monitor and apply radiation safety measures.

Significant advancements have been made with C-arm-type fluoroscopic units used for a variety of anatomic areas. For example, the mini C-arm (Fig. 10.20) provides a lower dose rate and greater equipment flexibility while providing quality images of extremities. The mini C-arm is available with flat-panel detector fluoroscopy, rotating detectors, both full FOV and magnification modes, and a touch screen display.

In fact, the smaller size and lighter weight of flat panels have led to portable C-arm systems that can be carried into any number of settings (Fig. 10.21).

Surgical procedures have multiple imaging needs and the O-arm system (Fig. 10.22) can provide both

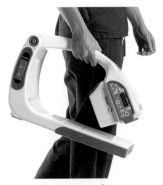

Fig. 10.21 A portable fluoroscopic C-arm system using a small field-of-view, flat-panel detector. (Courtesy SMART-C, Turner Imaging Systems.)

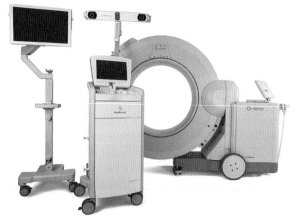

Fig. 10.22 O-arm unit. (From Lampignano J, Kendrick, LE. *Bontrager's Textbook of Radiographic Positioning and Related Anatomy.* 9th ed. St Louis: Mosby; 2018.)

static and dynamic images along with two- and three-dimensional (3D) images. The O-arm design places two flat-panel fluoroscopic detectors in an orthogonal (right-angle) orientation and permits fluoroscopy from two different views in real time. This viewing perspective is very important to surgeons for the placement of vascular lines and orthopedic devices such as pins, rods,

and fixation plates. Equipment movement is motor controlled, the gantry opens for easy patient access laterally, and specialized draping is used to maintain sterility when the gantry is closed. Fluoroscopic and radiographic images are obtained with flat-panel detector technology, which allows the surgeon to assess the outcome of the procedure before closing the patient.

A similar design uses an open architecture with two orthogonal digital receptors (Fig. 10.23). This system is not motorized and lighter in weight, making it easier to position around the patient. Additionally, because the digital receptors are not covered, the user can see their exact angle orientation relative to the patient.

RADIATION SAFETY

Radiation safety is just as important during fluoroscopic imaging as it is with radiographic imaging. It is the fluoroscopic operator's responsibility to be knowledgeable about the equipment and methods to reduce patient radiation dose. A few methods of minimizing radiation dose to the patient during fluoroscopic procedures include omission of the grid during fluoroscopy (when appropriate), minimal use of the magnification feature, and use of LIH when the x-ray exposure is not activated

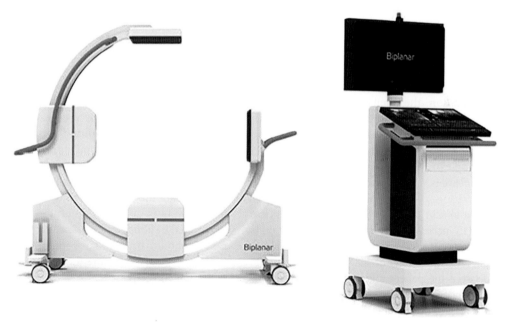

Fig. 10.23 An orthogonal C-arm system with open architecture similar to the O-arm design. (Source: Bjarnelu, CC BY-SA 4.0 <https://creativecommons.org/licenses/by-sa/4.0>, via Wikimedia Commons.)

while the operator reviews the image. In addition, maneuvering the equipment or patient to distribute the radiation exposure over a wider area of skin minimizes the absorbed dose.

If working with older image-intensified fluoroscopic units that use a continuous stream of x-rays, the exposure should be intermittently pulsed by the operator. Applying pressure to the exposure switch or pedal intermittently significantly reduces the exposure of both patients and personnel and reduces the heat load on the x-ray tube. Modern image-intensified and digital fluoroscopic systems use a controlled pulsed x-ray exposure, and the operator is not required to intermittently release the pressure. Operating the fluoroscope in the lowest pulsed mode along with a lower dose rate will minimize patient radiation dose.

Time, distance, and shielding are the standard radiation safety practices used during fluoroscopic imaging. Reducing the x-ray exposure time reduces the exposure to the patient and any personnel remaining in the room. The control panel timer produces an audible noise when 5 minutes of x-ray fluoroscopic time has been used. It is the operator's responsibility to minimize the x-ray fluoroscopy, and the radiographer should document the total amount of x-ray fluoroscopic time used during the procedure. Modern fluoroscopic units provide dose monitoring in addition to the cumulative fluorotimer. The DAP or KAP and cumulative air kerma (reference dose) provide radiation exposure data and need to be recorded in the patient's medical record. If these dose monitoring systems are not available, then the cumulative exposure time and number of acquired static images need to be documented. In addition, the intensity of the x-ray exposure at the tabletop should not exceed ~88 mGy/min (10 R/min) for routine fluoroscopic units equipped with ABC. However, in some advanced procedures a higher tabletop exposure is warranted. Whenever the patient's exposure is reduced, personnel exposure also is reduced.

The source-to-skin distance (SSD) should be no less than 38 cm (15 inches) for stationary fluoroscopic units and no less than 30 cm (12 inches) on a mobile C-arm fluoroscopic unit. Increasing the SSD and decreasing the distance between the patient and the radiation detector (OID) will decrease patient exposure. Increasing collimation and decreasing the number of static (radiographic) images will reduce patient exposure. If the fluoroscopic unit has features such as virtual collimation (x-ray field size can be adjusted without irradiating the patient) and the ability to save a sequence of fluoroscopic images without acquiring radiographic images, patient exposure will be further decreased. Additionally, personnel other than the operator should increase their distance from the patient to reduce exposure to scatter radiation from the patient.

In addition to all personnel in the room wearing lead aprons (recommended 0.5 mm of lead equivalent), two additional types of shielding are required during fluoroscopy. Because the receptor tray is positioned at the end of the table for operation of the under-table x-ray tube in a fixed fluoroscopic unit, a receptor tray slot cover with at least 0.25 mm of lead equivalent should automatically cover the opened space at the side of the table. Also, a protective lead curtain with at least 0.25 mm of lead equivalent must be placed between the patient and the operator to reduce exposure to the operator. Table 10.1 lists methods of reducing patient and personnel exposure during fluoroscopy.

Pay particular attention to the digital fluoroscopic system design regarding the location of the x-ray tube for fluoroscopy. The scatter curves (isodose) are noticeably different with each design. Remember, during fluoroscopy the patient is the source of occupational exposure, and maximizing distance to a practical level is a very effective as low as reasonably achievable (ALARA) practice.

QUALITY CONTROL

Quality control programs are vitally important for all ionizing radiation–producing equipment to monitor equipment performance and minimize patient dose. Fluoroscopic equipment is used extensively in health care and contributes significantly to the radiation dose received by the general population. Quality control is a team effort among the radiographer, radiologist, and medical physicist. Although some equipment monitoring and data may be collected by a radiographer, performance tests and their interpretation are typically performed by a medical physicist. However, the radiographer should be familiar with the monitoring and testing necessary to ensure that the fluoroscopic unit is operating correctly.

The radiographer, in particular, a quality control radiographer, may be responsible for the operational inspection of the equipment. This inspection should be conducted using a checklist of the items found in

TABLE 10.1 Methods of Reducing Patient and Personnel Exposure During Fluoroscopy

- Operating the fluoroscopic exposure intermittently or in the lowest pulsed mode along with a lower dose rate and the use of last image hold minimizes the patient radiation dose.
- Evaluate and use preset or default settings available to minimize the patient dose.
- Reducing the amount of x-ray fluoroscopic time reduces patient and personnel exposure.
- Increase collimation with virtual collimation, remove the grid, and minimize the use of magnification.
- Monitor and document the amount of total x-ray fluoroscopic time displayed in 5-minute increments on the control panel in addition to the number of acquired radiographic images. If provided, cumulative radiation dose data should be recorded.
- The intensity of x-ray exposure at the tabletop should not exceed 88 mGy/min (10 R/min) for units equipped with ABC or AERC.
- The SSD should be not less than 38 cm (15 inches) for stationary fluoroscopic units and not less than 30 cm (12 inches) on mobile C-arm fluoroscopic units.
- Personnel in the fluoroscopic room during procedures should increase their distance from the patient to reduce exposure to scatter radiation.
- Personnel should wear appropriate lead shielding during fluoroscopic procedures.
- The receptor slot cover must contain at least 0.25 mm of lead-equivalent shielding and cover the opened space on the side of the table.
- A protective curtain placed between the patient and operator must have at least 0.25 mm of lead equivalent.

ABC, Automatic brightness control; *AERC*, automatic exposure rate control; *SSD*, source-to-skin distance.

BOX 10.3 Fluoroscopic Equipment Inspection Checklist

Inspect	Ensure that
Bucky slot cover	When the receptor tray is parked at the foot of the table, the metal cover should expand and cover the entire opening.
Protective curtain	The curtain should be in good condition and move freely into place when the tower is moved to the operating position.
Tower: locks, power assist, control panel	The electromagnetic locks are in good working order, the power assist moves the tower about easily in all directions, and all control panel indicator lights are operational.
Exposure switch (dead-man switch)	The switch is not sticking and operates the x-ray tube only while in the depressed position. (Also test the switch with the tower in the park position; it should not activate the x-ray tube while parked.)
Collimator shutters	In the fully open position, the shutters should restrict the beam to the size of the input phosphor and be accurate to within ±3%.
Fluoroscopic timer	The timer should buzz audibly after 5 minutes of fluoroscopic "beam-on" time.
Monitor brightness	While exposing a penetrometer through a fluoroscopic phantom, the monitor image is adjusted to display as many of the penetrometer steps as possible.
Table tilt motion	The table tilts smoothly to its limit in both directions, and the angulation indicator is operational.

Box 10.3 at least every 6 months. The radiographer may also be responsible for an inspection of the imaging suite itself to examine the general physical condition of the room, unit, supporting electrical cables, and control booth, noting any wear or deterioration. This inspection of the physical condition should be placed on the same schedule and conducted along with the operational inspection.

The other important part of the quality control program is the performance inspection and equipment testing. Box 10.4 lists a few common fluoroscopic quality control tests. Although a quality control radiographer may perform some of these tests, an appropriately trained and licensed medical physicist should conduct and interpret this portion of the program and oversee the entire quality control monitoring program.

BOX 10.4 Quality Control Specific to Fluoroscopic Equipment

Quality Control Test	Description
Fluoroscopic system resolution	Tests the system's ability to display details of small objects (high-contrast resolution) and larger objects (low-contrast resolution)
Fluoroscopic ABC/AERC performance	Evaluates image quality for changes in exposure parameters such as high dose rate, pulsed modes, and FOV
Fluoroscopic phantom image quality	Evaluates the quality of the displayed fluoroscopic image, including image distortion or lag
Fluoroscopic exposure rates	Measures the intensity of the x-ray beam; fluoroscopic exposure rate should not exceed ~88 mGy/min (10 R/min)
Fluoroscopic alignment test	Ensures the radiation beam aligns with the center of the image intensifier or flat-panel detector within 2% of the SID
Patient dose monitoring system calibration, if present	Evaluates proper function of patient dose monitoring systems such as DAP meters
Display monitor performance	Evaluates the display characteristics of the monitor (described in Chapter 6)

ABC, Automatic brightness control; *AERC*, automatic exposure rate control; *DAP*, dose area product; *FOV*, field of view; *SID*, source-to-image receptor distance.

CHAPTER SUMMARY

- Fluoroscopy allows imaging of the movement of internal structures by its use of a continuous or pulsed beam of x-rays.
- Image intensification provides a brighter image for viewing. The exit radiation is absorbed by the input phosphor, converted to electrons, sent to the output phosphor, released as visible light, and converted to a digital signal for transmission to a computer and display monitor.
- Brightness gain is the product of flux gain and minification gain and results in a brighter image on the output phosphor.
- ABC maintains the overall appearance of the image by monitoring the current through the image intensifier or the output phosphor intensity and adjusting exposure factors if the monitored values fall below preset levels.
- Image intensifiers provide a multifield mode that magnifies the image. When operating the unit in the magnification mode, spatial resolution improves but patient exposure increases.
- Digital fluoroscopy can be accomplished by attaching a CCD to the output phosphor which creates a digital signal for image processing and display.
- The use of flat-panel detectors in place of an image intensifier offers several advantages, such as reductions in the size, bulk, and weight of the fluoroscopic tower; allowing easier manipulation of the tower; and greater access to the patient during the examination.
- Flat-panel detectors also replace spot filming and other recording devices, and because they are capable of operating in radiographic mode, additional radiographic images are not needed in many cases. The images, both dynamic and static, can also be readily archived with the patient record in a MIMPS.
- Image-intensified fluoroscopy uses a lower mA (0.5–5 mA), whereas digital fluoroscopy uses a higher mA (50–1200 mA). A higher mA is needed for the lower pulse width to maintain sufficient exposure to the IR for a diagnostic image (maintaining the needed SNR).
- Modern fluoroscopic units use a pulsed x-ray beam, whereas older image intensifiers operate as a continuous x-ray beam exposure unless the operator produces intermittent x-ray exposures.
- Modern fluoroscopic units have features such as AERC, the ability to select dose rates, virtual collimation, change filtration, and select predetermined set of exposure factors, in addition to pulsed fluoroscopy, frame averaging, pixel binning, electronic magnification, fluoro loop save, and dose monitoring.
- Flat-panel fluoroscopic systems use pixel binning to achieve manageable file sizes and pulse rates for optimum viewing.
- Pulsed fluoroscopy and frame averaging are effective methods to reduce fluoroscopic dosages without compromising image quality.

- Flat-panel fluoroscopic systems come in two basic designs that center around the location of the fluoroscopic x-ray tube relative to the patient. The isodose scatter radiation areas are different between the designs since the patient is the source of exposure to fluoroscopic staff.
- LCD monitors are the preferred display technology and offer superior resolution, brightness, and work in a different way than traditional television monitors.
- Several specialized fluoroscopic units are available for use outside the radiology department such as mobile C-arm, mini C-arm, and O-arm.

- Radiation safety practices include reducing the amount of fluoroscopic time and shielding the operator with the Bucky slot cover and a protective curtain placed between the patient and the operator. The SSD should be not less than 38 cm (15 inches) for stationary fluoroscopic units and not less than 30 cm (12 inches) on a mobile fluoroscopic unit, and the intensity of the x-ray exposure at the tabletop should not exceed ~88 mGy/min (10 R/min).
- Quality control procedures are important for monitoring the performance of the fluoroscopic unit.

REVIEW QUESTIONS

1. In image-intensified fluoroscopy, the mA range is typically _____.
   A. 0.5 to 5 mA
   B. 20 to 50 mA
   C. 100 to 300 mA
   D. 400 to 600 mA

2. During fluoroscopy, releasing the pressure applied to the pedal or switch terminates the radiation exposure and is known as the _____.
   A. fluoroscopic timer
   B. intensification switch
   C. activation switch
   D. dead-man switch

3. What component of the image intensifier converts the exit or remnant radiation into visible light?
   A. Output phosphor
   B. Photocathode
   C. Input phosphor
   D. Electrostatic focusing lenses

4. What component of the image intensifier converts the visible light into electrons?
   A. Output phosphor
   B. Photocathode
   C. Input phosphor
   D. Electrostatic focusing lenses

5. In image-intensified fluoroscopy, to view the images on a display monitor, the light from the output phosphor is converted to a digital signal by the _____.
   A. photocathode
   B. electrostatic lens
   C. CCD
   D. LCD monitor

6. Brightness gain is a product of _____.
   A. minification gain and ABC
   B. flux gain and ABC
   C. minification gain and flux gain
   D. ABC and mA

7. The numeric conversion factor value is equal to _____ of the brightness gain value.
   A. 0.001
   B. 0.01
   C. 0.1
   D. 1.0

8. A brightness gain of 40,000 would have a conversion factor of _____.
   A. 40
   B. 400
   C. 4000
   D. 40,000

9. A disadvantage of using the magnification mode during image-intensified fluoroscopy is _____.
   A. decreased spatial resolution
   B. increased patient exposure
   C. decreased brightness
   D. decreased contrast

10. The process of pixel binning is designed to achieve _____.
    A. reduced digital file sizes
    B. improved spatial resolution
    C. practical pulsed frame rates
    D. A and C

11. Which of the following fluoroscopic features will decrease patient radiation dose?
    A. Virtual collimation
    B. Pulsed fluoroscopy
    C. Frame averaging
    D. All of the above

12. When operating a stationary fluoroscopic unit, the SSD should not be less than _____.
    A. 25 cm (10 inches)
    B. 30 cm (12 inches)
    C. 38 cm (15 inches)
    D. 45 cm (18 inches)

13. During fluoroscopy, the x-ray exposure at the table-top should not exceed _____.
    A. 0.01 R/min
    B. 0.1 R/min
    C. 1.0 R/min
    D. 10 R/min

14. The Bucky slot cover must have a lead-equivalent thickness of _____.
    A. 0.10 mm
    B. 0.25 mm
    C. 0.50 mm
    D. 2.5 mm

15. Which of the following combinations reduces patient radiation exposure during fluoroscopy?
    A. Highest pulse mode and highest dose rate
    B. Highest pulse mode and lowest pulse rate
    C. Lowest pulse mode and highest dose rate
    D. Lowest pulse mode and lowest dose rate

16. In comparing flat-panel detector fluoroscopy with image-intensified fluoroscopy, which is NOT correct about flat-panel detector fluoroscopy?
    A. Spatial resolution is less than image intensified
    B. The size of the fluoroscopic tower is less
    C. Higher detective quantum efficiency
    D. Less image distortion artifacts

17. The input surface of a fluoroscopic imaging detector above the patient is referred to as the _____.
    A. photoemissive surface
    B. primary protective barrier
    C. electrostatic coupling lens
    D. Bucky cover

18. To improve fluoroscopic image quality that is noisy and demonstrates quantum mottling, an effective method is to _____.
    A. select pixel binning on the control
    B. reduce the pulsed fluoro frame rate
    C. increase the pulsed height
    D. increase the pulse interval

19. In a fluoroscopic system with the x-ray tube above the patient and the receptor below, the scatter radiation exposure to the operator is _____.
    A. greatest below the waist
    B. equal throughout the head, chest, and trunk areas
    C. more intense at the level of the chest and head areas
    D. of no concern because of the use of pulsed fluoroscopy

20. When performing dynamic fluoroscopy of fast-moving anatomy such as the vascular system, the application of pulsed fluoroscopy will require _____.
    A. frame averaging
    B. faster pulse rates and shorter pulse intervals
    C. higher pulse heights and slower pulse rates
    D. longer pulse widths and longer pulse intervals

Summary of Important Relationships

CHAPTER 1: RADIATION AND ITS DISCOVERY

The Dual Nature of X-ray Energy

X-rays act like both waves and particles.

Wavelength and Frequency

Wavelength and frequency are inversely related. Higher-energy x-rays have decreased wavelength and increased frequency. Lower-energy x-rays have increased wavelength and decreased frequency.

CHAPTER 2: FUNDAMENTALS OF RADIATION PRODUCTION

Filament

The filament is the source of electrons during x-ray production.

Target

The target is the part of the anode that is struck by the focused stream of electrons coming from the cathode. The target stops the electrons and creates the opportunity for the production of x-rays.

Tungsten

Because tungsten has a high atomic number (74) and a high melting point (3400°C [6152°F]), it efficiently produces x-rays.

Dissipating Heat

The heat produced when the x-ray exposure is activated is transferred to the electrical insulating, dielectric oil that surrounds the x-ray tube.

Rotating Anodes

Rotating anodes can withstand higher heat loads than stationary anodes because the rotation causes a greater physical area, or focal track, to be exposed to electrons.

Circuits

Circuits precisely control the flow and intensity of electrons as they travel through the circuit pathways and components. Electrons only work for us when they flow through circuits in electrical devices to create energy, and the x-ray tube is an example of this process.

High Voltage

X-ray production is a high-voltage process and can range from 50,000 to 150,000 Volts (50–150 kV), and because of this, the amperage necessarily must drop to milliamperage (mA) values. Higher kilowatts systems naturally offer more power and therefore higher mA and kilovoltage peak (kVp) values.

Transformers and Mutual Induction

Transformers regulate voltage on the principle of mutual induction. All transformers have an input side, the primary coil, and an output side, the secondary coil. An electrical current coming into a set of coils on the input side (primary side) will create an electrical current and voltage in the secondary coil windings, the output side. The ratio of wire windings between the primary and secondary sides determines whether the transformer is a step-up or step-down transformer.

Resistors

Negative electron charges moving along circuit pathways inherently impede the flow of electrons, known as resistance, primarily due to electron friction. Resistors regulate the amount of current passing through the cathode filament during exposure and are used to control amperage. Resistors allow for the specific selection of mA values such as 100, 200, or even 1000 mA.

Step-Up and Step-Down Transformers

Transformers operate on the principle of mutual induction, are used to control voltage values on the secondary side and are constructed with a set of primary copper wire windings that are electrically insulated and wrapped around a larger set of secondary windings, referred to as step-up transformers. Working in conjunction with the high-tension, step-up transformer, the autotransformer consists of a single coil winding that acts as both a primary and secondary coil. It supplies an induced voltage to the primary windings of the step-up transformer and permits the selection of kVp values by the operator. The cathode filament is controlled by the low-voltage side of the circuit. During exposure, high voltage flows through the x-ray tube at low milliamperage. Because the filament circuit uses low voltage, step-down transformers have more core windings on the primary side than on the secondary side and reduce the incoming voltage to a lower value.

Rectification

Electrical power supplied by the power utility to a modern x-ray system is typically three-phase, alternating current (AC). Because x-ray tubes perform most efficiently with direct current (DC), rectification is the process of changing AC to DC. Rectification diodes permit current flow in only one direction.

Capacitors

Capacitors are charge storage components and, when placed in the circuit with the invertors, result in a current waveform that has a very small voltage fluctuation, known as ripple. This provides a very efficient, high-quality x-ray beam with a higher average energy that minimizes patient x-ray exposure without negatively affecting image quality.

X-ray System Circuits

X-ray system circuits, by design, take incoming alternating current (AC) at voltage levels supplied by the power utility and increase it to kilovoltage peak (kVp) levels, and convert the AC to a direct current (DC) waveform with a voltage fluctuation (ripple) that is minimal.

CHAPTER 3: THE X-RAY BEAM

Production of X-rays

As electrons strike the target, their kinetic energy is transferred to the tungsten atoms in the anode to produce x-rays. Bremsstrahlung interactions and characteristic interactions both produce x-ray photons.

Bremsstrahlung Interactions

Bremsstrahlung interactions occur when a projectile (incident) electron completely avoids the orbital electrons of a tungsten atom and travels very close to its nucleus. The closer the projectile electron travels to the nucleus, the stronger the attraction. The stronger this attraction, the more energy the projectile electron loses and the stronger the resultant x-ray photon (higher energy). Projectile electrons that travel farther from the nucleus create x-ray photons with less energy. Most x-ray interactions in the diagnostic energy range are bremsstrahlung.

Characteristic Interactions

Characteristic interactions are produced when a projectile (incident) electron interacts with an electron from the inner shell (K-shell) of a tungsten atom. Characteristic x-rays can be produced in a tungsten target only when the kVp is set at 70 or greater because the binding energy of the K-shell electron is 69.5 kiloelectron volt (keV).

Thermionic Emission

When the tungsten filament gains enough heat (therm), the outer-shell electrons of the filament atoms are boiled off, or emitted, from the filament, which creates free electrons as ions.

Tube Current

Electrons flow only in one direction in the x-ray tube—from cathode to anode. This flow of electrons is called the *tube current* and is measured in milliamperage (mA).

Energy Conversion in the X-ray Tube

As electrons strike the anode target, more than 99% of their kinetic energy is converted to heat, whereas less than 1% of their energy is converted to x-rays.

Kilovoltage and the Speed of Electrons

The speed of the electrons traveling from the cathode to the anode increases as the kilovoltage applied across the x-ray tube increases. It is a direct relationship, but not proportional.

Speed of Electrons and Quality of X-rays

The speed of the electrons in the tube current directly affects the quality or energy of the x-rays that are produced but it is not a proportional relationship. The quality or energy of the x-rays in turn determines the penetrability of the primary beam (ease with which it moves through tissue).

kVp and Beam Penetrability

As kVp increases, beam penetrability increases; as kVp decreases, beam penetrability decreases.

Milliamperage, Tube Current, and X-ray Quantity

The quantity of electrons in the tube current and the quantity of x-rays produced are directly proportional to the mA.

Exposure Time, Tube Current, and X-ray Quantity

The quantity of electrons flowing from the cathode to the anode and the quantity of x-rays produced are directly proportional to the exposure time.

Quantity of Electrons, X-rays, and mAs

The quantity of electrons flowing from the cathode to the anode and the quantity of x-rays produced are directly proportional to milliamperage-seconds (mAs).

Line-Focus Principle

The line-focus principle describes the relationship between the actual focal spot, where the electrons in the tube current bombard the target, and the effective focal spot, which is the same area as seen from directly below the tube.

Anode Angle and Effective Focal Spot Size

Based on the line-focus principle, the smaller the anode target angle, the smaller the effective focal spot size.

Anode Heel Effect

X-rays are more intense on the cathode side of the tube; their intensity decreases toward the anode side.

Low-Energy Photons, Patient Dose, Image Formation

Low-energy photons serve only to increase patient dose and do not contribute to image formation.

Half-Value Layer

Half-value layer (HVL) is the amount of added filtration to the beam (usually in millimeters [mm] of aluminum) that reduces the beam intensity to half its original intensity. HVL is an effective and relatively convenient method for tracking x-ray system output over time as a function of usage.

CHAPTER 4: IMAGE FORMATION AND RADIOGRAPHIC QUALITY

Differential Absorption and Image Formation

A radiographic image is created when an x-ray beam passes through a patient and then interacts with an image receptor (IR), such as a digital IR. The variations in the absorption and transmission of the exiting x-ray beam structurally represent the anatomic area of interest.

X-ray Photon Absorption

During attenuation of the x-ray beam, the photoelectric effect is responsible for the total absorption of the incoming x-ray photon.

X-ray Beam Scattering

During attenuation of the x-ray beam, the incoming x-ray photon may lose energy and change direction as a result of the Compton effect.

Factors Affecting Beam Attenuation

Increasing tissue thickness, higher effective atomic number, and tissue density increases x-ray beam attenuation because more x-rays are absorbed by the tissue. Increasing the quality of the x-ray beam decreases beam attenuation because the higher-energy x-rays penetrate the tissue.

X-ray Interaction With Matter

When the diagnostic primary x-ray beam interacts with anatomic tissues, three processes occur: absorption, scattering, and transmission.

Displayed Image Gray Levels

Anatomic tissues that vary in absorption and transmission range between radiopaque and radiolucent to create a range of dark and light areas (shades of gray).

Electronic Signal Values

When the exit or remnant radiation interacts with the digital IR, it is converted to electronic signal values. The strength (intensity) of the signal value and the differences in adjacent signal values are a result of x-ray beam attenuation with the varying anatomic tissues.

Displayed Brightness and Digital Image Quality

A digital image must have sufficient brightness to visualize the anatomic structures of interest.

Differentiating Among Anatomic Tissues

The ability to distinguish among types of tissues is determined by the differences in brightness levels in the displayed image or contrast. Anatomic tissues that attenuate the beam similarly have low subject contrast. Anatomic tissues that attenuate the beam very differently have high subject contrast.

Sharpness of Anatomic Detail

The accuracy of the anatomic structural lines displayed in the digital image is determined by its spatial resolution.

Size Distortion

Radiographic images of objects are always magnified in terms of the true object size. The source-to-image receptor distance (SID) and object-to-image receptor distance (OID) have a geometric relationship and play an important role in minimizing the amount of size distortion of the radiographic image.

Shape Distortion

Shape distortion can occur from inaccurate central ray (CR) alignment of the tube, the part being radiographed, or the IR. Elongation refers to images of objects that appear longer than the true objects. Foreshortening refers to images that appear shorter than the true objects.

Number of Photons and Quantum Noise

Decreasing the number of photons reaching the IR may increase the amount of quantum noise within the radiographic image; increasing the number of photons reaching the IR may decrease the amount of quantum noise within the radiographic image.

Fluoroscopy

Dynamic imaging of internal anatomic structures can be visualized with the use of a flat-panel detector. The exit radiation interacts with the acquisition device, is processed, and is then transmitted to the display monitor for viewing.

Image Formation

The process of differential absorption for image formation remains the same regardless of the type of imaging system, radiographic or fluoroscopic. The varying x-ray intensities exiting the patient structurally represent the area of interest in the displayed image.

CHAPTER 5: DIGITAL IMAGE CHARACTERISTICS, RECEPTORS, AND IMAGE ACQUISITION

Pixel Size, Displayed FOV, and Matrix Size

The pixel size is directly related to the field of view (FOV) displayed and inversely related to the matrix size. Increasing the FOV displayed for the same matrix size will increase the size of the pixel and decrease spatial resolution, whereas increasing the matrix size for the same FOV displayed will decrease the pixel size and increase spatial resolution.

Pixel Bit Depth and Contrast Resolution

The greater the pixel bit depth (i.e., 16-bit), the more precise the digitization of the analog signal and the greater the number of shades of gray available for image display. Increasing the number of shades of gray available to display in a digital image improves its contrast resolution.

Pixel Density and Pitch and Spatial Resolution

Increasing pixel density and decreasing pixel pitch increases spatial resolution. Decreasing pixel density and increasing pixel pitch decreases spatial resolution.

Spatial Frequency and Spatial Resolution

The unit of measure for spatial frequency is line pairs per millimeter (lp/mm). Increasing the number of lp/mm resolved by the imaging system (higher spatial frequency) results in improved spatial resolution.

Digital Receptors, Dynamic Range, and Exposure Latitude

Digital IRs have a wide dynamic range; that is, they can accurately capture a wide range of x-ray intensities exiting the patient. The computer then processes the raw pixel data to compensate for an exposure error and create a diagnostic radiographic image. However, lower- or higher-than-necessary exposure techniques do not guarantee a quality digital image. Exposure latitude is the range of exposures that should be used to produce a diagnostic image.

Modulation Transfer Function and Anatomic Detail

Modulation transfer function (MTF) is a measure of the imaging system's ability to accurately display small anatomic objects having high spatial frequency. An imaging system that has a high MTF can display anatomic detail with improved visibility.

Detective Quantum Efficiency and X-ray Exposure

An IR with a higher detective quantum efficiency (DQE) requires less x-ray exposure to produce a quality radiographic image when compared to an IR with a lower DQE value.

Signal-to-Noise Ratio and Image Quality

Increasing the signal-to-noise ratio (SNR) increases the visibility of anatomic details, whereas decreasing the SNR decreases the visibility due to the presence of objectionable noise.

Contrast-to-Noise Ratio and Image Quality

Increasing the contrast-to-noise ratio (CNR) increases the visibility of anatomic details, whereas decreasing the CNR decreases the visibility.

Computed Radiography Image Receptors

The computed radiography raw image data are acquired in the photostimulable phosphor (PSP) layer of the imaging plate (IP). Most energy from the exit radiation intensities is stored in the PSP for extraction in the reader unit.

Sampling Frequency and Spatial Resolution

Increasing the sampling frequency results in more sampling points and decreased sampling pitch, which improves the spatial resolution of the digital image. Decreasing the sampling frequency results in fewer sampling points and increased sampling pitch and decreased spatial resolution.

Image Receptor Size and Matrix Size

For a fixed matrix size CR system, using a smaller IR for a given exposure FOV results in improved spatial resolution of the digital image. Increasing the size of the IR for a given exposure FOV results in decreased spatial resolution.

Indirect Conversion Detectors in Digital Radiography

Indirect conversion detectors involve a two-stage process of converting remnant x-ray intensities first to visible light and then to electrical charges. A scintillator-type material is used to absorb the x-ray energy, emits light in response, and then the light is converted to electrical signals. The electrical signals are then directed to amplifiers and the analog-to-digital converter (ADC) to produce a raw digital image. Flat-panel thin-film transistor (TFT) detectors are common in direct radiography (DR), but charge-coupled device (CCD) and complementary metal oxide semiconductor (CMOS) indirect conversion detectors are also used in digital radiography.

Direct Conversion Detectors in DR

Direct conversion uses amorphous selenium-coated (a-Se) detectors to directly convert the incoming radiation exiting the patient to electrical charges. Similar to indirect conversion detectors, the electronic charge is stored in a TFT array before it is amplified, digitized, and processed in the computer.

CHAPTER 6: DIGITAL IMAGE PROCESSING, DISPLAY, AND HEALTH INFORMATION MANAGEMENT

Corrections and Histogram Creation

Several operations occur on the raw image data to prepare for further processing in order to display a quality image. Software corrections can be applied to account for imperfections (bad or dead pixels) that only occur with DR-type IRs, and flat fielding is a process of correcting the nonuniformity of pixel values throughout the entire image. A histogram is created that represents the range of digital pixel values versus the relative prevalence of the pixel values in the invisible image. Scanning the entire CR IR to identify the exposure field brightness levels and the edges of the collimated image (exposure field recognition and segmentation) is necessary to identify only the image data representing the anatomic area.

Histogram Analysis

During histogram analysis, the exposure histogram is compared with a stored (reference) histogram for that anatomic part; values of interest (VOIs) are identified in preparation for image processing and display.

Applied Lookup Tables

It is important that the correct lookup table (LUT) be applied to the body part imaged. If an incorrect LUT is applied to the histogram of the body part imaged, its appearance could be jeopardized for display.

Lookup Tables

LUTs provide the means to alter the original pixel values to improve the brightness and contrast of the displayed image.

Image Repeat

A decision to repeat an image should be based on the quality of the displayed image and departmental standards in addition to the exposure indicator (EI) value.

Exposure Indicator

The EI provides a numeric value indicating the level of radiation exposure to the digital IR. These values may be vendor specific and have a direct or inverse relationship to the IR exposure. A universal standard exposure indicator, deviation index [DI], has been developed and provides the radiographer with important information about the IR exposure.

Deviation Index

DIs range from -3 to $+3$ and are labeled as standard deviations (SDs) above and below the target DI of 0. DIs greater than $+1.0$ SD are considered overexposed. A DI of $+3.0$ SD has excessive exposure by a factor of 2 or 100% more than the target exposure index (EI_t). DIs less than -1.0 SD are considered underexposed and a DI of -3.0 SD has insufficient exposure by $\frac{1}{2}$ or 50% of the EI_t.

Improper Image Receptor Exposures

Attempting to adjust the image data with postprocessing display functions would not correct for improper IR exposure and may result in noisy or suboptimal images that should not be submitted for interpretation.

Electronic Masking

Proper collimation before radiation exposure is important and should not be replaced with electronic masking. It is not within the standards of practice for radiographers to make decisions about removing information within the radiation-exposed field.

Window Level and Image Brightness

A relationship exists between window level and image brightness on the display monitor. Changing the window level on the display monitor allows the image brightness to be increased or decreased throughout the entire range.

Window Width and Image Contrast

A narrow (decreased) window width displays higher radiographic contrast, whereas a wider (increased) window width displays lower radiographic contrast.

Display Monitor

A high-resolution 5-megapixel (2048 $\times$ 2560 pixels) display monitor will provide improved visualization of the imaging system's high spatial resolution. In addition, a display monitor having diagonal dimensions of 53 cm (21 inches) is adequate for viewing images sized 35 $\times$ 43 cm (14 $\times$ 17 inches) with a recommended pixel pitch of 0.200 mm at a standard viewing distance of about 60 cm (24 inches).

Display Monitor Luminance

Luminance is a measurement of the light intensity (brightness) emitted from the surface of the monitor and is expressed in units of candela per square meter (cd/m^2). Primary display monitors should exhibit a minimum luminance of 1.0 cd/m^2 and a maximum luminance of 350 cd/m^2. A ratio of the maximum to minimum luminance, luminance ratio (LR), is recommended to be greater than 250 and a display monitor with an LR of 350 has improved image contrast.

Display Workstation

A display workstation is simply a desktop computer that allows for the retrieval and viewing of medical images from one of the modalities or storage components of the medical image management and processing system (MIMPS). Quality control (QC) display stations and interpreting stations have greater function and capability, such as more advanced image manipulation, windowing (level and width), annotation, patient demographic information, cropping, panning, and magnification (zoom). In addition to other standards of communication, Digital Imaging and Communications in Medicine (DICOM) specifies information included as a header on digital images (DICOM header), and the grayscale standard display function (GSDF) is the DICOM recommended standard for consistent display characteristics, such as grayscale appearance and image quality.

Health Information Management

Health information management (HIM) involves the management of the medical record and the data contained within. Health informatics and data management, components of the HIM system, are utilized in the acquisition, storage, retrieval, transmission, and display of digital images from multiple imaging modalities and throughout healthcare systems.

Patient Health Information

Patient health information is collected and stored in the hospital information system (HIS) and shared with the radiology information system (RIS). The electronic medical record (EMR) is a digital record with the ability to store, share, and manage protected health information (PHI) within a single healthcare organization. The electronic health record (EHR) is the system for patient PHI that can be shared outside the facility and among many healthcare systems.

Medical Image Management and Processing System

A MIMPS is a computer system designed for digital imaging that can receive, store, archive, distribute, and display digital images. The major components of MIMPS include the imaging modalities, digital communication networks, display workstations, and archival capabilities for storage and retrieval.

Digital Communication Networks

DICOM is an international communication standard for information sharing between MIMPS and imaging modalities to transmit, store, retrieve, print, process, and display medical imaging information. The Health Level Seven standard (HL7) is a communication standard for medical information. Connectivity and communication among these systems are necessary for radiology to realize the full potential of imaging informatics. Integrating

the Healthcare Enterprise (IHE) promotes the coordinated use of established standards such as DICOM and HL7 to address specific clinical needs in support of optimal patient care.

Teleradiology

Teleradiology is the practice of diagnostic image interpretation outside the facility (offsite) from where the imaging data are acquired. Communication needs between teleradiologists and the imaging professionals include providing timely and relevant patient information, ability to answer questions regarding the procedure, and maintaining standard quality control (QC) practices. The practice of teleradiology should maintain the same high standards, safety, and quality as onsite radiology services.

Transmission, Storage, and Archive

Transmission devices need to have the capacity to handle the volume of images delivered within a reasonable time frame and can check for errors. To improve transmission of the data to the various end users of the imaging data, compression (reversible or irreversible) may be used. Policies and procedures are also needed to effectively and appropriately archive (current and previous examinations) and store digital image data for years.

Security of Patient Health Information

Radiographers have routine access to PHI in the performance of their duties and must take responsibility for adhering to the department's policies and procedures. Patients must be confident that radiographers have the skills to perform their imaging procedures and believe that their PHI will be secure.

CHAPTER 7: EXPOSURE TECHNIQUE FACTORS

mAs and Quantity of Radiation

As mAs increases, the quantity of radiation reaching the IR increases. As mAs decreases, the amount of radiation reaching the IR decreases.

mA and Exposure Time

mA and exposure time have an inverse proportional relationship when maintaining the same mAs.

mAs and Digital Image Brightness

The level of mAs does not control image brightness when using digital IRs. During computer processing, image brightness is maintained when the mAs is too low or too high. A lower-than-needed mAs produces an image with increased quantum noise, and a higher-than-needed mAs exposes a patient to unnecessary radiation.

Exposure Indicator Value

An exposure indicator (EI) is displayed on the processed digital image to indicate the level of x-ray exposure received (remnant exposure) on the IR. If the EI value falls outside the manufacturer's suggested range, exposure to the digital IR, image quality, and patient exposure could be affected.

kVp and the Radiographic Image

Increasing or decreasing the kVp changes the amount of radiation exposure to the IR and the subject contrast produced within the image.

Exposure Errors in Digital Imaging

kVp and mAs exposure errors should be reflected in the EI value; however, image brightness can be maintained during computer processing.

kVp and the 15% Rule

A 15% increase in kVp has the same effect on exposure to the IR as doubling the mAs. A 15% decrease in kVp has the same effect on exposure to the IR as halving the mAs.

Increasing the kVp by 15% increases the exposure to the IR unless the mAs is decreased. In addition, decreasing the kVp by 15% decreases the exposure to the IR unless the mAs is increased.

kVp and Subject Contrast

A high kVp results in less absorption and more transmission in anatomic tissues, which results in less variation in the x-ray intensities exiting (remnant) the patient producing lower subject contrast. A low kVp results in more absorption and less x-ray transmission in the anatomic tissues but with more variation in the x-ray intensities exiting the patient resulting in higher subject contrast.

Kilovoltage, Scatter Radiation, and Displayed Image Contrast

At higher kVp, more x-rays are transmitted with fewer overall interactions; however, a greater proportion of the interactions are from Compton scattering (fog) than photoelectric absorption, which decreases the displayed image contrast. Decreasing the kVp will increase photoelectric absorption and increase the number of interactions, but the proportion of Compton scattering (fog) will decrease compared with photoelectric absorption, increasing radiographic contrast.

Focal Spot Size and Spatial Resolution

As focal spot size increases, unsharpness increases and spatial resolution decreases; as focal spot size decreases, unsharpness decreases and spatial resolution increases.

Source-to-Image Receptor Distance and X-ray Beam Intensity

As SID increases, the x-ray beam intensity becomes spread over a larger area. This decreases the overall intensity of the x-ray beam reaching the IR.

Source-to-Image Receptor Distance and mAs

Increasing the SID requires the mAs to be increased to maintain exposure to the IR, and decreasing the SID requires a decrease in the mAs to maintain exposure to the IR.

Source-to-Image Receptor Distance, Size Distortion, and Spatial Resolution

As SID increases, size distortion (magnification) decreases, and spatial resolution increases; as SID decreases, size distortion (magnification) increases, and spatial resolution decreases.

Object-to-Image Receptor Distance, Size Distortion, and Spatial Resolution

Increasing the OID increases magnification and decreases the spatial resolution, whereas decreasing the OID decreases magnification and increases the spatial resolution.

Minimizing Shape Distortion

A right-angle (orthogonal) relationship between the IR, part, and CR is preferred to minimize shape distortion. Shape distortion of the anatomic area of interest can occur from inaccurate CR alignment of the x-ray tube, the part being radiographed, or the IR. Any misalignment of the CR among these three factors alters the shape of the part recorded on the image.

Grids, Scatter, and Contrast

Placing a grid between the anatomic part and the IR absorbs scatter radiation exiting the patient and increases displayed image contrast.

Grids and IR Exposure

Adding, removing, or changing a grid requires an adjustment in mAs to maintain radiation exposure to the IR.

Beam Restriction and Image Receptor Exposure

Changes in beam restriction alter the amount of tissue irradiated and therefore affect the amount of exposure to the IR. The effect of collimation is greater when imaging large anatomic areas, performing examinations without a grid, and using a high kVp.

Tube Filtration, Radiation Quantity, and Average Energy

Increasing tube filtration decreases radiation quantity and increases the average energy of the x-ray beam. Decreasing tube filtration increases radiation quantity and decreases the average energy of the x-ray beam.

CHAPTER 8: SCATTER CONTROL

kVp and Scatter

The amount and energy of scatter radiation exiting the patient depends, in part, on the kVp selected. Examinations using higher kVp produce a greater proportion of higher-energy scattered x-rays compared with examinations using low kVp.

X-ray-Beam Field Size, Thickness of the Part, and Scatter

The larger the x-ray-beam field size, the greater the amount of scatter radiation produced. The thicker the part being imaged, the greater the amount of scatter radiation produced.

Volume of Tissue Irradiated and Scatter

The volume of tissue irradiated is affected by both the part thickness and the x-ray-beam field size. Therefore, the greater the volume of tissue irradiated, because of either or both factors, the greater the amount of scatter radiation produced.

Beam Restriction and Patient Dose

As beam restriction or collimation increases, the field size and patient dose decrease. As beam restriction or collimation decreases, the field size and patient dose increase.

Collimation and Scatter Radiation

As collimation increases, the x-ray field size and quantity of scatter radiation decrease; as collimation decreases, the x-ray field size and quantity of scatter radiation increase.

Collimation and Radiographic Contrast

As collimation increases, the quantity of scatter radiation decreases and radiographic contrast increases; as collimation decreases, the quantity of scatter radiation increases and radiographic contrast decreases.

Collimation and Exposure to the Image Receptor

As collimation increases, exposure to the IR decreases; as collimation decreases, exposure to the IR increases.

Scatter Radiation and Image Quality

Scatter radiation adds unwanted exposure (fog) to the IR and decreases image quality.

Grid Ratio and Radiographic Contrast

As the grid ratio increases for the same grid frequency, scatter cleanup improves and radiographic contrast increases; as grid ratio decreases for the same grid frequency, scatter cleanup becomes less effective and radiographic contrast decreases.

Focused Versus Parallel Grids

Focused grids have lead lines that are angled to approximately match the divergence of the primary beam. Thus focused grids allow more transmitted photons to reach the IR than parallel grids.

Grid Ratio and Exposure to Image Receptor

As the grid ratio increases, exposure to the IR decreases; as the grid ratio decreases, exposure to the IR increases.

Grid Ratio and Patient Dose

As the grid ratio increases, patient dose increases because of the increase in mAs; as the grid ratio decreases, patient dose decreases because of the decrease in mAs.

Upside-Down Focused Grids and Grid Cutoff

Placing a focused grid upside down on the IR causes the edges of the IR to be significantly underexposed.

Off-Level Error and Grid Cutoff

Angling the x-ray tube across the grid lines or angling the grid itself during exposure produces an overall decrease in exposure across the entire IR.

Off-Center Error and Grid Cutoff

If the center of the x-ray beam is not aligned from side to side with the center of a focused grid, grid cutoff can occur as a loss of exposure across the entire IR.

Off-Focus Error and Grid Cutoff

Using an SID outside the focal range creates a loss of exposure at the periphery of the IR.

Air Gap Technique and Scatter Control

Although limited in its usefulness, the air gap technique is an alternative to using a grid to control the scatter reaching the IR. By moving the IR away from the patient, more scatter radiation will miss the IR. The greater the gap, the greater the reduction in scatter reaching the IR.

CHAPTER 9: EXPOSURE TECHNIQUE SELECTION

Principle of Automatic Exposure Control Operation

Once a predetermined amount of radiation is transmitted through a patient, the x-ray exposure is terminated. This determines the exposure time and therefore the total amount of radiation exposure to the IR.

Radiation-Measuring Devices

Detectors are the automatic exposure control (AEC) devices that measure the amount of radiation transmitted through the patient (exit or remnant). The radiographer selects the combination of the detectors to use.

Function of the Ionization Chamber

The ionization chamber interacts with exit radiation before it reaches the IR. Air in the chamber is ionized, an electrical charge proportional to the amount of radiation is created, and this charge travels to the timer circuit where the exposure is terminated.

Automatic Exposure Control and mAs Readout

If the radiographic unit has an mAs readout display, the radiographer should take note of the reading after an exposure is made. This information can be invaluable.

kVp and Automatic Exposure Control Response

The radiographer must set the kVp as needed to ensure adequate penetration and enhance the subject contrast for the part examined. The kVp selected determines the length of exposure time when using AEC. A low kVp requires more exposure time to reach the predetermined amount of exposure. A high kVp decreases the exposure time to reach the predetermined amount of exposure and reduces the overall radiation exposure to the patient.

mA and Automatic Exposure Control Response

If the radiographer can set the mA when using AEC, it will inversely affect the time of exposure for a given procedure. Increasing the mA decreases the exposure time to reach the predetermined amount of exposure. Decreasing the mA increases the exposure time to reach the predetermined amount of exposure.

Function of Backup Time

Backup time, the maximum exposure time allowed during an AEC examination, serves as a safety mechanism when AEC is not used properly or is not functioning properly.

Setting Backup Time

The backup time should be set to 150% to 200% of the expected exposure time. This allows the properly used AEC system to appropriately terminate the exposure but protects the patient and tube from excessive exposure if a problem occurs.

Detector Selection

The combination of detectors affects the amount of exposure reaching the IR. If the area of radiographic interest is not directly over the selected detectors, that area will likely be overexposed or underexposed.

Patient Centering

Accurate centering of the area of interest over the detectors is critical to ensure proper exposure to the IR. If the area of interest is not properly centered to the detectors, overexposure or underexposure may occur.

Collimation and Automatic Exposure Control Response

Excessive or insufficient collimation may affect the amount of exposure reaching the IR. Insufficient collimation may result in excessive scatter reaching the detectors, causing the exposure time to terminate too quickly. Excessive collimation may result in an extremely long exposure time.

Type of Image Receptor and Automatic Exposure Control Response

The AEC system is calibrated based on the type of IR used. If an IR of a different type is used, the detectors will not sense the difference, and the exposure time will terminate at the preset value, which may jeopardize image quality.

Exposure Technique Charts and Radiographic Quality

Exposure technique charts are important for digital imaging because digital systems have a wide dynamic range and can compensate for exposure technique errors. Technique charts should be developed and used with all types of radiographic imaging systems to optimize for radiological protection. Meaning the radiation dose should be appropriate to the imaging procedure and avoid unnecessary exposure to the patient while producing quality images for diagnostic interpretation.

Variable kVp/Fixed mAs Technique Chart

The variable kVp chart adjusts the kVp for changes in part thickness while maintaining a fixed mAs (2-kVp change for every 1-cm [~0.5-inch] change in part thickness).

Fixed kVp/Variable mAs Technique Chart

The fixed kVp/variable mAs technique chart identifies optimal kVp values and alters the mAs for variations in part thickness (every 4- to 5-cm [1.6- to 2-inch] change in part thickness, the mAs should be adjusted by a factor of 2).

Exposure Technique Charts

A commitment by management and staff to use exposure technique charts is critical to the consistent production of quality radiographic images. Well-developed technique charts are of little use if radiographers choose not to consult them.

CHAPTER 10: DYNAMIC IMAGING: FLUOROSCOPY

Image-Intensified Fluoroscopy

Dynamic imaging of internal anatomic structures can be accomplished with the use of an image intensifier. The exit radiation is absorbed by the input phosphor, converted to electrons, sent to the output phosphor, released as visible light, and converted to an electronic signal that is digitized and processed by a computer and sent to the display monitor.

Brightness Gain

A brighter image is created on the output phosphor when accelerated electrons strike a smaller output phosphor.

Magnification Mode and Patient Dose

Operating the image intensifier in one of the magnification modes increases the operator's ability to see small structures but at the price of increasing the radiation dose to the patient.

Charge-Coupled Device

The CCD is a device that converts the light image from the intensifier's output phosphor to an electronic signal that is digitized and can be reconstructed on the display monitor.

Digital Fluoroscopic Systems

The use of flat-panel detectors in place of an image intensifier offers several advantages, such as a reduction in the size, bulk, and weight of the fluoroscopic tower; allowing for easier manipulation of the tower; and greater access to the patient during the examination. The flat-panel detectors also replace other recording devices, and, because they operate in radiographic mode, in many cases, additional radiographic images are not needed. The images, both dynamic and static, can also be readily archived with the patient record.

Flat-Panel Detectors in Fluoroscopy

Flat-panel detectors used in fluoroscopy require rapid readout speeds for dynamic imaging. Current dynamic versions are capable of up to 60 frames per second. Application-specific integrated circuits (ASICs) minimize noise, maximize readout speed, and allow for switching from low-dose to high-dose inputs (for static imaging).

Scatter Radiation

During fluoroscopy, the patient is the primary source of radiation exposure to fluoroscopic personnel. With the x-ray tube above the patient, the most intense scatter radiation to the operator is directed above the waist to include the upper trunk, neck, and head. With the x-ray tube beneath the patient, the scatter area to the operator is below the chest and toward the floor.

Fluoroscopic Features

Use of virtual collimation during last image hold (LIH), preset anatomic programs, and added filtration reduces the patient dose. Conversely, use of a grid increases the patient dose.

Pulsed Fluoroscopy

Operating the fluoroscope in a pulsed mode reduces the number of images each second, decreases the patient dose, and should match the dynamic motion of patient anatomy.

Pulsed Fluoroscopy and Dose Rates

Using pulsed fluoroscopy along with lower dose rates appropriate to the procedure reduces the patient radiation dose.

Frame Averaging

Frame averaging is an operation that averages multiple video image frames together in rapid succession for display and reduces overall patient dose and image noise.

Pixel Binning

During fluoroscopy, the DELs can work individually or as combined detector elements (DELs) through pixel binning. Pixel binning reduces the total number of DEL units that are working during fast fluoroscopic framing sequence, increases the collective SNR, reduces visible noise, and is a practical approach to the huge file sizes created with digital fluoroscopy.

Summary of Mathematical Applications

CHAPTER 3: THE X-RAY BEAM

Characteristic X-ray Photons

To find the energy of a characteristic x-ray photon, one must know the shell-binding energies of the element and the shells involved. The projectile electron must possess kinetic energy equal to or greater than the shell-binding energy to remove it from orbit. The photon energy is then equal to the difference in the binding energy of the shells involved.

Example:

A projectile electron removes a K-shell electron, and an L-shell electron fills the vacancy:
K-shell binding energy = 69.5 keV
L-shell binding energy = 12.1 keV
69.5 − 12.1 = 57.4 keV

The energy of the K-shell characteristic x-ray photon produced is 57.4 keV.

Calculating mAs

mAs = mA × seconds (1 second = 1000 ms)
Examples:
200 mA × 0.25 s (250 ms) = 50 mAs
500 mA × 2/5 s = 200 mAs
800 mA × 100 ms (0.1s) = 80 mAs

Calculating Heat Units

An exposure is made with a three-phase x-ray unit at 600 mA and 75 kVp over 0.05 s. How many heat units are produced from this exposure?
HU = mA × time × kVp × generator factor
HU = 600 × 0.05 × 75 × 1.35
3037.5 HU

CHAPTER 5: DIGITAL IMAGE CHARACTERISTICS, RECEPTORS, AND IMAGE ACQUISITION

Pixel Size and Displayed FOV

FOV = 17 inches (431.8 mm) and matrix size = 1024:

$$\frac{431.8}{1024} = 0.42 \text{ mm pixel size}$$

If the FOV was decreased to 12 inches (304.8 mm) for the same matrix size of 1024:

$$\frac{304.8}{1024} = 0.30 \text{ mm pixel size}$$

Decreasing the FOV displayed for a given matrix size will decrease the size of the pixels and increase spatial resolution.

Pixel Size and Matrix Size

Displayed FOV = 17 inches (431.8 mm) and matrix size = 1024:

$$\frac{431.8}{1024} = 0.42 \text{ mm pixel size}$$

If the matrix size was increased to 2048 for the same FOV displayed:

$$\frac{431.8}{2048} = 0.21 \text{ mm pixel size}$$

Increasing the matrix size for a given FOV displayed will decrease the size of the pixels and increase spatial resolution.

CHAPTER 7: EXPOSURE TECHNIQUE FACTORS

Adjusting mA or Exposure Time

$200 \, \text{mA} \times 0.100 \, \text{s} = 20 \, \text{mAs}$

To increase the mAs to 40, one could use the following formulas:

$400 \, \text{mA} \times 0.100 \, \text{s} \, (100 \, \text{ms}) = 40 \, \text{mAs}$

$200 \, \text{mA} \times 0.200 \, \text{s} \, (200 \, \text{ms}) = 40 \, \text{mAs}$

Adjusting mA and Exposure Time to Maintain mAs

$200 \, \text{mA} \times 100 \, \text{ms} \, (0.100 \, \text{s}) = 20 \, \text{mAs}$

To maintain mAs, use the following formulas:

$400 \, \text{mA} \times 50 \, \text{ms} \, (0.050 \, \text{s}) = 20 \, \text{mAs}$

$100 \, \text{mA} \times 200 \, \text{ms} \, (0.200 \, \text{s}) = 20 \, \text{mAs}$

Using the 15% Rule

To increase exposure to the IR, multiply the kVp by 1.15 (original kVp + 15%):

$75 \, \text{kVp} \times 1.15 = 86 \, \text{kVp}$

To decrease exposure to the IR, multiply the kVp by 0.85 (original kVp − 15%):

$75 \, \text{kVp} \times 0.85 = 64 \, \text{kVp}$

To maintain exposure to the IR, when increasing the kVp by 15% (kVp × 1.15), divide the original mAs by 2:

$75 \, \text{kVp} \times 1.15 = 86 \, \text{kVp}$ and mAs/2

When decreasing the kVp by 15% (kVp × 0.85), multiply the mAs by 2:

$75 \, \text{kVp} \times 0.85 = 64$ and mAs × 2

Inverse-Square Law Formula

$$\frac{I_1}{I_2} = \frac{(D_2)^2}{(D_1)^2}$$

If the intensity of radiation at an SID of 100 cm (40 inches) is equal to 4 mGy (400 mR), what is the intensity of radiation when the distance is increased to 180 cm (72 inches)?

$$\frac{4 \, \text{mGy}}{X} = \frac{(180 \, \text{cm})^2}{(100 \, \text{cm})^2}; \; 4 \, \text{mGy} \times 10,000 = 40,000$$

$$= 32,400 \, X; \; \frac{40,000}{32,400} = X; \; 1.24 \, \text{mGy} = X$$

Direct Square Law or Exposure Maintenance Formula

$$\frac{\text{mAs}_1}{\text{mAs}_2} = \frac{(SID_1)^2}{(SID_2)^2}$$

Optimal exposure to the IR is achieved at an SID of 40 inches (100 cm) using 25 mAs. The SID must be increased to 72 inches (180 cm). What adjustment of mAs is needed to maintain exposure to the IR?

$$\frac{25}{X} = \frac{(40)^2}{(72)^2}; \; 1600X = 129,600;$$

$$\frac{129,600}{1600}; \; X = 81 \, \text{mAs}$$

Optimal exposure to the IR is achieved at an SID of 120 cm (48 inches) using 15 mAs. The SID must be decreased to 90 cm (36 inches). What adjustment of mAs is needed to maintain exposure to the IR?

$$\frac{15}{X} = \frac{(120 \, \text{cm})^2}{(90 \, \text{cm})^2}; \; 14,400X = 121,500; \; =$$

$$\frac{121,500}{14,400} = X = 8.4 \, \text{mAs}$$

Magnification Factor

An anteroposterior projection (AP) of the knee is produced with an SID of 100 cm (40 inches) and an OID of 7.5 cm (3 inches). SOD is equal to 92.5 cm (37 inches). What is the MF?

$$SOD = SID - OID, \; MF = \frac{100}{92.5}; \; MF = 1.081$$

$$92.5 = 100 - 7.5$$

Adjusting mAs for Changes in the Grid

A quality radiographic image is obtained using 5 mAs at 70 kVp without using a grid. What new mAs is needed when adding a 12:1 grid to maintain the same exposure to the IR?

$$\frac{5 \, \text{mAs}}{X} = \frac{1}{5}; \; 1X = 25; \; X = 25 \, \text{mAs}$$

The new mAs produces an exposure comparable to the IR without the grid.

Exposure Conversions

A. Calculate the new exposure factor required to maintain a similar exposure to the IR as in the initial exposure technique.

Initial Exposure Technique		New Exposure Technique
25 mAs		_____ mAs
80 kVp	TO	68 kVp

Calculations:

a. Decrease from 80 to 68 kVp = 15% decrease (80×0.85)

b. Increase mAs $\times$ 2, 25 $\times$ 2 = 50 mAs

c. The new mAs needed to maintain a similar exposure to the IR as the initial technique is 50

B. Calculate the new exposure factor required to maintain a similar exposure to the IR as in the initial exposure technique.

Initial Exposure Technique		New Exposure Technique
25 mAs		_____ mAs
80 kVp	TO	68 kVp
12:1 grid		no grid

Calculations:

a. Decrease from 80 to 68 kVp = 15% decrease (80×0.85)

b. Increase mAs $\times$ 2, 25 $\times$ 2 = 50 mAs

c. Remove 12:1 grid (GCF 5) = decrease mAs, $50 \div 5 = 10$ mAs

d. The new mAs needed to maintain a similar exposure to the IR as the initial technique is 10

C. Calculate the new exposure factor required to maintain a similar exposure to the IR as in the initial exposure technique.

Initial Exposure Technique		New Exposure Technique
25 mAs		_____ mAs
80 kVp	TO	68 kVp
12:1 grid		no grid
40-inch (100 cm) SID		54-inch (135 cm) SID

Calculations:

a. Decrease from 80 to 68 kVp = 15% decrease (80×0.85)

b. Increase mAs $\times$ 2, 25 $\times$ 2 = 50 mAs

c. Remove 12:1 grid (GCF 5) = decrease mAs, $50 \div 5 = 10$ mAs

d. Increase SID from 40 to 54 inches $= \dfrac{10\ \text{mAs}}{X} = \dfrac{40^2}{54^2}$; $10 \times 2916 = 1600\,X$; $= 29{,}160 \div 1600 = 18.2 = X$

e. The new mAs needed to maintain a similar exposure to the IR as the initial technique is 18.2

CHAPTER 8: SCATTER CONTROL

Calculating Grid Ratio

What is the grid ratio when the lead strips are 2.4 mm high and separated by 0.2 mm?

$$\text{Grid ratio} = h/D$$

$$\text{Grid ratio} = \frac{2.4}{0.2} = 12 \text{ or } 12{:}1$$

Adding a Grid

If a radiographer produced a shoulder image with non-grid exposure using 3 mAs and then wanted to use a 12:1 ratio grid, what mAs should be used to produce the same exposure to the IR?

Nongrid exposure = 3 mAs

GCF (for 12:1 grid) = 5 (from Table 8.2)

$$\text{GCF} = \frac{\text{mAs with the grid}}{\text{mAs without the grid}}$$

$$5 = \frac{\text{mAs with the grid}}{3}$$

$$\frac{5}{1} = \frac{X}{3}; \; X = 15$$

$$15 = \text{mAs with the grid}$$

When adding a 12:1 ratio grid, mAs must be increased by a factor of 5 (in this case to 15 mAs).

Removing a Grid

If a radiographer produced a knee image using an 8:1 ratio grid and 10 mAs and on the next exposure wanted to use nongrid exposure, what mAs should be used to produce the same exposure to the IR?

Grid exposure = 10 mAs

GCF (for 8:1 grid) = 4 (from Table 8.2)

$$GCF = \frac{\text{mAs with the grid}}{\text{mAs without the grid}}$$

$$4 = \frac{10 \text{ mAs}}{\text{mAs without the grid}}$$

$$\frac{4}{1} = \frac{10}{X}; \; 4X = 10$$

2.5 = mAs without the grid

When removing an 8:1 ratio grid, mAs must be decreased by a factor of 4 (in this case to 2.5 mAs).

Decreasing the Grid Ratio

If a radiographer used 40 mAs with a 12:1 ratio grid, what mAs should be used with a 6:1 ratio grid to produce the same exposure to the IR?
Exposure 1: 40 mAs, 12:1 grid, GCF = 5
Exposure 2: _____ mAs, 6:1 grid, GCF = 3

$$\frac{mAs_1}{mAs_2} = \frac{GCF_1}{GCF_2}$$

$$\frac{40}{mAs_2} = \frac{5}{3}$$

$$5X = 120; \; X = 120/5; \; X = 24$$

$$mAs_2 = 24$$

Decreasing the grid ratio requires less mAs.

Increasing the Grid Ratio

If a radiographer performed a routine portable pelvic examination using 40 mAs with an 8:1 ratio grid, what mAs should be used if a 12:1 ratio grid is substituted?
Exposure 1: 40 mAs, 8:1 grid, GCF = 4
Exposure 2: _____ mAs, 12:1 grid, GCF = 5

$$\frac{mAs_1}{mAs_2} = \frac{GCF_1}{GCF_2}$$

$$\frac{40}{mAs_2} = \frac{4}{5}$$

$$4X = 200; \; X = 200/4; \; X = 50$$

$$mAs_2 = 50$$

Increasing the grid ratio requires additional mAs.

Summary of Radiation Protection Alerts

CHAPTER 1: RADIATION AND ITS DISCOVERY

ALARA Principle and Optimization for Radiological Protection

It is the radiographer's responsibility to minimize the radiation dose to the patient, to themselves, and to others in accordance with the as low as reasonably achievable (ALARA) principle. Optimization for radiological protection means the radiation dose should be appropriate to the imaging procedure and avoid unnecessary exposure to the patient while producing quality images for diagnostic interpretation.

Cardinal Principles for Minimizing Radiation Dose

Time: Limit the amount of time exposed to ionizing radiation.

Distance: Maintain a safe distance from the source of ionizing radiation exposure.

Shielding: Maximize the use of shielding from ionizing radiation exposure.

Beam Restriction

Limiting the size of the x-ray exposure field reduces the volume of tissue irradiated and reduces the radiation dose to the patient.

Primary Exposure Factors

The combination of kilovoltage (kVp) and milliampere-seconds (mAs) is selected based on a number of considerations, including the anatomic part being examined, patient age, condition, and pathology, and should be ideally suited to the circumstance to minimize radiation dose while producing optimum exposure to the image receptor (IR).

Avoid Unnecessary Duplicate Examinations

Radiographers must recognize and accept their role as a patient advocate and do what is necessary to avoid unnecessary duplication of examinations.

Screening for Pregnancy

Screening for pregnancy is another important task for minimizing unnecessary exposure to a developing fetus. When it is necessary to perform a radiographic examination on a pregnant patient, shielding materials may be used, in special circumstances, along with precise collimation to minimize the radiation dose administered to the fetus.

CHAPTER 3: THE X-RAY BEAM

Beam Filtration

Low-energy photons, created during x-ray production, are unable to penetrate the patient. Patients are protected from unnecessary exposure to this low-energy radiation by the placement of inherent and added filtration in the path of the x-ray beam.

CHAPTER 5: DIGITAL IMAGE CHARACTERISTICS, RECEPTORS, AND IMAGE ACQUISITION

Digital Receptors and Dynamic Range

Because digital IRs have a wide dynamic range, a quality image can be produced when using more radiation exposure than necessary. Radiographers must take extra precautions to not unnecessarily overexpose patients and select exposure techniques within the exposure latitude established by the department.

CHAPTER 6: DIGITAL IMAGE PROCESSING, DISPLAY, AND HEALTH INFORMATION MANAGEMENT

Image Repeat for Overexposure

It is important to note that repeating an image due to overexposure further increases the radiation dose to the patient and therefore should be clinically warranted.

Exposure Indicators

The radiographer should strive to select techniques that result in exposure indicator values falling within the indicated optimum range for the corresponding digital imaging system. However, the radiographer also needs to recognize the limitations of exposure indicators for providing accurate information. The radiographer should assess the exposure indicator along with image quality before considering a repeat image.

CHAPTER 7: EXPOSURE TECHNIQUE FACTORS

Excessive Radiation Exposure and Digital Imaging

Although the computer can adjust image brightness for technique exposure errors, routinely using more radiation than required for the procedure in digital radiography unnecessarily increases patient exposure. Even though the digital system can adjust overexposure, it is an unethical practice to knowingly overexpose a patient.

kVp/mAs

Whenever possible, a higher kilovoltage and lower mAs should be used to reduce patient exposure. Increasing kilovoltage requires a lower mAs to maintain the desired exposure to the IR and decreases the radiation dose to the patient. For example, changing kVp from 75 to 86 when imaging a pelvis is a 15% increase and would require half the mAs needed for the original 75 kVp. Higher kVp increases the beam penetration; therefore less radiation is needed to achieve a desired exposure to the IR.

Grid Selection

Decisions regarding the use of a grid and grid ratio should be made by balancing image quality and patient protection. To keep patient exposure as low as reasonable, grids should be used only when appropriate, and the grid ratio should be the lowest that would provide sufficient contrast improvement.

Beam Restriction

In performing a radiographic examination, the radiographer should be aware of the anatomic area of interest and limit the x-ray field size to just beyond this area. Collimating to the appropriate field size is a basic method for protecting patients from unnecessary exposure.

CHAPTER 8: SCATTER CONTROL

Appropriate Beam Restriction

In performing a radiographic examination, the radiographer should be aware of the anatomic area of interest and limit the x-ray field size to just beyond this area. Collimating to the appropriate field size is a basic method for protecting patients from unnecessary exposure.

Postexposure Electronic Masking or Cropping

Postexposure electronic masking or cropping the displayed image should never replace preexposure collimation because it does not reduce scatter production, reduce patient radiation exposure, or increase image contrast. All anatomy that has been irradiated should be included for interpretation by the radiologist.

Limit Field Size to the Anatomic Area of Interest

The radiographer should always be sure that the size of the x-ray field is restricted to the anatomic area of interest. Digital IRs are typically of a similar size, and, in many instances, larger than the anatomic area of interest. Therefore it is crucial for the radiographer to appropriately collimate for the imaging procedure so that the patient is not unnecessarily exposed to radiation.

Grid Selection

Decisions regarding the use of a grid and grid ratio should be made by balancing image quality and patient protection. To minimize patient exposure, grids should be used only when appropriate, and the grid ratio selected should be the lowest capable of providing sufficient contrast improvement. In examinations in which the anatomic part does not produce excessive scatter, a grid may not be necessary because the computer can vary contrast in the displayed image.

CHAPTER 9: EXPOSURE TECHNIQUE SELECTION

Kilovoltage Selection

Using a higher kVp with automatic exposure control (AEC) decreases the exposure time and the overall mAs needed to produce a diagnostic image, significantly reducing patient exposure. The kVp selected for an examination should display the desired subject contrast for the part examined while being as high as possible to minimize the patient's radiation exposure.

Monitoring Backup Time

To minimize patient exposure, the backup time should be neither too long nor too short. Backup time that is too short results in the exposure being stopped prematurely, and the image may need to be repeated because of poor quality. Backup time that is too long results in the patient receiving unnecessary radiation if a problem occurs and the exposure does not end until the backup time is reached. In addition, the image may have to be repeated because of poor quality.

Errors in Automatic Exposure Control Use

It is important for radiographers to evaluate image quality, the applied mAs, and the exposure indicator when using the AEC device. Errors in selecting the appropriate combination of AEC detectors, detector size, or positioning errors may not be visually apparent because of computer adjustment.

Patient Variability

Factors related to the patient affect the time of exposure reaching the IR and ultimately the image quality; such factors include pathology, contrast media, foreign objects, and pockets of gas. Increases or decreases in patient thickness result in changes in the time of exposure if the AEC system is functioning properly. It is up to the radiographer to determine whether a manual exposure technique is a better choice than the AEC device.

Anatomically Programmed Technique and Patient Exposure

When using a preprogrammed set of exposure factors, the radiographer must evaluate the appropriateness of the selected exposure technique factors. Adjustment of the preprogrammed exposure factors may be necessary for that patient or procedure.

CHAPTER REVIEW QUESTIONS ANSWER KEY

CHAPTER 1: RADIATION AND ITS DISCOVERY

1. B
2. C
3. D
4. A
5. D
6. C
7. B
8. D
9. A
10. C
11. C
12. B
13. A
14. D

CHAPTER 2: FUNDAMENTALS OF RADIATION PRODUCTION

1. B
2. D
3. A
4. D
5. D
6. C
7. C
8. C
9. D
10. B
11. A
12. A
13. D
14. A

CHAPTER 3: THE X-RAY BEAM

1. B
2. D
3. B
4. A
5. C
6. A
7. D
8. A
9. C
10. D
11. C
12. B
13. D
14. D
15. A
16. C
17. A

CHAPTER 4: IMAGE FORMATION AND RADIOGRAPHIC QUALITY

1. D
2. D
3. C
4. B
5. D
6. A
7. D
8. C
9. C
10. B
11. D
12. B
13. D
14. A
15. B
16. D
17. B
18. D

CHAPTER 5: DIGITAL IMAGE CHARACTERISTICS, RECEPTORS, AND IMAGE ACQUISITION

1. D
2. C
3. A
4. D
5. D
6. C
7. D
8. C
9. A
10. C
11. B
12. A
13. C
14. A
15. B
16. D
17. D
18. D
19. A
20. D
21. D

CHAPTER 6: DIGITAL IMAGE PROCESSING, DISPLAY, AND HEALTH INFORMATION MANAGEMENT

1. C
2. A
3. C
4. E
5. D
6. A
7. D
8. A
9. D
10. D
11. B
12. A
13. A
14. D
15. B
16. A
17. C

18. A
19. D
20. A

CHAPTER 7: EXPOSURE TECHNIQUE FACTORS

1. D
2. C
3. A
4. B
5. D
6. C
7. C
8. D
9. A
10. D
11. B
12. B
13. Calculate the new exposure factor required to maintain a similar exposure to the IR as in the initial exposure technique.

Initial Exposure Technique		New Exposure Technique
10 mAs		_____ mAs
70 kVp	TO	81 kVp

Calculations:
a. Increase from 70 to 81 kVp = 15% increase (70 × 1.15)
b. Decrease mAs × a factor of 2, 10 ÷ 2 = 5 mAs
c. **The new mAs needed to maintain a similar exposure to the IR as the initial technique is 5**

14. Calculate the new exposure factor required to maintain a similar exposure to the IR as in the initial exposure technique.

Initial Exposure Technique		New Exposure Technique
10 mAs		_____ mAs
70 kVp	TO	81 kVp
8:1 grid		12:1 grid

Calculations:
a. Increase from 70 to 81 kVp = 15% increase (70 × 1.15)
b. Decrease mAs by factor of 2, 10 ÷ 2 = 5 mAs
c. Change 8:1 grid (GCF 4) to 12:1 (GCF 5) =

d. Increase mAs,

$$\frac{5}{X} = \frac{4}{5}; \ 25 = 4X; \ \frac{25}{4} = 6.25$$

e. **The new mAs needed to maintain a similar exposure to the IR as the initial technique is 6.25**

15. Calculate the new exposure factor required to maintain a similar exposure to the IR as in the initial exposure technique.

Initial Exposure Technique		New Exposure Technique
10 mAs		_____ mAs
70 kVp	TO	81 kVp
8:1 grid		12:1 grid
180-cm SID		150-cm SID

Calculations:

a. Increase from 70 to 81 kVp = 15% increase (70 × 1.15)
b. Decrease mAs by a factor of 2, 10 ÷ 2 = 5 mAs
c. Change 8:1 grid (GCF 4) to 12:1 (GCF 5) =
d. Increase mAs,

$$\frac{5}{X} = \frac{4}{5}; \ 25 = 4X; \ \frac{25}{4} = 6.25$$

e. Decrease SID from 180 to 150 cm =

$$\frac{6.25 \text{ mAs}}{X} = \frac{180^2}{150^2};$$

6.25 × 22500 = 32400 X; =
140625 ÷ 32400 = 4.3 = X

f. **The new mAs needed to maintain a similar exposure to the IR as the initial technique is 4.3**

CHAPTER 8: SCATTER CONTROL

1. C
2. B
3. D
4. B
5. B
6. A
7. D
8. E
9. B

10. A
11. D
12. A
13. C
14. D
15. A
16. B
17. C
18. D
19. D
20. B
21. D

CHAPTER 9: EXPOSURE TECHNIQUE SELECTION

1. B
2. C
3. D
4. D
5. D
6. B
7. A
8. C
9. B
10. D
11. D
12. B
13. C
14. A
15. C
16. D

CHAPTER 10: DYNAMIC IMAGING: FLUOROSCOPY

1. A
2. D
3. C
4. B
5. C
6. C
7. B
8. B
9. B

10. D
11. D
12. C
13. D
14. B

15. D
16. A
17. B
18. C
19. C
20. B

GLOSSARY

A

15% rule Rule stating that changing the kVp by 15% has the same effect on image receptor exposure as doubling or halving the mAs.

absorbed dose The transfer of radiation energy into matter (e.g., tissue).

absorption As the energy of the primary x-ray beam is deposited within the atoms composing the tissue, some x-ray photons are completely absorbed. Complete absorption of the incoming x-ray photon occurs when it has enough energy to remove (eject) an inner-shell electron.

accelerating anode Attracts and sets the electron stream in motion at a constant velocity inside the image intensifier tube.

active layer The radiation-sensitive and light-sensitive layer of the film.

actual focal spot size The size of the area on the anode target that is exposed to electrons from the tube current. Actual focal spot size depends on the size of the filament producing the electron stream.

added filtration The filtration that is added to the port of the x-ray tube.

air gap technique Based on the simple concept that much of the scatter will miss the image receptor if there is an increased distance between the patient and the image receptor (increased OID).

air kerma (**k**inetic **e**nergy **r**eleased in **m**atter) Specifies the intensity of x-rays at a given point in air at a known distance from the focal spot or source of x-rays.

ALARA As low as reasonably achievable.

alternative algorithms A mechanism for the radiographer to reprocess the image data by selecting an alternative anatomical region or projection to improve its presentation at the display monitor.

ambient lighting The level of light in the room while viewing images.

anatomically programmed techniques A radiographic system that allows the radiographer to select a particular button on the control panel that represents an anatomic area; a preprogrammed set of exposure factors is displayed and selected for use.

anode A positively charged electrode within the x-ray tube composed of molybdenum, copper, tungsten, and graphite. It consists of a target and, in rotating anode tubes, a stator and rotor.

anode heel effect The x-ray beam has greater intensity (number of x-rays) on the cathode side of the tube, with the intensity diminishing toward the anode side. The heel effect occurs because of the angle of the target.

aperture diaphragm A flat piece of lead (diaphragm) containing a hole (aperture) for beam restriction.

artifact Any unwanted image on a radiograph.

artificial intelligence (AI) Uses pattern-recognition computer programs for image analysis.

attenuation Reduction in the energy or number of the primary x-ray beam as it passes through anatomic tissue.

automatic brightness control (ABC) A function of the fluoroscopic unit that maintains the overall appearance of the fluoroscopic image (contrast and density) by automatically adjusting the kVp, mA, or both.

automatic collimator/positive beam-limiting device Automatically limits the size and shape of the primary beam to the size and shape of the image receptor.

automatic exposure control (AEC) A system used to consistently control the amount of radiation reaching the image receptor by terminating the length of exposure.

automatic exposure rate control (AERC) Automatically adjusts the tube current (mA), voltage (kVp), filtration, and pulse width to maintain radiation exposure to the flat-panel detector.

automatic rescaling Occurs during histogram analysis and is used to maintain consistent image brightness despite overexposure or underexposure of the digital image receptor.

autotransformer Determines the induced voltage going to the primary side of the high-tension transformer.

B

backup time The maximum length of time for which the x-ray exposure continues when using an AEC system.

beam restriction/collimation Interchangeably used terms that refer to a decrease in the size of the projected radiation field.

beam-restricting device Changes the shape and size of the primary beam, located just below the x-ray tube housing.

bit 0 or 1 that refers to the computer's basic unit of information.

bit depth Number of bits.

body habitus The general form or build of the body, including size. The four types of body habitus are sthenic, hyposthenic, hypersthenic, and asthenic.

body mass index (BMI) A person's weight in kilograms divided by the square of height in meters. A high BMI (>30) can be an indicator of obesity.

bremsstrahlung interactions Occur when a projectile electron completely avoids the orbital electrons of the tungsten atom and travels very close to its nucleus. The very strong electrostatic force of the nucleus causes the electron suddenly to "slow down." As the electron loses energy, it suddenly changes its direction, and the energy loss reappears as an x-ray photon.

brightness The amount of luminance (light emission) of a display monitor.

brightness gain The product of both flux gain and minification gain; this results in a brighter image on the output phosphor.

Bucky Located directly below the radiographic tabletop, the grid is found just above the tray that holds the image receptor. More accurately called the Potter-Bucky diaphragm.

Bucky factor/grid conversion factor Used to determine the adjustment in mAs needed when changing from using a grid to nongrid (or vice versa) or when changing to grids with different grid ratios.

byte 8 bits combined.

C

caliper   A device that measures part thickness.

camera tube   A device used to convert the light emitted from the output phosphor to an electrical signal sent to the television monitor.

capacitors   Charge storage components and when placed in the circuit with the inverter, the stored charges are released in a sequential fashion that result in a current waveform with a very small voltage fluctuation, known as ripple.

cathode   A negatively charged electrode (within the x-ray tube). It comprises a filament and a focusing cup.

characteristic interactions   Produced when a projectile electron interacts with an electron from the inner (K) shell of the tungsten atom and ejects it. An outer-shell electron drops into vacancy and the energy difference is emitted as an x-ray photon.

charge-coupled device (CCD)   A light-sensitive semiconducting device that generates an electrical charge when stimulated by light and stores this charge in a capacitor.

circuit   A fixed path that electricity flows through and its purpose is to precisely control the flow and intensity of electrons as they travel through the circuit pathways and components.

coherent scattering   An interaction that occurs with low-energy x-rays, typically below the diagnostic range. The incoming photon interacts with the atom, causing it to become excited. The x-ray does not lose energy but changes direction.

collimator   Two sets of adjustable lead shutters located 3 to 7 inches below the tube that consist of longitudinal and lateral leaves or blades, each with its own control; this makes the collimator adjustable in terms of its ability to produce projected fields of varying sizes.

comparative anatomy   Concept stating that different parts of the same size can be radiographed using the same exposure factors, provided the minimum kVp value needed to penetrate the part is used in each case.

compensating filter   Special filters added to the primary beam to alter its intensity. These types of filters are used to image anatomic areas that are nonuniform in makeup and assist in producing more consistent exposure to the image receptor.

complementary metal oxide semiconductor (CMOS)   A scintillator device made up of a crystalline silicon matrix. Each detector element has its own amplifier, photodiode, and storage capacitor and is surrounded by transistors. Can be used to convert the light image from the intensifier's output phosphor to an electronic signal that can be reconstructed on the display monitor. Recent advances in CMOS technology, particularly the creation of crystal light tubes that prevent light spread and methods for increasing their size, make them applicable for radiographic imaging.

Compton effect   The loss of energy of the incoming photon when it ejects an outer-shell electron from the atom. The remaining lower-energy x-ray photon changes direction and may leave the anatomic part.

Compton electron/secondary electron   The ejected electron resulting from the Compton effect interaction.

computed radiography (CR) fading   When the imaging plate is not processed in a timely manner, the latent image dissipates over time because some of the signal (released energy) captured in the imaging plate is lost.

cone   An aperture diaphragm that has an extended flange attached to it. The flange can vary in length and is shaped as a cone. The flange can also be made to telescope, increasing its total length.

continuous fluoroscopy   The x-ray exposure continues without interruption while the exposure pedal or button is activated.

contrast enhancement   A postprocessing technique that alters the pixel values to increase image contrast.

contrast medium   A substance instilled into the body by injection or ingestion that is used when imaging anatomic tissues that have low subject contrast. Also called *contrast agent*.

contrast resolution   The ability of the image receptor to distinguish between objects having similar subject contrast.

contrast-to-noise ratio   A method of describing the contrast resolution with the amount of noise apparent in a digital image.

convergent line   If points were connected along the length of the grid, they would form an imaginary line.

convergent point   If imaginary lines were drawn from each of the lead lines in a linear focused grid, these lines would meet to form an imaginary point.

conversion factor   An expression of the luminance at the output phosphor divided by the input exposure rate; its unit of measurement is candela per square meter per milliroentgen per second.

crossed/crosshatched grid   A grid containing lead lines that are perpendicular to one another. Crossed grids remove more scattered photons than linear grids because they contain more lead strips, oriented in two directions.

cylinder   An aperture diaphragm that has an extended flange attached to it. The flange can vary in length and is shaped as a cylinder.

D

data management   A complex system-wide effort to ensure that people, equipment, and processes are in place to expand healthcare communication and improve patient outcomes.

density controls   A mechanism that allows the radiographer to adjust the amount of preset radiation detection values.

detective quantum efficiency (DQE)   A measurement of the efficiency of an image receptor in converting the x-ray exposure it receives to a quality radiographic image.

detector element (DEL)   A charge-collection device with a fixed dimension, expressed in microns and is the functional unit of the detector as far as signal collection.

detectors   The sensors, cells, or chambers within an AEC device that sense how much radiation has reached the imaging plate to terminate the exposure.

deviation index (DI)   A value that reflects the difference between the desired or target exposure to the image receptor and the actual exposure to the image receptor.

dielectric   nonconducting material and considered an insulator since it does not conduct electricity.

differential absorption   A process whereby some of the x-ray beam is absorbed in the tissue and some passes through (transmits) the anatomic part.

digital image processing   Various computer algorithms (mathematical computations) applied to digital data for the purpose of optimizing the image for display.

digital imaging   Constructing an image from numeric data.

Digital Imaging and Communications in Medicine (DICOM)   A communication standard for information sharing between picture archival and communication system (PACS) and imaging modalities.

diodes   Use solid-state, semiconductor materials that permit current flow in only one direction.

direct square law   A formula that provides a mathematical calculation for adjusting mAs when changing the source-to-image receptor distance (SID).

disaster recovery   A requirement to duplicate all files in a remote location so that recovery is possible in the event of a disaster and the primary files are lost.

display workstation   A desktop computer that allows for the retrieval and viewing of medical images from one of the modalities or storage components of the PACS.

distortion   Results from the radiographic misrepresentation of either the size (magnification) or the shape of the anatomic part.

dose area product (DAP)   A measure of exposure in air, followed by a computation to estimate absorbed dose to the patient. It is the same as kerma area product (KAP).

dosimeter   A device that measures x-ray exposure.

downtime procedure   Serves to create an organized strategy for upholding vital patient information and healthcare functions during electronic medical record (EMR) system disruptions.

dual energy subtraction   A technique that can remove superimposed structures so that the anatomic area of interest becomes more visible. Because the image is in a digital format, the computer can subtract selected brightness values to create an image without superimposed structures.

edge enhancement   A postprocessing technique that improves the visibility of small, high-contrast structures.

effective dose   An expression of the *relative risk to humans* (whole-body exposure) of exposure to ionizing radiation and measured in sieverts (Sv).

effective focal spot size   Focal spot size as measured directly under the anode target.

electromagnetic radiation   Radiation that has both electrical and magnetic properties. All radiations that are electromagnetic make up a spectrum.

electron transition   When an outer-shell electron drops into the open position and creates an energy difference.

electronic data set   Electronic signal values created by the ionization energies when the exit radiation interacts with an image receptor.

electronic health record (EHR)   The system for patient health information (PHI) that can be shared outside the facility and among many healthcare systems.

electronic magnification   The selection of a smaller field of view (FOV). When a smaller FOV is selected, an area smaller than the size of the detector is exposed by the x-ray beam, but the area is enlarged to fill the display monitor area magnifying the anatomic structures.

electronic medical record (EMR)   A digital record with the ability to store, share, and manage PHI within a single healthcare organization.

electronic masking   Also known as *shuttering*. A postprocessing function that can remove regions of the digital image.

electrostatic focusing lenses   Focuses and accelerates the electrons through the image intensifier toward the anode.

elongation   Images of objects that appear longer than the true objects.

equalization   A postprocessing function whereby underexposed areas (light areas) are made darker and overexposed areas (dark areas) are made lighter. The effect is an image that appears to have lower contrast so that dense and lucent structures can be better seen within the same image.

equivalent dose   Similarly known as dose equivalent, are radiation equivalents in man (rem) and sieverts (Sv).

exit radiation   When the attenuated x-ray beam leaves the patient, the remaining x-ray beam is composed of both transmitted and scattered radiation.

exposure   The amount of ionizations or electrical charge in a specified amount of air expressed by Roentgen (R).

exposure adjustment   A mechanism that allows the radiographer to adjust the amount of preset radiation detection values.

exposure indicator   A numeric value that is displayed on the processed image to indicate the level of x-ray exposure received on the digital image receptor.

exposure intensity   The amount and energy of the x-rays reaching an area of the image receptor.

exposure maintenance formula   A formula that provides a mathematical calculation for adjusting the mAs when changing the SID.

exposure technique charts   Preestablished guidelines used by the radiographer to select standardized manual or AEC exposure factors for each type of radiographic examination.

exposure time   Determines the length of time that the x-ray tube produces x-rays.

extrapolated   Mathematically estimated; the mathematical process used to create technique charts.

filament   A coiled tungsten wire that is the source of electrons during x-ray production.

filament current   Heats the tungsten filament. This heating of the filament causes thermionic emission.

fill factor   The percentage of the x-rays reaching the sensitive area of the detector element (DEL).

fixed kVp/variable mAs technique chart   A type of exposure technique chart that is based on the concept of selecting an optimal kVp value that is required for the radiographic examination and adjusting the mAs for variations in part thickness.

flat-panel detectors (FPDs)   Solid-state image receptors using a large-area active matrix array of electronic components ranging in sizes from 43 × 35 to 43 × 43 cm.

fluoro loop save   A feature that saves a fluoro sequence loop to memory (based on the equipment's memory capacity).

fluoroscopy   Allows imaging of the movement of internal structures. It differs from film-screen imaging in that it uses a continuous beam of x-rays to create images of moving internal structures that can be viewed on a television monitor.

flux gain   The increase in light intensities at the output phosphor by accelerating the electrons.

focal distance   The distance between the grid and the convergent line or point, sometimes referred to as *grid radius*.

focal range   The recommended range of SIDs that can be used with a focused grid. The convergent line or point always falls within the focal range.

focused grid   Grid that has lead lines that are angled, or canted, to approximately match the angle of divergence of the primary beam.

focusing cup   Made of nickel and nearly surrounds the filament. It is open at one end to allow electrons to flow freely across the tube from cathode to anode. It has a negative charge, which keeps the cloud of electrons emitted from the filament from spreading apart. Its purpose is to focus the stream of electrons.

fog   Scatter radiation (Compton interactions) that reaches the image receptor and creates unwanted exposure on the radiographic image.

foreshortening   Images that appear shorter than the true objects.

frame averaging   An operation that reduces overall patient dose and image noise by averaging multiple image frames together. Because the combining of frames reduces noise, less radiation is needed to maintain image quality; however, spatial resolution will be decreased.

frequency   The number of waves passing a given point per given unit of time. Frequency is represented by a lowercase *f* or by the Greek letter *nu* (*ν*), and values are given in Hertz (Hz).

G

grayscale   The number of different shades of gray that can be stored and displayed by a computer system.

grayscale standard display function (GSDF)   The DICOM recommended standard for consistent display characteristics, such as grayscale appearance and image quality.

grid   A device that has very thin lead strips with radiolucent interspaces, intended to absorb scatter radiation emitted from the patient.

grid cap   Contains a permanently mounted grid and allows the image receptor to slide in behind it.

grid cassette   An image receptor that has a grid permanently mounted to its front surface.

grid cutoff   A decrease in the number of transmitted photons that reach the image receptor because of some misalignment of the grid.

grid focus   The orientation of the lead lines to one another.

grid frequency   Expresses the number of lead lines per unit length inches, or centimeters, or both. Grid frequencies can range from 25 to 45 lines/cm (60–110 lines/inch).

grid pattern   The linear pattern of the lead lines of a grid. The two types of grid pattern are linear and crossed or crosshatched.

grid ratio   The ratio of the height of the lead strips to the distance between them.

H

half-value layer (HVL)   The amount of filtration that reduces the intensity of the x-ray beam to half of its original value is considered the best method for describing x-ray quality. The HVL also can be used as an indirect measure of the total filtration in the path of the x-ray beam. It is expressed in millimeters of aluminum (mm-Al).

health informatics   Informatics within radiology departments (also known as radiology informatics) involves data management for radiology services both within and outside the healthcare system.

health information management (HIM)   Involves the management of the medical record and the data contained within.

Health Insurance Portability and Accountability Act (HIPAA)   National standards for electronic healthcare transactions and national identifiers for providers, health insurance plans, and employers.

Health Level Seven standard (HL7)   A communication standard for medical information.

heat unit (HU)   The amount of heat produced from any given exposure.

histogram   Graphic display of the distribution of pixel values. Each image has its own histogram, and it is evaluated to determine the adequacy of the image receptor exposure to x-rays.

histogram analysis   The computer analyzes the histogram using processing algorithms and compares it with a preestablished (reference) histogram specific to the anatomic part being imaged.

hospital information system (HIS)   A facility's system to collect and store personal patient information gathered (e.g., demographic data, relevant history, physician orders) that will assist in their care.

I

image intensifier   An electronic vacuum tube that converts the remnant (exit) x-ray beam to light, then to electrons, then back to light, increasing the light intensity in the process.

image receptor (IR)   A device that receives the radiation leaving the patient.

imaging informatics   Involves data management for radiology services both within and outside the healthcare system, also known as radiology informatics.

imaging plate (IP)   Located in the CR image receptor, where the photon intensities are absorbed by the phosphor.

inherent filtration   The filtration that is permanently in the path of the x-ray beam. Three components contribute to inherent filtration: (1) the glass envelope of the tube, (2) the oil that surrounds the tube, and (3) the window in the tube housing.

input/output phosphor   Phosphors within the image intensifier. The input phosphor converts incoming radiation into visible light energy, and the output phosphor converts the electrons into a brighter image.

integrating the health enterprise (IHE)   Initiative by healthcare professionals and industry to improve the way computer systems in healthcare share information.

interspace material   Radiolucent strips between the lead lines of a grid; generally made of aluminum.

inverse-square law   The relationship between distance and x-ray beam intensity, which states that the intensity of the x-ray beam is inversely proportional to the square of the distance from the source.

inversion   A postprocessing technique that reverses the grayscale from the original image.

ionization The ability to remove (eject) electrons; a property of x-rays.

ionization/ion chamber A hollow cell that contains air and is connected to the AEC timer circuit via an electrical wire.

irreversible compression Image compression where there is some loss of image data (lossy) at the end user and may be used to decrease transmission time or storage spaces.

K

kerma area product (KAP) The product of the total air kerma (intensity of x-rays at a given point in air) and the area of the x-ray beam at the entrance of the patient. It is the same as dose area product.

kilovoltage (kVp) Potential difference applied across the x-ray tube at the time the exposure is initiated; kVp determines the speed at which the electrons in the tube current move.

L

last image hold (LIH) The last fluoroscopic image displayed without any radiation exposure.

leakage radiation Any x-rays, other than the primary beam, that escape the tube housing.

line-focus principle Describes the relationship between the actual and the effective focal spots in the x-ray tube. A smaller target angle produces a smaller effective focal spot.

linear grid Contains lead lines that run in only one direction.

long-dimension linear grid Contains lead strips that run parallel to the long axis of the grid.

lookup tables (LUTs) Provide a method of altering the image to change the display of the digital image in a variety of ways.

M

magnification An increase in the image size of the object compared with its true or actual size. Also known as size distortion.

magnification factor (MF) Indicates how much size distortion or magnification is shown on a radiograph. MF = SID divided by source-to-object distance (SOD).

magnification mode Image intensifiers have a multifold function to increase the size of the area of interest displayed on the television monitor. Changing the voltage of the electrostatic focusing lenses tightens the diameter of the electron stream, giving the appearance of magnification.

Milliampere-seconds (mAs) readout The actual mAs used for the image is displayed immediately after the AEC exposure, sometimes for only a few seconds.

matrix A digital image is displayed as a combination of rows and columns (array) of small, usually square, "picture elements" called pixels.

medical image management and processing system (MIMPS) A networked computer system designed for digital imaging that can receive, store, archive, distribute, and display digital images, previously known as picture archival and communication system (PACS).

megapixels (MP) Millions of pixels. Radiologists typically interpret images using 5MP LCD monitor displays or greater.

milliamperage (mA) The unit used to measure the tube current.

minification gain Increased light intensities as a result of the reduction in size of the output phosphor image compared with that of the input phosphor image.

minimum response time The shortest exposure time that the AEC system can produce.

modulation transfer function (MTF) A measure of the imaging system's ability to display contrast of anatomic objects varying in size.

moiré effect An artifact that can occur when a stationary grid is used during computed radiography imaging if the grid frequency is similar to the scanning frequency. Also known as the *Zebra pattern*.

mutual induction The process of an electrical current coming into a set of coils on the input side (primary side) will create an electrical current and voltage in the secondary coil windings, the output side.

N

Nyquist frequency A standard formula for converting analog data into discreet digital units to accurately represent the analog signal or imaging data in digital radiography. To accurately reproduce an image from the continuous analog signal, the sampling rate must be at least two times the highest spatial frequency in the exit x-ray intensities (signal).

O

object-to-image-receptor distance (OID) Distance created between the object radiographed and the image receptor.

off-focus radiation Occurs when projectile electrons are reflected and x-rays are produced outside the focal spot.

optimal kVp The kVp value that is high enough to ensure penetration of the part but not too high to diminish radiographic contrast.

orthogonal Right-angle relationship between the CR and the image receptor.

P

parallel/nonfocused grid A grid with lead lines that run parallel to one another.

photocathode Converts the visible light in the image intensifier into electrons.

photoelectric effect Complete absorption of the incoming x-ray photon occurs when it has enough energy to remove (eject) an inner-shell electron. The ionized atom has a vacancy, or electron hole, in its inner shell, and an electron from an outer shell drops down to fill the vacancy.

photoelectron The ejected electron resulting from ionization during the photoelectric effect.

photoemission A process of emitting electrons in response to light stimulus.

photon A small, discrete bundle of energy.

photostimulable luminescence (PSL) The emission of visible light from the photostimulable phosphor when stimulated by a high-intensity laser beam.

photostimulable phosphor (PSP) The phosphor layer of the imaging plate composed of barium fluorohalide crystals doped with europium.

phototimer Uses a fluorescent (light-producing) screen and a device that converts light to electricity in an AEC device.

pixel The smallest component of the matrix. Also known as *picture elements*.

pixel binning A process that combines and reduces the total number of DEL units that are working during a fast fluoroscopic framing sequence.

pixel density The number of pixels per unit area.

pixel pitch The pixel spacing or distance measured from the center of a pixel to an adjacent pixel.

pulse height The level of mA per pulse.

pulse interval The time in milliseconds between successive mA pulses.

pulse rate The number of pulses (frames) per second of operation.

pulse width The length of the radiation exposure for each pulse (frame).

pulsed fluoroscopy The x-ray exposure has gaps of exposure between each image frame.

Q

quantum A small, discrete bundle of energy.

quantum noise Visible as brightness or density fluctuations on the image as a result of too few photons reaching the image receptor to form the image. *Quantum mottle* is the term typically used when referring to noise on a film image.

R

radioactivity Unstable atoms spontaneously emitting particles and energy from the nucleus in an effort to attain stability.

radiology information system (RIS) Similar to the HIS but specific to radiology. If the patient is scheduled for a radiology procedure, patient electronic information (demographics, relevant history, digital images, and interpretations) is stored and becomes a part of the radiology workflow.

rectification Changing alternating current (AC) to direct current (DC).

region of interest Postprocessing function that provides calculation of selected pixel values within the area of interest to provide quantitative information about the tissue.

remnant radiation When the attenuated x-ray beam leaves the patient, the remaining x-ray beam is composed of both transmitted and scattered radiation. Also known as *exit radiation*.

resistance Electric friction that inherently impedes the flow of electrons along its pathway.

resistors Regulate the amount of current passing through the cathode filament during exposure and are used to control amperage.

reversible compression Image compression where there is no loss of image data (lossless) at the end user.

rotor A device in the x-ray tube that causes the target to rapidly rotate during x-ray production.

S

sampling frequency How often the analog signal is reproduced in its discrete digitized form.

sampling pitch The distance between the sampling points.

saturation The image receptor is extremely overexposed, cannot be properly processed, and the quality is severely degraded.

scattering Some incoming photons are not absorbed; instead they lose energy during interactions with atoms comprising tissue.

scintillator A phosphor material that converts the exit radiation into visible light.

secondary electron The ejected electron resulting from the Compton effect interaction. Also known as a *Compton electron*.

shape distortion Images of objects that appear longer or shorter than the true objects.

short-dimension linear grid Contains lead strips running perpendicular to the long axis of the grid.

signal-to-noise ratio (SNR) A method of describing the strength of the radiation exposure compared with the amount of noise apparent in a digital image.

size distortion or magnification An increase in the image size of an object compared with its true, or actual, size.

smoothing A postprocessing technique that suppresses image noise (quantum noise). However, spatial resolution is degraded.

source-to-image receptor distance (SID) The distance between the source of the radiation and the image receptor.

source-to-object distance (SOD) The distance from the x-ray source (focal spot) to the object being radiographed.

space charge The electrons liberated from the filament during thermionic emission that form a cloud around the filament.

space charge effect The tendency of the space charge not to allow more electrons to be boiled off the filament.

spatial frequency Variation in anatomic details imaged as white to black brightness levels that can be defined by the unit of line pairs per millimeter (lp/mm).

spatial resolution The smallest detail that can be detected in an image; the term typically used in digital imaging.

stator An electric motor that turns the rotor at very high speed during x-ray production.

step-down transformers Have more core windings on the primary side than on the secondary side and reduce the incoming voltage to a lower value.

step-up transformers Have fewer core windings on the primary side than on the secondary side and increase the incoming voltage to a higher value.

stitching A postprocessing operation to combine multiple images into one image for viewing anatomic areas such as for a scoliosis series.

subject contrast A result of the absorption characteristics of the anatomic tissue radiographed along with the quality of the x-ray beam.

T

target A metal that abruptly decelerates and stops electrons in the tube current, allowing the production of x-rays.

teleradiology The practice of diagnostic image interpretation outside the facility (offsite) from where the imaging data are acquired.

temporal resolution The inherent resolution on an image as a function of image acquisition time. Increasing the time of exposure during image acquisition can increase motion unsharpness and therefore decrease temporal resolution, even if it is not visible on the displayed image.

thermionic emission The boiling off of electrons from the cathode filament.

tissue density Matter per unit volume or the compactness of the anatomic particles comprising the anatomic part.

total filtration The sum of the x-ray tube's added and inherent filtration.

transformer Regulates voltage in an x-ray system. The ratio of wire windings between the primary and secondary sides determines whether the transformer is a step-up or step-down transformer.

transmission The incoming x-ray photon passes through the anatomic part without any interaction with the atomic structures.

trough filter A double-wedge compensating filter added to the primary beam to produce more consistent exposure to the image receptor.

tube current The flow of electrons from cathode to anode, measured in milliamperes (mA).

V

values of interest (VOI) Determines the range of the histogram data set included in the displayed image.

variable kVp/fixed mAs technique chart A type of exposure technique chart based on the concept that kVp can be increased as the anatomic part size increases. The baseline kVp is increased by 2 for every 1-cm increase in part thickness, and the mAs is maintained.

vendor neutral archives (VNAs) Allows for images and data from different systems and in different formats to be stored using a singular system on a common infrastructure.

virtual collimation Lines on the last image hold indicating the position of the collimator plates that allows for collimation without exposing the patient to additional radiation.

voltage ripple The amount of consistency in voltage waveforms during x-ray production.

W

wafer grid A type of stationary grid placed on top of the image receptor.

wavelength The distance between two successive crests or troughs.

wedge filter The most common type of compensating filter. The thicker part of the wedge filter is lined up with the thinner portion of the anatomic part that is being imaged, allowing fewer x-ray photons to reach that end of the part.

window level Sets the midpoint (center) of the range of brightness visible in the digital image.

window width The range or number of shades of gray visible on the digital image.

X

x-ray emission spectrum The range and intensity of emitted x-rays.

INDEX

Page numbers followed by '*f*' indicate figures, '*t*' indicate tables, and '*b*' indicate boxes.